K

D0895346

OKANAGAN UNIVERSITY COLLEGE
LIBRARY
BRITISH COLUMBIA

The
Scientific Basis
of
Integrative Medicine

The Scientific Basis of Integrative Medicine

Leonard A. Wisneski, M.D.
Lucy Anderson, M.S.W.

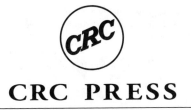

CRC PRESS

Boca Raton   London   New York   Washington, D.C.

Library of Congress Cataloging-in-Publication Data

Wisneski, Leonard A.
    The scientific basis of integrative medicine / by Leonard A. Wisneski, Lucy Anderson.
      p. ; cm.
    Includes bibliographical references and index.
    ISBN 0-8493-2081-X (alk. paper)
    1. Integrative medicine. 2. Psychoneuroimmunology. 3. Mind and body. I. Anderson,
Lucy. II. Title.
    [DNLM: 1. Psychoneuroimmunology. 2. Mind-Body and Relaxation Techniques. WL
103.7 W815s 2004]

R733.W576 2004
616.07′9--dc22
                                                  2004050335

This book contains information obtained from authentic and highly regarded sources. Reprinted material is quoted with permission, and sources are indicated. A wide variety of references are listed. Reasonable efforts have been made to publish reliable data and information, but the author and the publisher cannot assume responsibility for the validity of all materials or for the consequences of their use.

Neither this book nor any part may be reproduced or transmitted in any form or by any means, electronic or mechanical, including photocopying, microfilming, and recording, or by any information storage or retrieval system, without prior permission in writing from the publisher.

The consent of CRC Press does not extend to copying for general distribution, for promotion, for creating new works, or for resale. Specific permission must be obtained in writing from CRC Press for such copying.

Direct all inquiries to CRC Press, 2000 N.W. Corporate Blvd., Boca Raton, Florida 33431.

Trademark Notice: Product or corporate names may be trademarks or registered trademarks, and are used only for identification and explanation, without intent to infringe.

Visit the CRC Press Web site at www.crcpress.com

© 2005 by Leonard A. Wisneski

No claim to original U.S. Government works
International Standard Book Number 0-8493-2081-X
Library of Congress Card Number 2004050335
Printed in the United States of America 1 2 3 4 5 6 7 8 9 0
Printed on acid-free paper

Dedication

To my loving and supportive wife Judith, who renews my enthusiasm for life each and every day; to my daughters Amy and Hope, who have given me the opportunity to parent two wonderful souls and are a constant reminder of the eternal youth within my being; and to my brother Harris, who, from a young age, taught me the meaning of diligence, scholarship, and love of knowledge.

In loving memory of my mother Faye, who taught me the meaning of love and true service.

L.A.W.

For Nicholas, whom I adore, and for Anne Anderson, who taught me loving kindness.

In loving memory of Lila Anderson, whose insights and invaluable guidance are woven through these pages.

L.A.

Foreword

Welcome to this exciting and much needed textbook in the field of integrative medicine. It may change your view of disease and conventional medicine.

The revolutions of the past two decades in molecular biology and molecular genetics have done an outstanding job of informing physicians and scientists of the molecules, DNA, RNA, peptides, enzymes, proteins, and other components that comprise the human body. We now understand how, and to a great degree, which hormones, neurotransmitters, cytokines, and antibodies are produced in various states of health and disease.

To a great extent, we biomedical types remain isolated within narrow areas of knowledge and often think only about our own disciplines and subdisciplines. We have accumulated facts and figures about our chosen fields at a mind-numbing pace, and we have excelled at using this information to develop treatments and procedures that are largely directed at treating the symptoms manifested by full-blown pathologies. *The Scientific Basis of Integrative Medicine* goes a considerable distance in providing physicians and biomedical researchers with the opportunity to reassemble all those disparate molecules and biological mechanisms into a logical integrated whole from which a real understanding of the causes of disease may arise. This is particularly true for grasping the perturbations in normal physiology that lead to the difficult-to-manage chronic diseases—persistent conditions that do not respond to the usual armamentarium of pharmaceuticals or invasive procedures so that the only sanity-saving measure is to refer the patient to the next subspecialist who is no better equipped than we are to provide relief to the patient.

Len Wisneski and Lucy Anderson's approach in this text is to connect those seemingly separate biological systems to give us a rational roadmap to use to locate the underlying mechanisms of many multifaceted disease processes. In so doing, they make it more likely that practitioners and healers will understand better what the primary targets of their treatment modalities should be and what the relationship of each disorder is to the others. In other words, the content of these chapters allows us to identify the sources of a number of cascading pathologic events and how they magnify underlying disease processes.

The authors educate us using a conversational, patient-centered approach that is not overly preachy or dogmatic. Their extensive documentation of scientific studies and their results lends credibility to their interpretation of their findings and conclusions. The first five chapters provide a strong scientific foundation for our understanding of human physiology, psychoneuroimmunology, stress, and relaxation . The last three chapters open our minds to the less organic and corporeal realm of our existence and health as influenced by our environment. At the very least, we might all heed this advice to listen to and respect the desire of those patients who wish to invoke spiritual aspects in the healing process.

Len Wisneski, a practicing M.D., also sets an example by showing us that it is indeed alright to collaborate with healers from other backgrounds and traditions, especially when the greater goal of the best possible outcome for the patients is achieved (rather than protecting the sanctity and exclusiveness of the M.D. club).

In summary this book achieves the following three major goals. It shows us how the body's organs and cells are not isolated systems but work together in an integrated fashion to maintain our health. It explains how many diseases arise as a result of stressors that perturb homeostasis and that addressing these *initial* stressors is necessary for healing to occur, and it opens our minds to consider energetic healing modalities that heretofore were taboo in the western medical establishment.

Read, enjoy, and expand your healing horizons.

Michael D. Lumpkin, Ph.D.
Chairman and Professor of Physiology & Biophysics
Georgetown University School of Medicine

About the Authors

Leonard A. Wisneski, M.D., FACP, is Clinical Professor of Medicine at George Washington University Medical Center and adjunct faculty in the Department of Physiology and Biophysics at Georgetown University, where he is a founding member of the Complementary and Alternative Medicine Curriculum Planning Committee. He was vice chairman of the NIH Consensus Panel on Acupuncture and is chairman of the NIH Advisory Board on Frontier Sciences at the University of Connecticut. He was Medical Director of Integrative Medicine Communications (IMC) and Chief Medical Editor of *The Integrative Medicine* 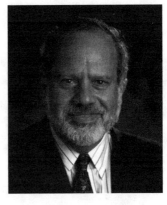 *Consult* newsletter. He holds fellowship positions in the American College of Physicians, the American College of Nutrition, and the American Institute of Stress. He has published over 30 scientific articles and has been in the clinical practice of endocrinology and integrative medicine for over 25 years.

Lucy Anderson is a medical author, editor, and journalist. She has researched and written medical and mental health conference reports, reviews, monographs, and newsletters as well as CME reports and biomedical corporate training materials. She wrote numerous articles for *The Integrative Medicine Consult* newsletter, including monthly reviews of both the allopathic and complementary treatment issues of a designated medical condition. She is the content editor for American Epilepsy 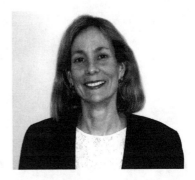 Society's journal, *Epilepsy Currents*. Her nonmedical publications include *Taking Charge* (Bantam Books, 1976). Lucy has a BA from Stanford University and an M.S.W. from the University of California, Berkeley.

Acknowledgments

We are forever grateful to Lesley Carmack and Lila Anderson whose wisdom and profound understanding of subtle energy compelled us to write about the physiology of spirituality.

Deepest thanks to Judith Homer Wisneski who helped in numerous practical ways and whose gentle stillness supported us both.

To our outstanding medical illustrator, Rob Flewell, CMI, whose courage to conceptualize new medical drawings, technical excellence, and witty sense of humor delighted us no end.

Our gratitude to Dr. William Tiller for reviewing sections of Chapter 8 and ensuring that our layperson's interpretation of physics was, indeed, accurate as well as to Dr. Richard Wurtman at MIT and Dr. Raphael Mechoulam at Hebrew University in Israel for taking the time to share their insight and knowledge of endogenous ligands, which we feel are critical to the human relaxation system. We would like to thank Dr. Elmer Green, the father of biofeedback and a remarkable scientist, who is willing to think outside the boundaries of conventional medicine. He was one of the first researchers to scientifically study healing and spirituality.

For Holly and Doug Hobbie, whose rare artistic and literary talents gave us some well-chosen wording and whose friendship is sustaining.

We thank Johanna Povrick-Znoy, who spent hours preparing the extensive reference sections.

For Jonathan Thomas, who gave us the image of the Rosetta stone, we wish you insight and courage.

At CRC, we thank Barbara Ellen Norwitz, our editor, Mimi Williams, our project editor, and Pat Roberson, our project coordinator, for their indispensable guidance.

We gratefully acknowledge the scholarship and diligence of the vast number of scientists and clinicians upon whose research this book is based. In particular, we want to pay tribute to those individuals who have had the courage to explore new frontiers of medical science.

The Scientific Basis of Integrative Medicine

Although all of the stories that are included in this book are true and based on factual situations, some information and identifying details have been changed to protect the identity of the individuals described. The purpose of this book is to educate. The authors and publisher shall have neither responsibility nor liability to any person or entity with respect to any loss, damage, or injury caused or alleged to be caused directly or indirectly by the information contained in this book. The information presented herein is in no way intended as a substitute for medical counseling and treatment.

Leonard A. Wisneski, M.D. and Lucy Anderson, M.S.W.

Beyond the Mind–Body Connection: An Introduction

The most divine art is that of healing; it must occupy itself with the soul as well as the body.

Pythagoras, 5th century B.C.

In 1978, Steven, a strapping 40-year-old, appeared at my office for a physical examination. He looked and felt vibrant but came at his wife's urging. Steve had a very low hematocrit—an indication of serious disease. An endoscopic exam revealed extensive gastric carcinoma. A subsequent operation confirmed that Steve was studded with cancer throughout his abdomen and into the surrounding lymph nodes. Then, as now, there was no definitive treatment, especially for such an advanced cancer.

In the recovery room, beset with fear, Steve asked, "Lenny, how long do I have to live?" His eyes were wide and his pupils were dilated; he was frantically pumping adrenaline. Steve was hanging on my every word. I did the old vaudeville routine, "How long do you want?" "Ten years," he said. "You got it," I replied. And he did get it. Steve got sick in the winter of 1987 and died within 6 months. Steve not only went into remission for years; he was healthy and vital until months before he died.

This incident with Steve profoundly altered my perspective on practicing medicine and my beliefs about the nature of the healing process, particularly regarding the power of the mind to heal. Consequently, for over 20 years now, I have engaged in the study of psychoneuroimmunology (PNI) or, as I prefer to call it, *integral physiology*. Integral physiology has to do with the synthesis of conventional physiology and how our individual psyches (i.e., mind, emotions, and spirituality) interact with the world around us to induce positive or detrimental changes in our bodies. In a broader sense, the concept applies to the health of society as a whole.

In the past two decades, biomedical research has changed our understanding of body systems. It is now known that there is a complex network of feedback, mediation, and modulation among the central and autonomic nervous systems, the endocrine system, the immune system, and the stress system. These systems, which were previously considered pristinely independent, in fact, interact on myriad levels. PNI is concerned with the various interactions among these body systems and provides the underpinnings of a scientific explanation for what is commonly referred to as the mind–body connection.

In 1964, George Freeman Solomon wrote "Emotions, immunity, and disease: a speculative theoretical integration." In this paper, Solomon first used the term *psychoimmunology* and introduced the concept of a medical link between our emotions and immune systems (Solomon and Moos, 1964). In 1975, Ader expanded on Solomon's work and coined the term *psychoneuroimmunology*. During that same year, Ader and his colleagues published the startling results of their research on the conditioned immune response in a rat population (Ader and Cohen, 1975). The rats in the experimental group were injected with cyclophosphamide (an immuno-suppressive agent) while simultaneously being given drinking water flavored with saccharin. The rats were later given only the saccharin-flavored water but no cyclo-phosphamide. To the researchers' surprise (not to mention the rest of the medical community), the rats continued to evidence immune suppression. This was the first documented example of pavlovian conditioning of the immune response.

In Ader's groundbreaking research, he used a pharmaceutical agent to induce the conditioned immune response. Subsequent studies have expanded on the theory to include investigations of conditioning stimuli that are neither physical nor chem-ical but are instead cognitive (e.g., perceptions, thoughts, or emotional states). What has been learned is that these cognitive stimuli can just as easily mediate changes in the immune system. Two examples:

- Lymphocyte activity in men is diminished immediately following the death of a spouse from breast cancer (Schleifer et al., 1983).
- A study of 75 medical students showed a significant reduction in natural killer-cell activity during final examinations as compared with the previ-ous month (Kiecolt-Glaser et al., 1984).

Twenty years later, *Lancet* published a study by Ader and Cohen (1975) that concludes with the following statement: "The association between stressful life experiences and changes in immune function do not establish a causal link between stress, immune function, and disease. This chain of events has not been definitively established." In this book, we will illustrate that the integration among body systems and that causal link can now be established. The first few chapters of the book will cover this information in some detail.

What are the practical implications of the understanding that a mind–body system exists? It is a summons to bring holism to the practice of medicine; to do away with the unbalanced cold logic of clinical dispassion; and to bring to medical treatment the balance of nurturing, caring, and empathy as well as to instill hope, when appropriate. Over 100 years ago, the Dean of the Johns Hopkins University School of Medicine, Sir William Osler, said that the care of the patient with tuber-culosis has more to do with what is in the head than what is in the chest. Somehow, in all our enthusiasm for scientific precision and methodology, we have lost sight of that important message. And in doing so, we have lost sight of the art and heart of medicine, of the healing process, and of the mystery of life itself.

When I was supervising the training of medical students, I had a few students who deeply concerned me because of their lack of empathy and an inability to understand their patients' feelings of vulnerability or frustration at being dependent upon the medical staff around them. Upon occasion, I required these students to spend time as a "patient" in the cardiac care unit. Just like any other cardiac patient, the students had to wear a hospital gown, were isolated in a room, and hooked up to a heart monitor. They could overhear nurses speaking about them and were totally dependent on the nurse's help to use the bathroom, wash, or eat. They experienced feelings of powerlessness, helplessness, dependency, and victimization. Many of these students later told me that it changed their lives and their whole perspective of being a physician. They had learned the art and heart of medicine simply by becoming a patient themselves. Perhaps every person working in the healthcare field would do well to spend a day being the patient.

In this book, we first establish the scientific basis for the mind–body connection and begin to understand why Steve lived only as long as his requested time. We will learn that stories like Steve's are not all that unusual and begin to understand how this can happen. We will document the puissant interactions of the endocrine, immune, nervous, and stress systems that can so profoundly influence our lives. Once this information is clearly established, we will turn our attention to issues beyond the mind–body connection and examine what it is that the dimension of spirituality (i.e., that which informs but transcends the five senses) can add to healing. We will look at issues such as hope and faith and what they have to do with healing. If we are more emotionally present with our patients, can we influence their healing process or outcome? What does deeply caring or loving have to do with health and healing—not only in patients' lives but also in the lives of those called to the healing profession?

If Western medicine is to have a truly cohesive physiological system, it must incorporate a unified theory that can account for the existence of energy fields within as well as outside of the human body. This book looks at how various forms of energy (e.g., light, sound, electromagnetism, and prayer) translate into chemical and electrical signals that orchestrate our physical health. Some of these forms of energy can be called "subtle energy," that is, types of energy that typically are not detectable by the five senses or current scientific instrumentation. Integral physiology serves as a bridge between Western medical knowledge and the equally valuable, but less well-recognized, Eastern systems of medicine. Eastern medical concepts concern endogenous energy systems, such as *Qi* or life force that, according to Chinese medicine, flow throughout the body. A clear understanding of these issues will usher in a new form of medicine. I call it *integral medicine* because it combines important Western biological knowledge with forms of healing that incorporate the mental and emotional, if not the spiritual, capacities of humans to heal.

Jeff Levin writes the following in the last paragraphs of his book, *God, Faith, and Health*: "I believe that a new generalist perspective, which is on the rise, will be based on something akin to a 'unified field theory' of the determinants of health and healing. This perspective will not be grounded principally in genetics and molecular biology, as the mainstream medical research establishment presumes. Instead, it will be founded on an integrated, body–mind–spirit perspective—a view of all sentient life as part of a continuous bioenergetic spectrum, or to use a metaphor borrowed from author Ken Wilber, a 'spectrum of consciousness.' This will be the next era or historical epoch of Western medicine" (Levin, 2001).

In the final chapters of this book, we introduce a paradigm that we called "integral physiology," curiously, a schematic much akin to Levin's "unified field theory," which presents an integrated perspective of healthcare. It takes us on a pilgrimage well beyond the mind–body connection and research in the field of PNI—it brings the subtle-energy dimension into the mix. The bridge that we are constructing between Eastern and Western medical knowledge is like a Rosetta stone of integral physiology. In Chapter 8, we use the image of the Rosetta stone of ancient Egypt as an allegory for deciphering the pieces of information that incorporate the physical, mental, emotional, and spiritual aspects of our lives and of our health. Someday, we will have the scientific means to prove the principles inherent to a system of medical treatment that incorporates a fully integral physiology and the technology to employ it to benefit physical, emotional, and spiritual health. And someday, research on human subtle energy will be the next exciting frontier in medicine.

The fragility of life confronts us, often personally and certainly existentially. We have been inspired to give this book a deeper voice, a voice that neither of us thought would be expressed here but, rather, in a sequel to this book. We were wrong. It is clearly time to begin to describe the power and importance of the spiritual in overall health and in the healing process. In the final chapter (Chapter 8), we present some initial blueprints for construction of a "bridge" that will connect science and spirituality, leading medicine toward a fully integrated view of physiology.

While this book addresses many technical issues, it is not intended solely for the physician, but also for the interested healthcare practitioner. The technical parts are necessary to responsibly convey the contributions that Western medicine has offered to the deciphering of our "Rosetta stone." We would encourage the nonphysician reader not to get too bogged down in understanding every technical aspect or physiological explanation. Such readers can later return to the text to work on the more purely scientific understanding. The overriding message will be apparent, even if the medical details are not entirely understood. And to the physician, we encourage you to read it all. Although you might be familiar with, for example, the pineal gland or the neuroendocrinology of the stress response, topics are presented here from a new viewpoint and emerge to convey a candidly innovative perspective of healing.

Please note that throughout the book when the text states "I" or "my," it is intended to designate Len's voice and opinions.

INTRODUCTION REFERENCES

Ader, R. and Cohen, N., Behaviorally conditioned immunosuppression, *Psychosomatic Medicine*, (4), 333–340, 1975.

Kiecolt-Glaser, J.K., Garner, W., Speicher, C.E., Penn, G., and Glaser, R., Psychosocial modifiers of immunocompetence in medical students, *Psychosomatic Medicine*, 46 (1), 7–14, 1984.

Levin, J., *God, Faith, and Health: Exploring the Spirituality–Health Connection*, John Wiley & Sons, Inc., New York, NY, 2001.

Schleifer, S.J., Keler, S.E., Camerino, M., Thornton, J.C., and Stein, M., Suppression of lymphocyte stimulation following bereavement, *JAMA*, 250 (3) 374–377, 1983.

Solomon, G.F., Moos, R.H., Emotions, immunity, and disease: a speculative theoretical integration, *Archiv. General Psychiatry*, 11, 657–674, 1964.

ADDITIONAL RESOURCES

Ader, R., Ed., *Psychoneuroimmunology*, 1st ed., Academic Press, New York, NY, 1981.

Ader, R., Cohen, N., and Felten, D., Psychoneuroimmunology: interactions between the nervous system and the immune system, *Lancet*, 345 (8942), 99–103, 1995.

Ader, R., Felten, D.L., and Cohen, N., Eds., *Psychoneuroimmunology*, 2nd ed., Academic Press, San Diego, CA, 1991.

Ader, R., Felten, D.L., and Cohen, N., Eds. *Psychoneuroimmunology*, 3rd ed. (2 vol.), Academic Press, San Diego, CA, 2001.

Table of Contents

1 A Review of Classic Physiological Systems

CONTENTS

In this chapter, we will examine body systems that permit our mind and emotions to interact or communicate with the environment and, thus, to induce positive or detrimental physiological changes. The classic body systems that we will address are the *nervous system* (including the *enteric* system), the *endocrine system*, and the *immune system*. However, in addition to these classic body systems, we suggest that there are two other fundamental human body systems: the *stress system* and the *relaxation system*. The stress system will be introduced in this chapter and covered more thoroughly in Chapter 3. The relaxation system (see Chapter 5) will be presented for the first time in a medical text. It is necessary to acquire a general understanding of each system in order to grasp how the systems interact to influence the mind–body connection. Right away, we see that it is almost impossible to describe any one system in an isolated manner.

Each of these systems is ultimately a conduit for energy communication. What do we mean by that? Think about how you hear. The speaker's larynx vibrates and sets forth a wave of air molecules, which impinge upon your tympanic membrane. The molecules are converted to mechanical energy by three little bones (i.e., the malleus, incus, and stapes) in your ear. Next, electrical energy is produced and transmitted across your cortex, where it is understood as intelligible sound in the temporal lobe. Likewise, you look at the person who is speaking, but actually what you are seeing is light energy impinging upon the cerebral cortex (i.e., the brain), allowing you to interpret movements within time. In both instances, there is no material/material interaction. It is purely energy.

Energy communications similarly affect our emotions. We realize the implications of energy communication as we think about our relationships. How we feel in relationship to others accounts for the majority of the physiological reactivity that we experience. This may be most dramatically experienced when a harmonious relationship is disrupted by a major altercation. Simply being in the same room with that individual evokes an energy tension. As with our hearing or seeing, any emotional tension is transmitted by the body's systems. Some types of energy communication can be quite subtle, such as the transmission of "energy" that occurs with intercessory prayer (i.e., praying for others' well-being). Dr. Larry Dossey's commentary on a recent intercessory prayer study included the following thought-provoking statement: "We should be cautious in calling events *miraculous* or *mystical*, because the subsequent course of history may reveal that these terms reflect little more than our own ignorance" (Dossey, 2000). We will review extensively the topic of energy medicine in Chapter 7. As we look at the technical aspects of the electrical and chemical functioning of the various body systems, it will be useful to keep in mind that there are also types of energy transmission, such as prayer, that are less well understood but now have scientific studies confirming their impact on humans.

SECTION 1: THE NERVOUS SYSTEM

The nervous system is lightning fast, but it has a very poor memory. It serves as the Paul Revere of our bodies. It indicates, largely through electrical signals, that there is incoming information. The nervous system transmits information to the proper part of the brain to be assimilated and then sends it back out to the particular portion of the body it intends to influence. The nervous system has two main divisions: the central nervous system (CNS) and the peripheral nervous system (PNS). The CNS consists of the brain and the spinal cord. The PNS is comprised of the somatic nervous system and the autonomic nervous system (ANS), and the latter is further divided into the sympathetic and parasympathetic systems. The neuron is the basic unit of communication in the nervous system. Several of the structures of the brain that we will review here are also an integral part of the endocrine system. The enteric nervous system (ENS), which is reviewed later in this chapter, is a more recently identified system, and it involves the nervous system of the gut.

The heart also is currently being studied as another nervous system. It is known that upper chambers of the heart, called the *atria*, secrete a hormone called *atrial natriuretic hormone*, which decreases blood pressure and volume. The field related to systems interaction and the heart is called *cardioneuroimmunology*. I would speculate that in the coming few years, researchers will find that the heart does have its own nervous and immune systems.

THE CENTRAL NERVOUS SYSTEM

The Brain

We begin with an overview of the anatomy of the brain. The brain weighs approximately 3 pounds and contains about 100 billion neurons, which ultimately means enormous possible conduits of energy. The brain is supported by bone and meninges, which are connective tissue membranes.

The cerebrospinal fluid (CSF) is the clear, extracellular fluid that surrounds the entire brain and the spinal cord as well as filling the cavities (ventricles) within the brain. Most people have less than a cupful of CSF. It is secreted by tissue that lies within the ventricles. One of the crucial functions of the CSF is to protect the brain from injury. The brain literally floats in the CSF, which also minimizes compression of the spinal cord by its own weight. CSF nourishes the brain and provides an avenue for waste removal (waste returns to the blood via sinuses). Because the CSF is replaced numerous times each day, it provides a steady mechanism for frequently flushing out the CNS (Travis, 1999). The CSF carries messages that affect the endocrine, immune, and stress systems (see Chapter 2, Systems Integration).

While the CSF can exchange particles with the blood and can then pass those substances along to the neurons, the cells that make up the blood–brain barrier require that all blood-borne substances pass through them before entering the brain. The blood–brain barrier is quite a strict gatekeeper, permitting mostly healthy substances to reach the brain. Plasma proteins, for example, happily are invited in. However, there is another route by which particles enter the brain, which is lipid solubility. Natural lipid soluble substances (e.g., dietary components or vitamins) as well as some drugs (e.g., morphine) enter the brain by this pathway. The complications and diseases stemming from such substances are well known.

The Hemispheres

The right cerebral hemisphere responds primarily to signals from the left side of the body. The right side of the brain largely involves nonverbal processes, such as music or mathematics. It is concerned with more abstract thinking, loose associations, three-dimensional forms, insight, and imagination. This is the artistic part of us. The left cerebral hemisphere responds primarily to signals from the right side of the body. The left hemisphere largely is concerned with verbal or rational processes, such as spoken or written language and logic. However, each of the cerebral hemispheres functions separately, and depending upon your line of work, you may use one side of your brain a great deal more than the other.

If we slice the brain open, there is a large strip of material that connects the two hemispheres. It is called the *corpus callosum*. The corpus callosum is very rich in myelinated (promotes fast moving messages) nerve fibers (approximately 200 million to 300 million axons). Its job is to transmit information from one hemisphere to the other so that the hemispheres can communicate with one another.

Using one hemisphere at the expense of the other does not allow us to experience our full capabilities. What we need to learn to do is to dance on the corpus callosum. We need to learn to be centered between both brains. We need to learn to use our minds, combining both hemispheres in a dual brain mode, in a whole brain mode, in a holistic manner. Dancing on the corpus callosum is the way to gain more harmony in our lives.

The Lobes

The brain is divided by deep fissures into the right and left hemispheres. Each hemisphere is then divided into four lobes: frontal, parietal, temporal, and occipital (see Figure 1.1). Each of the lobes has discrete functions attributed to it, but there is a great deal of systems interaction within a lobe. For example, the temporal lobe, which involves musical activity, must interact with the parietal lobe, which involves mathematical ability, in order to perform a piece of music. Furthermore, a lobe does not perform entirely the same function in each hemisphere or side of the brain. For example, the portion of the frontal lobe that is most involved in speech articulation lays predominantly only in the left hemisphere.

Following is a brief description of each of the four lobes and their primary functions.

Frontal Lobe

The frontal lobe takes up one-third of the hemispheric surface of the brain. The frontal lobe has a lot to do with personality and how you basically think. It is involved with rationalization and inhibitions. It is the portion of the mind that allows us to plan and order things in a timely sequence. As mentioned, it is the center for articulation, but it also controls muscle contraction and discrete body movements from within the somatomotor cortex.

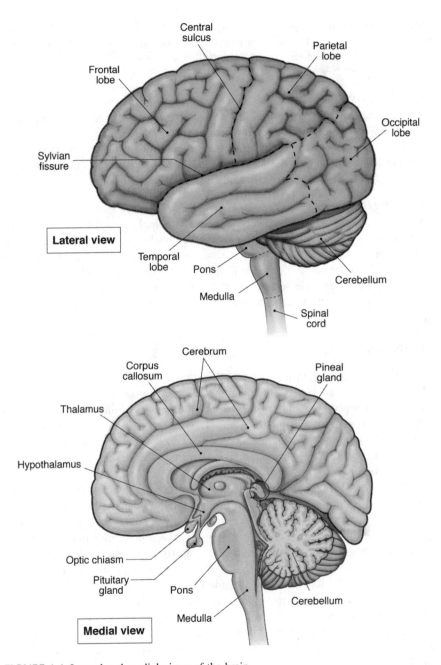

FIGURE 1.1 Lateral and medial views of the brain.

Parietal Lobe

The parietal lobe is centrally located at the upper rear portion of the two hemispheres, although it is basically impossible to delineate its precise boundaries. The parietal lobe assimilates incoming information from any of the five senses. It houses the somatosensory cortex, or primary sensory area, where all ascending somatosensory pathways (mainly from the skin and joints) terminate. Nerve pulses related to touch, pressure, heat, cold, and pain travel from the site of the sensation and are processed in the somatosensory cortex.

Occipital Lobe

The occipital lobe, which houses the primary visual cortex, records information about light and receives information from the visual receptors of the eye. The occipital lobe is capable of associative memory and for memory of what you have seen. However, damage to the lobe can cause loss of vision in all or part of the visual field. It is the most intensely studied portion of the brain.

Temporal Lobe

The temporal lobe, which is located near each temple, houses the auditory cortex, our processing center for hearing. The lobe is responsible for memory processes and complex associations related to things that you have seen. Some portions of the temporal lobe influence emotional behavior. The temporal lobe is also involved in the integration of multiple sensory functions (e.g., speech, vision, and touch) that can influence some of our more artistic qualities, such as remembering songs and things of that nature.

The Hindbrain

The cerebellum and brainstem are found in the hindbrain. The cerebellum is the CEO of the nervous system, modulating the entire system. It is crucial for the unconscious coordination of movements, maintenance of equilibrium, integration of skeletal muscle activity, and quality of muscle tone. The brainstem, which is attached to the cerebellum, includes the pons and the medulla. The brainstem connects the cerebral hemispheres with the spinal cord, carrying information that has been processed by the brain to the rest of the body.

The reticular formation is a network of interneurons extending the length of the brainstem and into the midbrain, taking in information carried by sensory, motor, and visceral pathways. It filters out repetitive stimuli and helps to maintain alertness. Motor portions of the reticular formation are involved in maintaining muscle tone and coordinating skeletal muscle activity. Neurons from the reticular formation make up the reticular activating system (RAS). This is a very interesting system because it is the core of consciousness. The ascending midbrain portion of the RAS extends to the hypothalamus and then to the thalamus. Directly or indirectly, it receives information from and is stimulated by every major somatic and sensory pathway. It modulates the level of cortical activity (by a gating mechanism that enhances or diminishes neuronal activation) and, therefore, the level of consciousness (Goetz and Pappert, 1999).

The Midbrain

The midbrain is the most superior portion of the brainstem. It houses the superior colliculi, which hold visual reflex centers, and the inferior colliculi, which contain auditory reflex centers. These reflex centers involve responses, such as blinking in response to a bright light or startling in response to a loud noise.

The Forebrain

The forebrain is undoubtedly the most highly developed region of the brain. It includes two olfactory lobes (relating to the sense of smell), the cerebrum, the thalamus, the hypothalamus, the pineal and pituitary glands, and the limbic system. Much of the forebrain is also integrally involved with the endocrine system.

The cerebral cortex or cerebrum covers both the hemispheres and is made up of gray matter and unmyelinated nerve fibers that are capable of receiving, encoding, and processing information. The cerebrum integrates sensory input and motor responses. It is responsible for higher mental functions, visceral functions, behavioral reactions, perception, and some types of motor activity.

The thalamus, which also is gray matter, is one of the main regulators of sensory (except the sense of smell) input from different areas of the body to the cerebrum. It is thought to be the place in the CNS at which sensations are first consciously experienced. The thalamus then channels the neuronal input to the appropriate area of the cortex, where it will be interpreted and processed.

The hypothalamus is a very small area of the brain, about the size of a walnut, and weighs about 4 grams. It is an incredibly powerful command center and relay station. It monitors internal organs, including the endocrine system and the visceral nervous system. It is actually a link between the nervous and endocrine systems because it regulates the hormonal secretions of the pituitary, the adrenal cortex, the gonads, and the thyroid either by direct or indirect hormonal stimulation. It regulates the adrenal medulla by direct neural stimulation. The hypothalamus regulates thirst, hunger, body temperature, sexual activity, and emotional behavior as well as allergic and immune responses. It relays sensory messages, such as pain, and governs many autonomic functions so that you do not have to think about breathing or regulating your temperature or your blood flow. You can just relax and read your book because you are on automatic pilot with the hypothalamus.

The hypothalamus contains several highly specialized nuclei. In the hypothalamus, there is a structure called the *suprachiasmatic nucleus*. It is a very small structure, which is composed of approximately 10,000 neurons. Destruction of this nucleus eliminates the body's ability to maintain its circadian rhythm (i.e., daily changes in physiological processes, such as sleep patterns) or biological clock.

If you take one of these human nuclei from the suprachiasmatic nucleus and put it in a petri dish, it will exhibit its own independent electrical firing. This firing can continue for several weeks in the dish. But what is really interesting is that it maintains a circadian rhythm, with a periodicity that never deviates more than tiny amounts from the 24-hour cycle (Hastings, 1998). The suprachiasmatic nucleus is our biological clock. If we take one of us, put us in total isolation, the suprachiasmatic nucleus will keep going. We really do not entirely understand it. There is a whole field of chronobiology that has been developed over the past 20 years. It concerns our circadian rhythms and biological clock. We will be discussing this more in Chapter 6, which covers the pineal gland.

The pituitary gland, which is about the size of a pea, hangs on a stalk from the hypothalamus and is controlled by the hypothalamus. Medical students have always been taught that the pituitary gland is the "master gland," but it really is not the master gland. The pituitary stores hormones and secretes them according to instructions given by the hypothalamus. That is not a master gland. The pituitary and the hypothalamus combined are, however, a major neural–endocrine control center.

Until about 240 million years ago, vertebrates had a third eye on the top of their head. Lampreys still have one just beneath the skin. This third eye was historically a photosensitive organ, and today it appears in a modified form as the pineal gland, still with photosensitive qualities. Ancient literature refers to the third eye, the pineal gland, as the seat of wisdom or light, which, as we will see in the latter chapters of the book, would make sense.

The pineal gland is the "master gland," and in the chapter on the pineal gland (Chapter 6), we will explain in great detail why it is our master gland. The pineal gland lies on top of the third ventricle posterior to the corpus callosum. It weighs about 100 to 150 mg and is 7 mm in length and 5 mm in width. Its name derives from the Latin word *pinea*, or pinecone, because of its cone-shaped appearance. The pineal gland is an external and internal transducer of energy. It regulates neuroendocrine functions, transfers environmental information to the appropriate internal structures, and helps to regulate the immune system. It modulates the circadian rhythm, keeping our biological clock in balance.

The limbic system is an amazing system. As depicted in Figure 1.2, it surrounds the hypothalamus. Consisting of scattered but interconnected regions of gray matter, it is our emotional brain. It receives all incoming sensory input and is capable of output to motor, endocrine, and visceral systems. The limbic system is also central to our memory, and as we will see, emotion and memory are integrally related. The limbic system is made up of various processes, including the cingulate gyrus, fornix, and mamillary body. But the processes that we will concern ourselves with here are those of the amygdala and the hippocampus, as well as the thalamus and hypothalamus, which we just reviewed.

The amygdala, which means "almond" after its shape, is our center for incoming sensory input for fear, rage, aggression, and sexual feelings. What happens if you were asked, for instance, to give a lecture? If you were afraid of speaking in front of a lot of people, your adrenal gland would be producing both cortisone and adrenaline. (Adrenaline is an older but still commonly used term for epinephrine; however, most research and many physicians now refer to it as epinephrine.) Increased cortisone and adrenaline production would cause you to start sweating, your heart would be beating fast, and perhaps your voice would go into soprano once in awhile. You would probably get exhausted within 40 minutes, or maybe less. On the other hand, you might really enjoy public speaking and remain quite calm. The amygdala says: "audience, audience in front of you, everyone looking at you." It then looks to the hippocampus to see if there is a trauma memory pattern. If so,

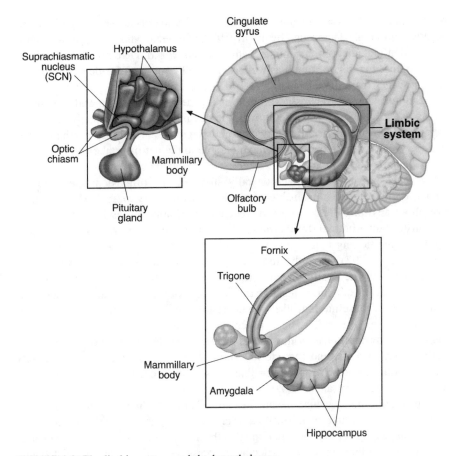

FIGURE 1.2 The limbic system and the hypothalamus.

a fear response, or what was initially described by Walter Cannon in 1914 as the "fight or flight" response, is triggered (Cannon, 1914). It is, therefore, the amygdala that determines whether or not there should be a fear or stress response and, if necessary, activates the nervous system's response via projections that link it directly with the fight-or-flight response center.

Research on the amygdala shows that there is severe impairment in the recognition of fear with patients whose amygdala has been destroyed. Studies reveal that the amygdala is involved in gaze direction and interpretation of facial expressions (Adolphs et al., 1994; Allman and Brothers, 1994). Scientists at the University of Wisconsin at Madison are carrying out research on the amygdala to learn about its association with negative emotions. They place wire meshes, which are capable of registering the electrical activity of 128 different brain sites, on the heads of subjects. The subjects are then shown a variety of pictures. Results of magnetic resonance imaging (MRI) of the brain demonstrate that our right prefrontal cortex governs negative or inhibiting feelings and that the left prefrontal cortex governs positive, more extrovert-type emotions (Robbins, 2000). There is evidence that this prefrontal portion of the brain has a memory for the representation of elementary positive and negative emotions (Davidson and Irwin, 1999). Subjects who are depressed show deficits that include both the brain's inability to allow positive emotion to dominate as a response to outside stimuli as well as an inability of the left side to turn off the fear messages from the amygdala.

Children who are depressed produce the same results of right and left frontal cortex variation as well as difficulty with processing the correct affective face as it is presented to them in pictures (Davidson and Slagter, 2000). This research indicates that the young brain is perhaps more vulnerable to the detrimental effects of severe stress than the adult brain.

When a person becomes chronically stressed, and often depressed, the left frontal cortex becomes incapable of turning off the amygdala's fear response to just about anything. This pattern of reaction inevitably brings hopelessness and despair to the individual. Furthermore, it could well be the physiological setup of the fear conditioning that occurs in posttraumatic stress disorder (Yehuda, 2000; Baker et al., 1997). Notably, the prefrontal cortex dominance pattern also is associated with the health of the immune system. Individuals who have greater right-side activity and more negative affect have lower levels of natural killer (NK) cell activity at baseline than their counterparts with predominant left-sided pre-frontal cortexes (NK cells will be discussed later in this chapter in Section 4 on the immune system). These individuals have greater decreases in their NK levels during exam periods, and they do not show as great an increase in NK activity after exposure to positive film clips than those with greater left prefrontal cortex activity (Davidson et al., 1999).

The hippocampus, which means "sea horse" after its shape, lies just next to the amygdala. Its job is to remember. What is crucial to understanding the whole theory of integral physiology is to bear in mind that the hippocampus is a huge filing cabinet for your personal memories. In particular, it stores memories that are associated with trauma and deeply imprints them in the memory.

This is very new data. Encoded traumatic memories are very hard to change because they crystallize. It takes a lot of work to change them, and this is the key, in my mind, to the healing process. It is possible, however, to erase traumatic memories or to override them with the cognitive functions of the higher-ordered brain. We will revisit this topic in later chapters.

THE PERIPHERAL NERVOUS SYSTEM

The PNS comprises 31 pairs of spinal nerves and 12 pairs of cranial nerves leading into and out of the spinal cord and the brain. The afferent (sensory) division of the PNS carries impulses *to* the CNS and the efferent (motor) division carries impulses away *from* the CNS. The efferent division of the PNS consists of the somatic nervous system and the ANS.

The Somatic Nervous System

The somatic nervous system (sometimes called the *voluntary nervous system*) involves the transport of information from the CNS to the skeletal muscle. It is concerned with motor pathways and our external world. This is the fast-moving part of the PNS.

The Autonomic Nervous System

The ANS is a network that synthesizes visceral (i.e., internal organs or their covering, especially those of the abdomen), humoral (i.e., elements, such as antibodies), and environmental information. This synthesis permits it to establish an integrated autonomic, neuroendocrine, and behavioral response to external and internal stimuli. Nerves branch out at each segment of the spinal cord to innervate the various visceral motor organs (see Figure 1.3). Autonomic means self-regulating, so these organs are all capable of functioning without our conscious thought. Mostly, that is what happens; the ANS just hums along by itself. However, we are capable of consciously altering certain visceral responses, such as heartbeat rate.

The ANS connects the CNS with numerous motor organs: the smooth muscles (i.e., not the skeletal muscles) of the heart, gastrointestinal system, and of the blood vessels as well as the adrenal, pancreas, and salivary glands. These are sometimes referred to as visceral or effector organs. What is less well known is that the ANS is also wired into the thymus, spleen, bone marrow, lymph nodes, and to the enteric nervous system. Curiously, all of these structures are a part of the immune system. What we are seeing here are new pathways, new tracks by which information may be conveyed and by which systems may communicate with one another.

There are two divisions of the ANS: the sympathetic, which leads to arousal, and the parasympathetic, which calms the body. The sympathetic nerves can cause the release of adrenaline (i.e., epinephrine), a hormone that is involved in the "fight or flight" response in our bodies. The amazing cacophony of intricate neural wiring that will respond to stimuli in the sympathetic nervous system is all regulated by that little walnut-sized hypothalamus. The PNS is set into motion by neurons in the midbrain, pons, and medulla via the vagus nerve (the major parasympathetic nerve), which allows the message to travel through the body.

THE ENTERIC NERVOUS SYSTEM

In 1917, Ulrich Trendelenburg, a German scientist, first introduced the term *peristaltic reflex* after illustrating this reflex with a segment of a guinea pig's gut, which he had isolated in an organ bath. If you tried to perform the same experiment with a heart vessel, no peristaltic reflexive action would occur, so this was an amazing finding. Trendelenburg showed that the gut has a nervous system all its own, yet his work somehow was lost from scientific practice and study. Then in 1921, an Englishman named J.N. Langley published his renowned book, *The Autonomic Nervous System*. Although until the past 10 years or so medical students have rarely been given this information, Langley stated that there were three divisions of the ANS: the sympathetic, the parasympathetic, and the enteric, which is located on the walls

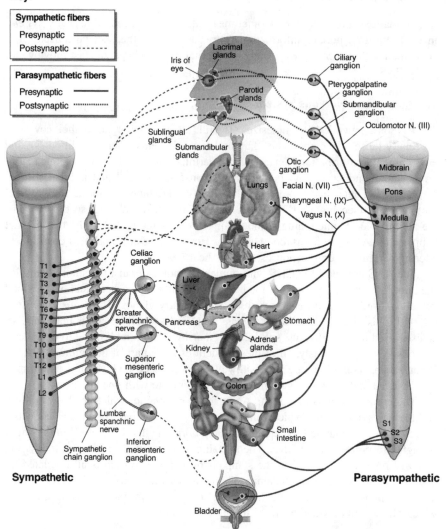

FIGURE 1.3 The autonomic nervous system.

of the gut. His opinion that the enteric system was a third division was based on his discoveries that the majority of enteric nerve cells received no direct connection or innervation from the brain or the spinal cord, in contrast to the rest of the PNS. Perhaps because of the rush of excitement resulting from the discovery of neurotransmitters, all of Langley's work was disregarded, and the neurons of the enteric system were considered simply to be part of the postganglionic parasympathetic system, which it is, but only in a relatively minor way. However, all of this information was recently brought to light by a physician, Dr. Michael Gershon, in his book *The Second Brain* (Gershon, 1998).

The enteric system, which contains approximately the same 100 billion neurons as does the spinal cord, closely resembles the CNS in its functioning (Goyal and Hirano, 1996). However, it has sensory receptors that can pick up information without any assistance from the CNS and then can activate a set of nerves that it alone controls. But the CNS does maintain contact with the enteric system via a network of sympathetic and parasympathetic fibers, allowing the ENS to integrate information into its own "brain" that comes from the CNS.

The scientific community adheres to the premise that there are two neurotransmitters that run the parasympathetic system, acetylcholine and norepinephrine. Stemming back to work begun in the 1950s, Gershon postulated that serotonin, previously considered only a CNS neurotransmitter, was also an enteric neurotransmitter. In 1981, his colleagues, not being able to deny the results of their own research, finally accepted this fact. Since that time, Gershon and others have determined that serotonin, in addition to being an enteric system neurotransmitter, is also a signaling molecule that is secreted by specialized, non-nerve cells in the gut lining. Serotonin works within the mucosa to stimulate sensory nerves that carry out peristaltic and secretory reflexes. The ENS is now known to contain at least seven different receptors that respond to serotonin (Gershon, 1998).

In addition to serotonin, there are numerous other neurotransmitters that have been identified from enteric neurons. The ENS also secretes neuropeptides identical to those secreted by the neurons in the brain, including norepinephrine, acetylcholine, endorphins, enkephalins, substance P, somatostatin, and vasoactive intestinal polypeptide (VIP). These various ENS neurotransmitters have discrete functions (Goyal and Hirano, 1996).

All of this is very interesting when you consider how we refer to our "gut feelings." One day when I was a college student, I was walking through town. I sensed a gang of boys approaching behind me. I sensed it because I felt it in the pit of my stomach. When I turned around, sure enough, a group of kids were coming after me. Similarly, when I do rounds in the hospital, I might say to a nurse or another doctor that I have a gut feeling that the patient in bed number 4 is not going to make it. I literally feel it in my gut. When we talk about our gut feelings, it is my contention that we are actually referring to our intuition (a far less acceptable term to use in the medical setting). Our gut has a brain of its own that seemingly can facilitate or collaborate with our mind or our intuition.

As a result of the work of Gershon and others, the scientific community is beginning to understand that medical problems in the enteric system may actually be localized there (i.e., as a result of heredity or other reasons) and not just a result of "nerves." In other words, the theory that the brain is responsible for all enteric abnormalities no longer holds water. Acceptance of this premise has opened the way to research and discoveries on treatment for gastrointestinal diseases, such as irritable bowel syndrome.

THE TRIUNE BRAIN

To top it off, we have three brains! We cannot contend with one, and we have three to worry about. Paul MacLean published his theory of the triune brain in 1985, showing that the forebrain of humans anatomically and chemically has common features with reptiles, early mammals, and late mammals (see Figure 1.4) (MacLean, 1985). He explains that in the evolutionary transition from reptiles to mammals, there were three key developmental factors. These include nursing, in conjunction with maternal care; auditory communication, for maintaining maternal–offspring contact; and play. These developmental changes, he theorized, correlated with the evolutionary development of the thalamocingulate division of the limbic system, which does not appear in reptiles and concerns emotion. In support of this theory, other researchers conducted an experiment that involved damage to the limbic, thalamic, and cingulate portion of female rat brains by seizure-inducing injections of lithium and pilocarpine. After giving birth, the injected rats displayed a complete absence of maternal behavior, supporting MacLean's triune theory that those brain portions are critical to the development of emotion (Peredery et al., 1992).

The first of our triune brains, then, has to do with our reptilian nature, which is controlled by the brainstem. The reptilian response to a stimulus is different from the fright one might experience before giving a lecture. It is more like the experience of stepping on a nail. You don't calmly say, "I perceive I just stepped on a nail. Perhaps it would be good to lift my foot now." No. It is a rapid, automatic response, generally accompanied by an expletive. There are long reflex arcs through the

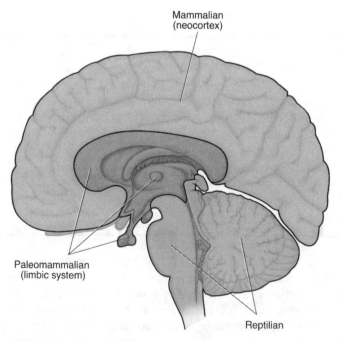

Mammalian
(neocortex)

Paleomammalian
(limbic system)

Reptilian

FIGURE 1.4 The triune brain.

brainstem that convey the information. So even before you feel the nail, the information is transmitted up to the brain. Think about how reptiles react. They do not reflect; they are not worried about feelings. They simply react. This is the reptilian brain.

The development of the thalamocingulate division of the limbic system is our second and mammalian brain. This is the brain that is concerned with feelings and emotions and is much like that of our pet dogs or cats. Pets exhibit emotions: they feel good; they purr; they bark; they get angry. They just put out their feelings. However, pets have absolutely no sense of time, no sense of prioritized thinking, and no ability to dream of the future. Therefore, animals are not really subject to the acculturation processes that humans are.

The third brain is the human brain, which is affiliated with the limbic system but controlled by the prefrontal neocortex. MacLean saw the human brain as key to the development of familial acculturation. The human brain is capable of higher cognitive processes, of perceiving time, and of pondering the spiritual self.

So these are the three brains: the reptilian, the mammalian, and the human brain. The triune brain is sometimes inaccurately described as simply an evolutionary process culminating in the human brain. However, our brains should more correctly be thought of as a dynamic interaction of the evolutionary trends of the three. We each employ all three of our brains in the course of a day. As we develop as individuals, we have the daunting task of effectively integrating our three minds.

NEURONS AND NEUROTRANSMITTERS

There are two interconnected modalities that the brain uses to communicate with the outside world as well as with the rest of the body: chemical and electrical. Electrical impulses, carried by neurons, move information to various locations, but they communicate with each other in a chemical language via neurotransmitters. In Section 2, entitled "The Endocrine System," we will review more fully the chemical, or hormonal, modes of communication.

As already mentioned, the neuron is the basic unit of communication or information processing in the nervous system. A neuron or nerve cell is made up of a cell body, dendrites, and an axon. Dendrites increase the available area for a neuron to receive incoming information. The axon is typically the structure by which the cell sends out information. A nerve is a cluster of processes (mostly axons) from many neurons. The axon is wrapped in a fatty coating called a *myelin sheath*, which is like a coat of insulation that preserves electrical impulses. It allows the impulses to traverse down the nerve in a rapid and smooth fashion. The sympathetic nervous system is myelinated, and the parasympathetic is unmyelinated. Multiple sclerosis, for instance, occurs when the myelin sheath is disturbed or destroyed, preventing the electrical impulses from being transmitted properly.

There are three types of neurons: sensory (which send information *to* the CNS), motor (which relay information *away* from the CNS to muscles or glands), and interneurons (which are situated between a sensory and a motor neuron and help to integrate information). For example, receptors in the eye that are sensitive to light are linked to sensory neurons that can relay the information to the CNS. After processing this information, if the brain determines that a motor response is needed, it sends the message via the motor neurons, and your body moves.

When a neuron is at rest, there is a steady voltage difference across its plasma membrane. This is called the *resting potential*. When the neuron receives a strong enough signal, an action potential is created. This is a get-up-and-go message, causing a brief reversal in voltage across the plasma membrane. Action potentials arise and move rapidly along sensory and motor neurons because of the myelin sheath.

Each neuron has an input or presynaptic zone and an output or postsynaptic zone. When the action potential reaches the postsynaptic output zone, it either just stops or it may release a neurotransmitter that passes the message along. Neurotransmitters are substances released on excitation from a presynaptic neuron of the CNS or PNS. They can be either excitatory, causing the receiving neuron to continue passing the electrical impulse, or inhibitory, stopping the chain of electrical firings. The neurotransmitter 'jumps' between the axon terminal of the presynaptic neuron to the receptor molecules located on the postsynaptic neuron to pass along information. The region of communication between two neurons is called a *synapse*, which is illustrated in Figure 1.5.

A signal coming from the CNS to any skeletal muscle takes a nonstop route. A signal coming from the CNS to an ANS organ passes the message along via nerve cell bodies called *ganglions*. The first nerve cell is called the *preganglionic nerve*, and the second nerve to receive the message is called the *postganglionic nerve*. The neurotransmitter for sympathetic and parasympathetic preganglionic and for the parasympathetic postganglionic neurons is acetylcholine. The neurotransmitter for sympathetic postganglionic neurons is norepinephrine. The postganglionic nerve carries the message along to the outlying effector organs. Thus, sending messages to the ANS is a little like playing "telephone" as a kid: the message might get there intact, but it might get changed along the way.

Do you ever wonder if your neurons can be replaced? Is there such a thing as neurogenesis? When I was in medical school, we were taught that humans were born with something like 100 billion neurons, and when any one neuron died, that was the end. Recently, Fred Gage, from the Salk Institute for Biological Studies in La Jolla, California, and his colleagues in Sweden have shown that neurons can be produced in the adult human being, not just the child, which completely blows a major theory. The neurons Gage researched were produced in the dentate gyrus of the hippocampus. The rate of proliferation was not high, about 500 new neurons a day, but they did have the morphologic and phenotypic characteristics of neurons (Eriksson et al., 1998). Although the biological significance of this neurogenesis is yet to be fully determined, it is very interesting to keep in mind for later, when we talk about the healing response, because, as you will remember, the hippocampus is the center of traumatic memory.

Neurotransmitters can bind with receptor proteins on the membrane of a neuron, a muscle (this is called the *neuromuscular junction*), or a gland, and as we said,

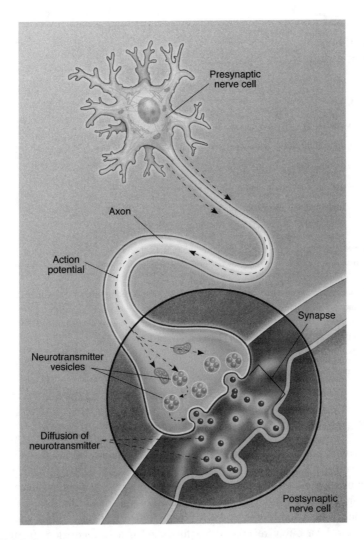

FIGURE 1.5 Synapse.

they can excite or inhibit them. See Table 1.1 for a list of neurotransmitters. Some of these substances (e.g., norepinephrine, epinephrine, dopamine, and serotonin) are also released directly into the bloodstream, and then they are considered hormones (see Section 2 on the endocrine system in this chapter).

In medical school, I learned that one neuron was capable of secreting only one neurotransmitter. That made it very easy to pass my physiology test. Today's medical students do not have it so easy, because it is now known that one neuron can secrete several neurotransmitters.

Neuromodulators can make the postsynaptic neuron more sensitive or less sensitive to the neurotransmitter that is present. Endorphins, which are naturally occurring substances in our body, are important neuromodulators because they are powerful painkillers.

TABLE 1.1
Neurotransmitters

Class I:

Acetylcholine (ACh)

Class II: Amines

Norepinephrine, epinephrine, dopamine, serotonin, and histamine

Class III: Amino acids

Inhibitory—glycine and γ-aminobutyric acid (GABA)

Excitatory—aspartate and glutamate

Class IV: Polypeptides—there are over 60 peptides, some are listed here:

A. Hypothalamic: corticotropin-releasing hormone (CRH), thyrotropin-releasing hormone (TRH), somatostatin (growth hormone), growth-hormone-releasing hormone (GRH), and gonadotropin-releasing hormone (GnRH)

B. Pituitary peptides: adrenocorticotropic hormone (ACTH), β-endorphin, vasopressin, oxytocin, and α-melanocyte-stimulating hormone

C. Peptides that act on the gut and brain: enkephalins, substance P, cholecystokinin (CCK), vasoactive intestinal polypeptide (VIP), insulin, glucagon, and neurotensin

D. Peptides from various other tissues: angiotensin II, bradykinin

E. Lipids: anandamide, sn-2 arachidonylglycerol (2-AG), noladin ether

YOUR THOUGHTS AND CNS NEUROTRANSMITTERS

It is my contention that the brain is capable of secreting any hormone it so chooses, at any given point in time. We are just beginning to understand this phenomenon. It is also my opinion that cortical activity, which means a thought, produces a series of hormones (neuropeptides) that flood into other portions of the brain, frequently the limbic system. The limbic system is asking, "Do I see anything I want to pick up here? Do I have any receptors that fit?" And if a receptor does fit, there is a response throughout the body.

A field of research called *psychoendocrinology* is concerned with hormones and the behavioral effects attributed to them. Neuropeptides are any of the molecules composed of short chains of peptides (e.g., endorphins, enkephalins, and vasopressin) that are found in the brain tissue. Typically, they localize in axon terminals at synapses. Peptides are small proteins. *Neuro* means they come from neurons. Neuropeptides are a type of neurotransmitter, but some function as hormones. Neuropeptides that function as hormones produce chemical signals instead of electrical signals. These hormones can communicate with another structure or another system. For instance, when we think a particular thought, receptors in the limbic system (the limbic system is rich in receptors) affect numerous functions, including sexual behavior, sleep, temperature regulation, breathing, blood pressure, addiction, habituation, memory, and learning. Influenced by thoughts, the brain secretes and releases neuropeptides. The core limbic structures, long considered the emotional center of the brain, are infused with receptors, not only for opioids, such as endorphins and enkephalins, but also for the majority of the neuropeptides. The neuropeptides are secreted when you have a thought process that impinges on this limbic system. If there are receptors in the limbic system for these particular hormones, there will be an alteration of the response.

Neuropeptides can alter or influence behavior and physiological function. For example, calcitonin, a neuropeptide produced in the CNS, is typically thought of as being produced in the thyroid gland. But it is produced in the brain also (Rizzo and Goltzman, 1981; van Houten et al., 1982). What is it doing in the brain? Recent research has shown that there is a whole calcitonin-based system for pain relief that is similar to the endorphins (e.g., Ormazabal et al., 2001; Xu et al., 2000; Yamazaki et al., 1999). It has been there for millions of years, and we are just discovering it.

Another example of a neuropeptide that has significant behavioral impact is DDAVP (desmopressin acetate), which is a synthetic version of a hormone called *antidiuretic hormone* (ADH) or *vasopressin*. ADH is a major stress hormone, secreted by the anterior pituitary during physical stress. For example, you go wandering in the desert and it is a hot day, and you forgot your water bottle. But, you do not care and continue to walk. The thirst mechanism exclaims, "Oh my, what are you doing?" and the pituitary begins to release ADH. Your kidneys get the message loud and clear: "Hold on to your water!" (The kidney tubules reabsorb the water so that less is lost as urine.) ADH is a major stress hormone that keeps you going until you get to the next oasis. ADH also helps you remember, "Do *not* do this again!" So, it also enhances memory.

Experiments with DDAVP have been conducted. Male subjects treated with DDAVP demonstrated better memory than control subjects, but the hormone has no effect on women (Beckwith et al., 1984). Male subjects who were given 60 μg of DDAVP by nasal inhaler had enhanced recall of narrative passages (Beckwith et al., 1987). However, in other DDAVP research, low-verbal subjects had greater improvement in *immediate* memory, and high-verbal subjects had increased *delayed* memory, demonstrating that the impact of vasopressin on memory relates not only to gender but to individual verbal ability as well (Till and Beckwith, 1985).

YOUR THOUGHTS AND IMMUNE CELLS

The nerve cells in the brain are capable of instigating an immune response. Not long ago, any medical doctor would have disagreed with that statement. We will devote a whole chapter to understanding this and other system-integration issues. The important concept to grasp now is that these very cells that we have elaborated are secreting hormones and consequently allowing communication across major systems.

We Are on the Planet like a Work of Art

There are basically three directions of information transmission to the command center, which is our hypothalamus. Moving via chemical and electrical pathways, our thoughts go to the hypothalamus from the cortex; our emotional reactions go to the hypothalamus from the limbic system; and, as described, our states of awareness go to the hypothalamus from the reticular formation.

I want to digress briefly to convey a belief that is very important to me. If someone has been meditating, maybe for 10 years, he or she begins to get a sense of eternity, a sense of accepting the fact that we are on the planet like a work of art. We are like flowers—we are seeded, we grow, we blossom, and part of life is that we start to refold, and then we are gone. That is the way it is; that is the way it has always been. When we deeply understand this truth, there is a sense of serenity that comes to our lives. This, I think, is going to be the key to future research in consciousness and awareness, and how it interfaces with physiology. I think that research will increasingly show that when our higher awareness center (i.e., the reticular formation) is capable of affecting input into the hypothalamus, it will not only override our fear system (i.e., the amygdala) but our thoughts as well. And when the reticular formation becomes the command center, everything settles down into a state of physiologic relaxation, healing, and harmony.

So, input to the hypothalamus is via the cortex for thoughts, the limbic system for emotions, and the reticular formation for "states of awareness or levels of consciousness." (I put this in quotes because it is not proven yet.) We will let the hypothalamus worry about which one to listen to. Another route to experiencing higher states of consciousness comes by working on quieting our state of mind, using a technique that I call limbic therapy. Limbic therapy begins with an understanding of brain waves. Brain waves are the fluctuations of electrical potential in the brain. They appear in different patterns, depending upon how much electrical current is emanating from the nerve cells.

When brain patterns are recorded on an electroencephalogram (EEG), the brain waves characteristically resonate between 14 and about 38 to 40 cycles per second. One cycle per second is called a *hertz* (Hz). Figure 1.6 depicts the appearance of various EEG brain waves and correlates them with their common states of awareness. States of awareness in which you are fully alert and in which there is intense activity of the nervous system are called *beta*. In the beta state, your brain waves have a frequency of 15 to 30 cycles per second. The alpha state, from 8 to 14 Hz, includes normal waking hours and when you are in a relaxed state of mind. You are able to be alert, but you are also very restful. You are not ruminating over memories of things you have to do, things you may not want to do, or arguments you may have had. Neither are you feeling very hungry, because that brings you back into beta. It is a feeling of restful peace. Theta, which is 4 to 7 Hz, is a state of approaching

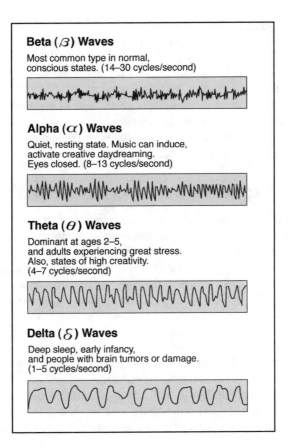

Beta (β) Waves

Most common type in normal, conscious states. (14–30 cycles/second)

Alpha (α) Waves

Quiet, resting state. Music can induce, activate creative daydreaming. Eyes closed. (8–13 cycles/second)

Theta (θ) Waves

Dominant at ages 2–5, and adults experiencing great stress. Also, states of high creativity. (4–7 cycles/second)

Delta (δ) Waves

Deep sleep, early infancy, and people with brain tumors or damage. (1–5 cycles/second)

FIGURE 1.6 Brain waves.

sleep and a state that is called *hypnogogic reverie* or *hypnogogia*. Meditation is an alpha and sometimes a theta state. If you move from color images while meditating to black-and-white images, you are into theta. If you are into delta (3.5 Hz), you are preparing to leave the planet or you are in very deep sleep. You are not thinking about anything.

It is my theory that theta is a state of mind in which the healing of old emotional traumas may occur, which is why I call it limbic therapy. It is a state that allows us to get into the traumatic memories that have been encoded in the hippocampus and either greatly decrease their impact or actually erase them. We will be revisiting this issue many times.

In the next section, we will take a look at the endocrine system.

Essential Points

- An understanding of the parts of the brain will aid you in understanding much of the rest of the book.
- The pineal, and not the pituitary, is the master gland.

- The amygdala is our fear center.
- The hippocampus encodes and crystallizes memories.
- The gut has a brain of its own.
- The triune-brain theory challenges us with the daunting task of integrating our reptilian, mammalian, and human brains.
- The neuron is the nervous system's basic unit of communication. Neurotransmitters facilitate this communication.
- Neuropeptides can have behavioral effects, and thoughts can influence the health of the immune system.

SECTION 2: THE ENDOCRINE SYSTEM

The endocrine system is a system of internal structures that secrete hormones (mostly into the bloodstream) to regulate metabolism and perform myriad other bodily functions. The endocrine system is not as zippy as the nervous system. It turns an electrical signal into the elaboration of a single hormone or of several hormones, which then travel to various places in the body, communicating and directing physiological activity. The glands of the endocrine system include the pituitary, hypothalamus, thyroid, parathyroid, pancreas, adrenals, gonads (ovaries and testes), thymus, and the pineal gland (see Figure 1.7). In addition, there are various other organs with hormonal functions that are not technically considered to be endocrine glands, such as the previously discussed enteric system. In the first half of the 20th century, scientists did not think of the brain as an endocrine organ. After nearly 15 years of work, two researchers, Guillemin and Schally, identified the first hypothalamic secretion of hormones. In 1976, they both won the Nobel Prize for their efforts. Scientists continue to discover new hormones and neurotransmitters.

HORMONES AND THEIR PROPERTIES

Hormones are the mode of communication for the endocrine system, and they include various types of proteins as well as steroids. For a hormone to have an effect, the cell must have a receptor site specific to that hormone. If the hormone does not exactly fit into the receptor (which is similar to the paradigm of a triangle fitting into a triangle or a circle into a circle), the hormone has absolutely no effect on that cell. Not every cell has a receptor for every hormone, although many cells have receptor sites for more than one hormone. Sometimes the receptors for a given hormone are predominantly localized on one organ, but increasingly, receptors for such hormones are being found in other organs as well as the brain.

The body produces its hormones or neurotransmitters, which are referred to as endogenous ligands. However, different pharmaceutical agents and other *exogenous* substances also fit into a receptor. These are important terms with which to be familiar. In some instances, the drug mimics the endogenous ligand; in other instances, it can produce a much stronger or different reaction. When either a drug *or* an endogenous ligand produces a known effect, it is called an *agonist*. When a drug or endogenous ligand exhibits the ability to block a receptor, it is called an *antagonist*. A reverse or inverse agonist is a drug or endogenous ligand that produces

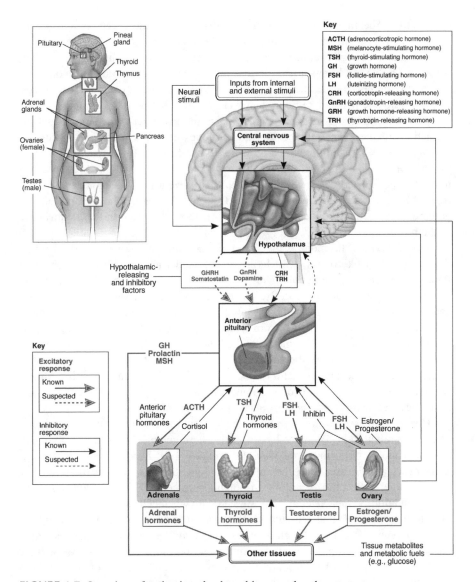

FIGURE 1.7 Overview of endocrine glands and hormonal pathways.

symptoms opposite to those that are known. Sometimes one receptor can interact with all three types of ligands. In Chapter 5, which addresses the relaxation system, you will read about the benzodiazepine receptor that accepts all three types of ligands. Keep in mind that multiple receptors also may be activated by the same ligand via a number of mechanisms. Different ligands for the same receptor probably elicit diverse magnitudes of response and use several signaling pathways under varied conditions (Pauwels, 2000).

Peptide hormones consist of proteins (e.g., insulin), glycoproteins (e.g., luteinizing hormone), peptides (e.g., oxytocin), or amines (e.g., epinephrine, formerly called *adrenaline*). The interaction between the hormone and the receptor activates an enzyme, called *adenyl cyclase*, within the cell. The adenyl cyclase diffuses into the cytoplasm and, through chemical reactions, produces cyclic adenosine monophosphate (cAMP). The cAMP brings about the reaction that is attributed to the hormone. It is the energy source—a little like filling the car with gas so that it can run. This process is quite rapid and is far more rapid than that of steroid hormones.

Hormone molecules that are steroids (e.g., cortisol) act on receptors that are located within the cell membrane. Steroid hormones are synthesized from cholesterol and are lipid or fat soluble, which as you will recall, means that they do not have to cross the blood–brain barrier. They diffuse through the cell membrane to receptors that affect designated genes within the DNA. This event instigates messenger RNA (mRNA) synthesis within the cytoplasm. The mRNA then synthesizes proteins. It is these proteins that produce cAMP and bring about the reaction that is attributed to the hormone.

Another type of hormone is the group of eicosanoid hormones (prostaglandins, thromboxanes, leukotrienes, C30 hydroxyfatty acids, and lipoxins), which are a family of oxygenated fatty acids. They are transported through the bloodstream like endocrine hormones and act locally. The eicosanoids are derived from arachidonic acid, an essential fatty acid, and have short half-lives. Each locally acting hormone system mainly affects the tissue from which it is produced. We will be discussing a class of arachidonic acid hormones, called the *cannabinoids*, in Chapter 5, which covers relaxation. They are the endogenous ligands that fit into the same receptors as the exogenous substance of tetrahydrocannabinol (THC) or marijuana. In addition, lymphocytes produce a type of hormone called *cytokines*. These are not classic hormones. We will review them in Section 4 on the immune system.

Hormonal messages are not always passed via the classic means of release of neurotransmitter and acceptance by receptor. These chemical messengers may also communicate in more localized ways (see Figure 1.8). For instance, when some messengers are diffused into the interstitial fluid, that is, the fluid between two neurons, they latch onto receptors on neighboring cells. This is called *paracrine* communication. *Autocrine* communication occurs when cells secrete hormones that bind to the same cell that secreted it. This may sound like a minor point. Indeed, you may even be thinking, "Well, that doesn't sound too significant because, after all, the powerful neuropeptides are the important hormones." Wrong. As we will see in the next chapter, what occurs by paracrine and autocrine communication is eminently important to the overall function of the organism.

We will now review each of the organs of the endocrine system.

THE PITUITARY GLAND

The pituitary gland, which is about the size of a pea, has been called the *master gland* because it produces hormones that regulate the activity and function of other endocrine glands. Even by the 1950s, scientist knew that the pituitary was not a master gland, but the myth persists today. It influences numerous metabolic processes, including growth. The posterior pituitary stores and secretes hormones that are synthesized by the hypothalamus (see Table 1.2). It secretes vasopressin (or

Autocrine

Paracrine

Endocrine

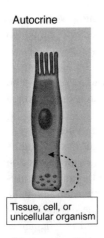

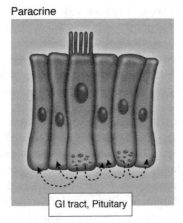

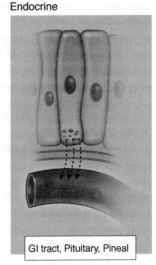

Tissue, cell, or
unicellular organism

GI tract, Pituitary

Neurotransmitter

GI tract, Pituitary, Pineal

Neuroendocrine

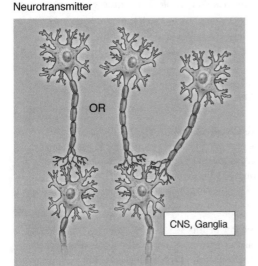

OR

CNS, Ganglia

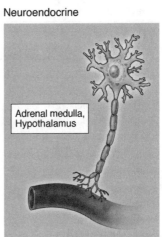

Adrenal medulla,
Hypothalamus

FIGURE 1.8 Transmission of endocrine messages.

TABLE 1.2
Hormones of the Posterior Pituitary

Antidiuretic hormone (ADH) or vasopressin (VAP)	conserves water, modulates ACTH release
Oxytocin	produces lactation, reduces stress in women

arginine vasopressin [VAP]), which is frequently referred to as ADH because one of its major physiological effects is retention of water by the kidneys, as we discussed previously. It conserves water for the body's use. The synthesis of ADH or VAP is controlled by the hypothalamus. Very importantly, VAP also potentiates the release

of adrenocorticotropic hormone (ACTH) by the hypothalamus, which would serve
to enhance the stress response. The posterior pituitary also secretes oxytocin, which
acts on the uterus and affects milk ejection during lactation. New research shows
that oxytocin is a significant factor in the stress response of women, but not for men.
It buffers the fight-or-flight response in women, encouraging instead a desire to tend
children and gather with other women. We will review this research in Chapter 3
on stress.

Neurons secreting posterior pituitary hormones do so directly into blood vessels
in the posterior pituitary, and they are then transported to the target tissue. This is
in contrast to the anterior pituitary, which primarily secretes hormones on instruction
from the hypothalamus (circulating hormones can also influence the anterior pituitary). These hormones then influence other glands, such as the thyroid, adrenals,
and gonads. The pituitary is also influenced by autocrine and paracrine signals arising
from its own cells. These signals, called *cytokines*, will be reviewed in Chapter 2.
The anterior pituitary secretes six hormones (see Table 1.3), three glycoproteins and
three polypeptides.

TABLE 1.3
Hormones of the Anterior Pituitary

	Three Glycoproteins
Luteinizing hormone (LH)	gametogenesis; production of male and female hormones
Thyroid-stimulating hormone (TSH)	stimulates the thyroid gland; stimulates production of thyroid hormone by the thyroid gland
Follicle-stimulating hormone (FSH)	stimulates the production of eggs or ova in females and sperm in males; also stimulates the ovary to produce estrogen
	Three Polypeptides
Adrenocorticotropic hormone (ACTH)	stimulates secretion of adrenal steroid hormones, including cortisol; stimulates the adrenal gland
Growth hormone (GH)	affects protein synthesis and cell division; critical for growth, especially of the cartilage and bone
Prolactin (PRL)	affects the mammary glands, lactation; stimulates the proliferation of cytokines

---

Briefly, LH and FSH are involved in reproduction, and TSH acts on the thyroid.
PRL affects the mammary glands and is most important for lactation. In Chapter 2,
Systems Integration, we will see that prolactin is a modulator of the immune system,
stimulating the proliferation of cytokines. GH affects protein synthesis and cell
division, and as the name implies, it is critical for growth, especially of the cartilage
and bone. Finally, ACTH facilitates the release of adrenal steroid hormones (see
section on adrenal glands) by stimulating receptor sites in the adrenal cortex. ACTH
is particularly important for controlling cortisol secretion. You will learn more about

ACTH and cortisol in Section 3 on the stress system, and it will be revisited in Chapter 3, Stress System.

Pro-Opiomelanocortin (POMC) and the Pituitary

There are a number of peptide proteins that are produced both by the nervous system and by the pituitary that derive from a big, primordial hormone called *pro-opiomelanocortin* (POMC). POMC is made in a variety of tissues, including the brain, lymphocytes, and the anterior and posterior pituitary. POMC is a precursor peptide that weighs 31,000 daltons and has 265 amino acids. In the mid-1970s, opiate receptors were discovered, and it was learned that some of the endogenous opioid ligands (hormones in this instance), such as β-endorphins, are present within the POMC molecule. In addition to β-endorphins, ACTH, lipoproteins, and melanocyte-stimulating hormone (MSH) are all synthesized from POMC. All of these peptides possess behavioral effects, and many are involved in the stress response, including ACTH, β-endorphin, and enkephalins. (See more in Section 3 on the stress system.)

HYPOTHALAMUS

The hypothalamus releases and inhibits hormones that are carried via vessels from the hypothalamus to the pituitary. It is the structure from which tropic hormones (i.e., hormones that cause secretion of other hormones) approach, influence, and stimulate various tissues. This is also the pathway by which other endocrine glands can exert their own feedback control on the hormones that the pituitary and hypothalamus secrete. The hypothalamus is our control center, integrating the chemical input from the CNS, the CSF, and from the general circulation. The hormones of the hypothalamus are listed in Table 1.4.

TABLE 1.4
Hormones of the Hypothalamus

Corticotropin-releasing hormone (CRH)	stimulates the secretion of corticotropin, which is a hormone that tells the pituitary to secrete ACTH during stress; in addition to the hypothalamus, it is present in the limbic system, cortex, adrenal medulla, pancreas, gut, and placenta
Thyrotropin-releasing hormone (TRH)	stimulates the release of thyrotropin from the anterior pituitary, which stimulates and sustains hormonal secretions from the thyroid
Growth-hormone-releasing hormone (GRH)	stimulates the secretion of growth hormone from the pituitary
Somatostatin (or growth-hormone-inhibiting hormone)	inhibits the release of numerous hormones, including GH, thyrotropin, corticotropin, insulin, glucagon, gastrin, and secretin
Gonadotropin-releasing hormone (GnRH)	regulates the growth and function of the ovaries and testes; it stimulates the secretion of FSH and LH from the pituitary
Prolactin-inhibiting hormone (dopamine)	is released to stop prolactin secretion, which stimulates milk production in a woman after giving birth

---

THYROID

The thyroid gland produces thyroid hormones (i.e., thyroxine and triodothyronine) which requires iodine for synthesis and cannot be produced in adequate amounts without it. Thyroid hormones stimulate cells to consume oxygen; increases the rate of cell metabolism (i.e., the rate that cells release energy from carbohydrates); regulates lipid, protein, and carbohydrate metabolism; stimulates bodily heat production; and is essential for normal growth. The functions of the thyroid are controlled by TSH secretion from the pituitary, and a balance in thyroid hormone level is necessary for proper development and to maintain health. The hypothalamus and pituitary are involved in a direct inhibitory feedback loop that adjusts the rate of thyroid secretion to keep it at a balanced level. The thyroid gland also produces calcitonin, a hormone that lowers calcium levels in the blood by inhibiting bone resorption (i.e., inhibits calcium from leaving the bone and increases calcium excretion in the urine). Calcitonin decreases the amount of calcium that the intestines absorb; as mentioned, it modulates pain perception in the brain (e.g., Ormazabal et al., 2001; Xu et al., 2000; Yamazaki et al., 1999). Calcitonin is probably going to prove to be one of the most important anti-aging hormones; however the research is not yet there to illustrate this theory definitively (Kalu, 1984; Yamaga et al., 2001).

PARATHYROID

The parathyroid glands are four small glands located behind the thyroid gland. Special cells, called *chief cells*, in the parathyroid secrete parathyroid hormone (PTH), which is involved in calcium and phosphate metabolism. PTH is the major regulator of blood calcium levels and performs actions opposite to calcitonin. PTH activates vitamin D to maintain a constant level of calcium in the blood. This is necessary for nerve and muscle function, blood coagulation, and formation of bone and teeth.

PANCREAS

The pancreas is an organ that has both exocrine and endocrine capabilities. The exocrine portion produces digestive enzymes. The endocrine portion involves the secretion of insulin, glucagon, and somatostatin. Insulin is important for metabolism and regulates glucose by *lowering* it. If there is more glucose than can be used by the body, it is converted by insulin to glycogen. Glycogen resides in the liver and muscle cells. Insulin facilitates storage of triglycerides in adipose tissue. Glucagon, like insulin, is important for metabolism and regulates blood glucose by *raising* it. A normal blood glucose level is essential, as it is the energy source for the entire nervous system. Somatostatin helps regulate carbohydrate metabolism and inhibits the release of numerous hormones, including insulin.

ADRENALS

The adrenal glands are our stress glands. There are two adrenal glands, one resting atop each kidney. The adrenal glands act like brake liners. When the rubber hits the road, when you start getting stressed, it is the stress hormones that go into action to keep your body in a somewhat resilient state. The adrenal gland consists of two endocrine organs: the adrenal medulla and the adrenal cortex. The hypothalamus communicates with the adrenal medulla via an electrical route and with the adrenal cortex via a hormonal route (Table 1.5).

TABLE 1.5
Hormones of the Adrenal Cortex (Corticosteroids)

Mineralocorticoids	aldosterone, which regulates mineral electrolytes, thus maintaining blood volume and pressure and facilitating nerve impulse conduction and muscle contraction
Glucocorticoids	cortisol and corticosterone, which break down proteins and convert them to glucose; cortisol ensures that the glucose in the bloodstream is adequate to meet the needs of the brain; during stress, it reduces glucose delivery to some parts of the body, slowing the uptake of glucose from the blood and using it for tissues like skeletal muscles, with the brain always being supplied first; glucocorticoids also break down fat that can be used for energy; the effect of these hormones is long lasting, as they are removed slowly from body tissue
Androgenic steroids	two androgens (the synthetic version is the well-known anabolic steroids)— dehydroepiandrosterone (DHEA) and androstenedione (which can be converted to testosterone)—and small amounts of estrogen

The main hormonal secretions of the adrenal medulla are the catecholamines, primarily epinephrine but also norepinephrine. Epinephrine and norepinephrine (which also act as neurotransmitters) are secreted during stress. The result is a multiorgan response. Epinephrine is a vasodilator, causing increased heart rate and force of myocardial contraction; dilation of the smooth muscles of blood vessels; and elevation of the level of available sugars and fatty acids in the blood, which gives immediate energy reserves for the fight-or-flight response. While both hormones increase alertness, epinephrine evokes anxiety and fear. Norepinephrine is a vasoconstrictor that affects brain regions concerned with emotions (it is found in elevated amounts in depressed persons), dreaming and awaking, control of food intake, and regulation of body temperature.

Gonads

The gonads are the testes in males and the ovaries in females. In both sexes, they have two functions, which is gametogenesis (creation of germ cells) and the production of sex hormones. The main feminizing sex hormones are the estrogens, and the main masculinizing hormones are the androgens, particularly testosterone. Gametogenesis is dependent upon hormonal secretions of GnRH from the hypothalamus as well as LH and FSH from the anterior pituitary.

THYMUS

The thymus has the appearance of a lymph node and lies behind the breastbone. The thymus is crucial to the immune system because it is the location where white blood cells, called *lymphocytes*, undergo important steps in maturation and, consequently, become T lymphocytes. The thymus is the master trainer of the T lymphocyte portion of the acquired immune system. Cells of the thymus are capable of producing hormones, including thymosin, thymulin, and thymopoietin. Thymic hormones have independent neuroendocrine effects and can increase the secretion of other hormones, including ACTH, corticosterone, GH, and prolactin (Ader et al., 1991).

When I was in medical school, it was thought that the thymus atrophies some time after puberty. If you take chest x-rays, the thymus will no longer appear after childhood. Studies were performed that showed that the thymus does not atrophy. Rather, it involutes, and it takes a computed tomography (CT) scan of the chest to pick up the image (see Figure 1.9). Correlating to the involution process, there is a progressive decline in thymic hormone secretion throughout adulthood (Bellinger et al., 2001). The thymic cortex progressively shrinks because it changes from a dense tissue full of blood into fatty tissue with fewer thymocytes (i.e., mature and immature T lymphocytes found in the thymus) (Bellinger et al., 2001). When we are young, the thymus is busy educating cells in an effort to establish a strong immune system in the body. It then becomes smaller because most of its work is completed. But it is still there, ready to secrete hormones and train lymphocytes if we become quite ill and need it.

PINEAL GLAND

The pineal gland orchestrates both the endocrine and immune systems. It truly is the master gland, as it transmits information from the environment to our body systems and helps us regulate ourselves with the outside world. In today's world, that can sometimes be a problem, an issue that we will address in other chapters.

The pineal gland secretes a hormone called *melatonin* that is crucial to our biological rhythm. The pineal is photosensitive, which means that it is influenced by light. Light stimulates the suprachiasmatic nucleus (which we will discuss in detail in Chapter 6, The Pineal) to tell the specialized secretory cells of the pineal gland, called *pinealocytes*, to slow secretion of melatonin. At night, or in the absence of light, higher levels of melatonin are secreted by the pinealocytes into the CSF, which carries it to the bloodstream and helps to promote sleep. Melatonin has various other functions, such as modulating reproductive development (by inhibiting gonadotropin-releasing hormone), influencing mood, and regulating hunger and satiety. There is a whole chapter on the pineal, so you will be learning a lot about this little gland and why it is our master gland.

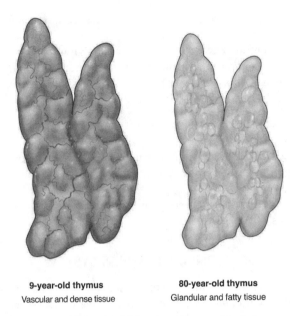

9-year-old thymus
Vascular and dense tissue

80-year-old thymus
Glandular and fatty tissue

FIGURE 1.9 Thymus of a 9-year-old child and an 80-year-old adult.

THE GUT

Endocrine cells in the stomach secrete the hormone gastrin, which stimulates the secretion of hydrochloric acid (HCl) into the stomach. The hormone somatostatin stops the secretion of this acid. The duodenum secretes secretin, a peptide in the lining of the small intestine that stimulates the pancreas to secrete bicarbonate, which neutralizes stomach acids, thus allowing the intestinal enzymes to function.

RECEPTORS AND HEALTH

Ideally, the endocrine system produces a harmonious cascade of chemicals that keep our bodies humming along, fit and content. The receptors, capable of receiving an endogenous hormone may be similar or identical to those that link up with an exogenous drug. Conversely, when there is an exogenous drug that is influencing behavior, there must be a receptor to receive it. THC, the active agent in marijuana, for example, is now known to have endogenous THC receptors in the brain and in spleen tissue. Similarly, specific receptors have been found in the brain for the chemical benzodiazepine. Benzodiazepine receptors are capable of receiving drugs, such as Librium and Valium, which also can influence behavior. Do pharmaceutical companies develop drugs that are the only substances that can fit into a given receptor? No. Every time there is a receptor located for an exogenous drug, there has to be an endogenous ligand that will fit into this receptor as well. Furthermore, and importantly, it is likely that there are natural (i.e., not synthetic) exogenous substances that fit into that same receptor. These natural agents, frequently, have a more favorable side-effect profile but may take much longer to exhibit efficacy. Far fewer research dollars are designated for natural exogenous substances than pharmaceutical agents, so consequently, less is know about their pharmacokinetic properties.

In the chapter on the relaxation system (Chapter 4), we will learn more about the benzodiazepines and other hormones that facilitate our relaxation response. The existence of a relaxation system that mirrors our stress system (i.e., the fight-or-flight response) is presented for the first time.

ESSENTIAL POINTS

- Hormones are the basic unit of communication for the endocrine system.
- The organs of the endocrine system secrete hormones that govern myriad functions.
- The same receptor can accept both endogenous ligands and exogenous substances.

SECTION 3: THE STRESS SYSTEM

Now that we have reviewed both the nervous and endocrine systems, we can begin to understand the contribution to and integration of these two systems in the stress response. We will also see that stress has a powerful role in instigation and modulation of the immune system. This discussion is a preview of the next chapter on systems interactions, and it will make the reading of the next section on the immune system a richer experience.

As shown in Figure 1.10, the human stress system has both a neural and an endocrine pathway, which means that the same stimulus activates both systems simultaneously. When there is a stressful stimulus, the message is conveyed, via the cerebral cortex and limbic system, to the hypothalamus. The stimulus can be either physical or cognitive, including upsetting emotions, memories, or thoughts. The electrical response is faster than the chemical one, but throughout the process, the chemical highway sustains the responses.

The hypothalamus–pituitary–adrenal (HPA) axis governs the chemical highway. The HPA axis is highly sensitive to stimuli of various sorts. The hypothalamus conveys the stress message to the pituitary. The pituitary can receive that message from the hypothalamus via either a neural or an endocrine (i.e., CRH) route, or both. VAP and CRH, in a synergistic manner, potentiate the release of ACTH by the pituitary, which in turn causes the adrenal cortex to release corticosteroids, primarily cortisol. If you read a study performed with rodents, the hormone comparable to cortisol is called *corticosterone*.

Corticosteroids convert fat and protein to useable energy for the stress experience. The blood flow is diverted from organs that are not essential to the stress response and directed toward the organs and systems that are critical to the response, providing them with the glucose, fatty acids, and oxygen necessary for effective action. This event causes the hormones related to such nonessential functions as reproduction, growth, and appetite to be inhibited. Simultaneously, endorphins are released, which reduces the experience of pain during trauma. Ideally, the stress stimulus is not harmful and is a short-term event. In such situations, the circulating cortisol inhibits further

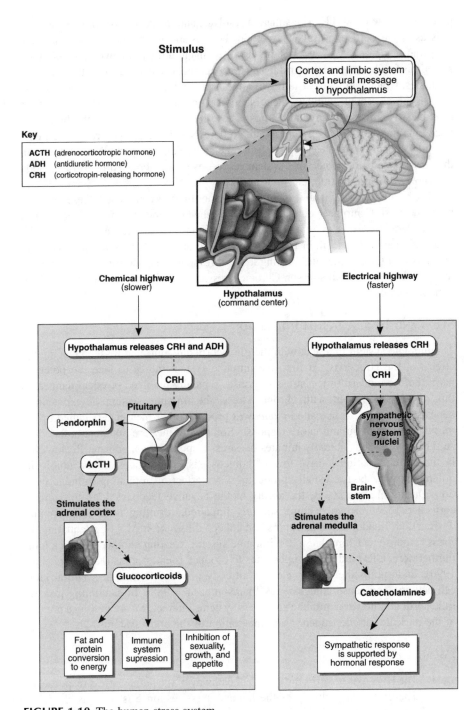

FIGURE 1.10 The human stress system.

pituitary release of ACTH. The situation resolves, and the body goes back to normal. It is as if the cortisol is set at a certain thermostatic temperature, and when that temperature is reached, it switches off. However, in circumstances involving long-term stress, this feedback loop is overridden by higher cortical centers, and the stress reaction continues, which can be devastating to long-term health.

On the electrical pathway, the ANS nuclei in the brainstem receive the stress alert messages from the hypothalamus. These messages come from the brainstem nuclei via neural (i.e., electrical) signals to the ANS. The ANS controls the adrenal medulla, causing it to release epinephrine (i.e., adrenaline). Epinephrine initiates all the classic sympathetic nervous system responses (e.g., increased heart rate, blood pressure, sweat production, etc.).

The beautiful part of it all is that the one, same stimulus causes both these response highways to shift into gear in tandem, allowing the body the maximal response when needed. However, this system was largely designed for the earliest humans, who frequently had to flee from or fight a predator. We modern-day humans are like cave dwellers in a three-piece suit, kicking a stress response into motion simply with our thoughts and no external stressor. Chronic stress, as we will see, has serious implications for health.

STRESS AND IMMUNE SYSTEM INTERACTION

The immune system interacts with the glucocorticoids during stress, enhancing the effects of the HPA axis. At first, the immune system rallies to face the potential harm (before modern times, stress responses typically involved physical danger, so this makes sense), but with chronic stress, the immune system often becomes depressed. Immune cells called *monocytes* produce other messengers called *cytokines* that evoke an inflammatory response. Some cytokines are potent stimulators of ACTH, so your body actually initiates the stress response when you are ill. However, in the body's continual drive toward homeostasis, the corticosteroids inhibit the inflammatory response, usually producing a net effect of mitigating immune function. During chronic stress, the ability of the negative feedback loop to decrease cortisol production can become severely impaired, resulting in serious immune dysfunction. In addition, endorphins and enkephalins inhibit ACTH, attenuating the stress response and stimulating the immune system, creating another feedback loop. Furthermore, CRH induces lymphocytes to produce β-endorphins (Kavelaars et al., 1990). Endorphins themselves elevate antibody production, enhance natural killer cell activity, and cause analgesia (Williamson et al., 1988). In examining just this little portion of how the immune and stress systems interact, we are getting a preview of the intricate interdependence and integration of the body systems.

ESSENTIAL POINTS

- The HPA axis governs the chemical pathway of the human stress response.
- The electrical pathway of the human stress response is responsible for initiating all the classic sympathetic nervous system responses.
- The stress system is related to each of the other major body systems.

SECTION 4: THE IMMUNE SYSTEM

The immune system is a series of dedicated glandular structures and cells whose purpose is to help recognize self from nonself. In other words, the immune system distinguishes your body from any foreign materials or invading organisms, including bacteria, viruses, cancer cells, or foreign materials (e.g., tissue transplants) (see Huston, 1997, for a general review). A molecule that is nonself or foreign is called an *antigen*. The immune system is the eliminator. It eliminates anything that is thought to be alien or unfamiliar to the body. It is the police patrol, called out to maintain homeostasis. The immune system has to preserve a delicate balance between mounting an aggressive response to outside invasion and not having that aggression turn against the body itself. When this process goes awry and the body loses tolerance to itself, it is called *autoimmunity*. In addition to skin, the immune system is typically thought of as having two divisions: the innate and the acquired immune systems. The two systems, however, are inextricably interwoven (see Delves and Roitt, 2000a, 2000b, for reviews).

As you read about the cells of the immune systems, note that there are four functions of the immune response that repeatedly occur:

- Recognition
- Recruitment
- Response
- Attenuation

These four functions will be pointed out to you. However, keep this pattern in mind as you read the entire section on immunity.

THE LYMPHATIC SYSTEM

The lymphatic system, which includes the spleen, thymus, tonsils, and various lymph nodes, supports the immune system (see Figure 1.11). The lymphatic system filters and removes foreign particles. Lymph nodes store B and T lymphocytes for activation when an antigen is present. Lymph nodes are distributed throughout the body and filter the lymph before it is sent out into the blood circulation again. They can remove bacteria, viruses, and cancerous cells. There are other cells, called *macrophages*, that are also present in lymph nodes and contribute significantly to the immune response. Lymph is blood plasma that has filtered through capillary walls. It is called *interstitial fluid* until it enters the lymph capillaries, and then it is called *lymph*. There is a whole lymph flow system that is still somewhat enigmatic.

THE INNATE IMMUNE SYSTEM

Natural or innate immunity exists from birth and is a more generalized system than the acquired system. The innate system is nonspecific to antigen and is initiated immediately. It includes skin, mucus, secretions (such as sweat and gastric acid), certain intestinal bacteria, urine, cytokines (which are capable of modulating leukocytes), leukocytes (other than B and T lymphocytes that are part of the acquired

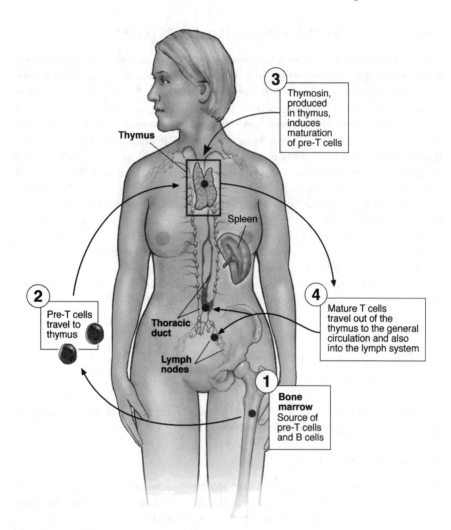

FIGURE 1.11 The lymphatic system.

system), fever, inflammation, and other factors that prevent foreign materials from invading the body. This system destroys unwanted organisms without having to create antibodies, although sometimes it influences the production of them. The innate immune response is often activated by chemical properties inherent in the antigen.

If a foreign body invades the system, a variety of cells respond and are transported by the bloodstream, although they function primarily in tissue. Leukocytes are white blood cells that vary in function. Some are phagocytes that are capable of consuming and destroying antigens or other types of harmful microorganisms. They simply engulf and ingests the foreign matter. Other leukocytes produce antibodies, secrete or neutralize histamine, or promote or inhibit inflammation. Leukocytes are either granulocytes (e.g., neutrophils, basophils, or eosinophils) or nongranulocytes (e.g., lymphocytes and monocytes).

Neutrophils

Neutrophils are the most common leukocyte. They play a significant role in inflammatory reactions, but only live a day or two. They are the first-response team and are capable of phagocytosis. They quickly begin an immune response but are essentially destroyed by their effort. Neutrophils also can be harmful, contributing to tissue damage through inflammation that, for example, can worsen myocardial injury.

Basophils

Basophils are the least common of the leukocytes. Basophils contain vasoactive amines (substances that can exert a dilating effect on blood vessels and increase the permeability of small vessels), such as serotonin. They secrete histamine (which dilates blood vessels, increasing blood flow to damaged tissue) and heparin (which inhibits blood clot formation).

Eosinophils

Eosinophils are valuable because they increase during allergic reactions. They are weakly phagocytic, kill parasites, and secrete leukotrienes, prostaglandins, and some cytokines.

Monocytes

Monocytes, which are the largest of the white blood cells, are phagocytes with the capability of engulfing fairly large particles. Antigens have receptors that the monocyte can recognize (this is the *recognition* phase). The monocytes literally eat up the foreign material. Monocytes are formed in bone marrow and then circulate in the bloodstream.

Macrophages

Macrophages are monocytes that are found in tissue and are thought to stay with you for most of your life. Macrophages are primordial looking, amoeba-like structures. They circulate for about 40 hours and then lodge in tissue and increase in phagocytic activity and, thus, in size. They are present in the liver and spleen, where they phagocytize invading organisms before tissue damage occurs, and in the lymph nodes, where they cleanse the lymph. They come into areas of damaged tissue and help clean up the mess by devouring bacteria and cellular debris. They restore homeostasis. Furthermore, while it is digesting, believe me, does it remember! Macrophages can remember thousands of antigens and can respond very quickly if this type of bacteria dares to enter the system again. They mediate nonspecific antigen destruction, eliminating tumor and bacteria cells in the absence of an antibody, but they can also have receptors for antibodies. Sometimes the macrophage presents a portion of partially digested antigen to B or T lymphocytes and alerts them to the situation. In this case, they are called *antigen-presenting cells*.

Osteoclasts

Osteoclasts evolve from macrophages that have gathered in the bone marrow. Osteoclasts are involved in the resorption and removal of bone. This slow, lumbering cell may hang out in the bone until the brain calls it into circulation. It actually may be another method of cellular communication, a Paul Revere if you will, albeit a somewhat slow one.

Microglia

Microglia are cells whose job it is to make sure that no foreign invader protein gets into the nervous system. They become mobile and literally start eating up invading cells (and therefore are phagocytes). Microglia are fundamental to the removal of dead neurons, proliferating and then removing the dead cells (Streit and Kincaid-Colton, 1995). They keep the place safe for democracy. They are fundamental in the maintenance homeostasis.

Cytokines

Cytokines are nonantibody proteins that are secreted by various immune cells when an antigen is present. Cytokines are intercellular mediators that influence and sometimes regulate immune responses and even the production of other cytokines. Monocytes, macrophages, neutrophils, T lymphocytes, and natural killer cells all produce cytokines (Table 1.6).

TABLE 1.6
Cytokines

Interleukins (IL)	a family of cytokines that stimulates T lymphocytes and alters various immune responses; some of the interleukins interact with the endocrine and nervous systems
Interferon (INF)	cytokines that adhere to virally infected cells, providing a line of defense
Tumor necrosis factor (TNF)	cytokines produced by macrophages and T lymphocytes during an acute inflammatory response; they are capable of stimulating interferon production

---

IL-6 is a cytokine that is secreted during active inflammation and chronic stress and will be further reviewed in Chapter 3. The secretion of IL-1 by a macrophage, upon exposure to an antigen, causes T lymphocyte activation (this is the *response* phase). Once activated, the T lymphocyte secretes another interleukin, IL-2, in response to both the message from IL-1 as well as to the stimulation from the antigen itself. IL-2 is capable of further stimulating the proliferation of T lymphocyte cells (this is the *recruitment* phase). The attenuation phase concludes the immune response. It is caused by secretion of hormones, such as cortisol, which have the capability to suppress the active immune response.

IL-1 does some very interesting things in addition to inducing T-cell proliferation. It incites slow-wave sleep, inhibits food intake, and mediates fever (Krueger et al., 1987; Rothwell, 1989, 1991). Furthermore, when challenges to the immune system increase HPA activity levels, both IL-1 and IL-2 stimulate the release of the stress hormone ACTH from the pituitary, which stimulates cortisol secretion (Bernton et al., 1987; Lotze et al., 1985; Fágárásan and Axelrod, 1990). We will discuss this issue in more detail in Chapter 2, Systems Integration.

So, the two cytokines, IL-1 and IL-2, stimulate a hormone from the pituitary gland. This is groundbreaking information—information that immunologists and endocrinologists found astounding, as it did not fit conventional theory. However, it had me dancing with glee because it was solid medical evidence of what I (as well as colleagues) had intuited about systems interaction. This was the first example of physiological systems truly interacting with one another. I will show you other examples, but this is the first.

Natural Killer (NK) Cells

Natural killer (NK) cells are large, granular lymphocytes that locate and destroy viruses and cells that spontaneously become malignant. They function without prior sensitization to, or recognition of, the antigens. The NK cell's most significant effect is in preventing primitive cancers from metastasizing. NK cells originate in the bone marrow. They are crucial to the body's natural resistance and are instigated early in host defense. The NK cell's effectiveness is enhanced by the presence of INF-γ. In almost every person, the sheer number of NK cells is adequate. Problems occur when the cells become weak and incapable of destroying tumor cells. Therefore, NK cells are measured by their activity or function level. A variety of stress-related factors and diseases can reduce their activity level. Figure 1.12 demonstrates the various routes by which immune information is conveyed.

Researchers have shown that creative visualization and relaxation training can cause the activity level of NK cells to increase. In one study, ten patients with metastatic cancer who were given both relaxation and imagery training showed increased immune response (Gruber et al., 1993). In another study, 45 subjects aged 60 to 88 were given relaxation training and demonstrated increased ability to destroy herpes cells (Kiecolt-Glaser et al., 1984). The effect did not appear with subjects who were assigned to social contact groups instead of the relaxation group. So, what we are seeing here is that the immune system is capable of getting stronger simply by the action of our thoughts.

THE ACQUIRED IMMUNE SYSTEM

Acquired immunity is more specific and occurs when an antigen enters the body. There are two types of lymphocytes or immune cells involved in acquired immunity: B lymphocytes and T lymphocytes. The cell-mediated immune response, which defends against virus, fungi, protozoa, cancerous cells, tissue transplants and functions in allergic reactions, involves T lymphocytes. The humoral immune response, which defends against bacteria and toxins, involves the secretion of antibodies by plasma cells that are derived from B lymphocytes. During fetal development, the cells that migrate to the thymus to mature are the T lymphocytes, whereas B

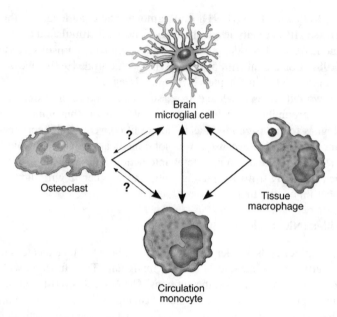

FIGURE 1.12 Information circulation.

lymphocytes mature in the bone marrow (B for bone and T for thymus, according to their sites of maturity). In spite of the reduction in size in the thymus during puberty, T lymphocytes continue to develop in the thymus throughout life. Both T and B lymphocytes develop receptors specific to each type of antigen encountered and can retain a memory for them.

Cell-Mediated Immunity and T Lymphocytes

T lymphocytes are not involved in the production of antibodies. The process of maturation of T lymphocytes to functional cells is a complex, hormonally guided process of rigorous selection (Vacchio et al., 1998). The thymus gland is the main regulator and the schooling site for T lymphocytes; this is referred to as *thymic education*. After maturing in the thymus, T lymphocytes enter the circulation and are distributed throughout the lymphatic system but are found most abundantly in the lymph nodes. The T lymphocyte is the most prevalent lymphocyte, accounting for approximately 70 to 80% of lymphocytes circulating in the body.

T lymphocytes differentiate into five distinct varieties:

1. *Cytotoxic T cells*, which are capable of destroying virus-infected or foreign cells.
2. *Killer T cells*, which recognize and obliterate specific antigens. They look for their target antigen, and like smart bombs, they blast a hole in the cell membrane. The cell essentially explodes, and the contents are lost.

3. *Helper T cells*, which prepare the antigen so that it is easier for the B cells to destroy them. They also assist in T-cell maturation.
4. *Suppressor T cells*, which suppress the immune response of both T and B cells when the antigen is destroyed. They act by suppressing the helper cells or by inhibiting activated lymphocytes.
5. *Memory T cells*, which have the capacity to remember previous exposure to an antigen and, thus, to hasten the immune response. They reside in the lymphatic system until called into action. This is called the *secondary immune response*.

To mount a fight on an infectious agent, macrophages and other cells present antigens to T lymphocytes that have *not* been activated. At the same time, the antigen-stimulated macrophage releases IL-1, which stimulates helper T-cell activity. The helper T cell then releases IL-2, which stimulates T lymphocyte proliferation and subsequently cytotoxic T-cell proliferation. It is the cytotoxic T cells that do the job of destroying the intruder. T cells that do not attach to macrophages eventually die by apoptosis, or programmed cellular death. Only about 5% of all T cells reach maturity. This is called the *primary immune response*.

Humoral Immunity and B Lymphocytes

The primary function of B lymphocytes is to fight invasion by producing antibodies rather than by directly attacking the antigen itself, as do T cells. They are considered a humoral response because B cells are mostly stored in the lymphatic system. A macrophage presents a portion of partially digested antigen to the B lymphocyte, and the antigen attaches to receptors on the surface of the macrophage. B lymphocytes and helper T cells that bear receptors specific to that antigen become activated by the antigen-presenting macrophage. As with cell-mediated immunity, helper T cells release IL-1 but also secrete a B-cell growth factor that causes the B lymphocyte to begin to rapidly divide. The B cell then releases antibodies specific to the offending antigen, which tags the antigen for destruction by other components that are present in the immune system. The rapid division of B lymphocytes results in differentiation into plasma cells and memory B cells.

When a B cell encounters an offending antigen, it transforms into a plasma cell, which secretes substances called *immunoglobulins* (IgG, IgA, IgM, IgD, and IgE). These are antibodies. They bind to the pathogen and, along with other immune system components, inactivate it. IgG is the most common, comprising 75 to 85% of the total serum immunoglobulin. Typically, a blood test is used to measure these antibodies, but IgA, for example, is produced in and can be measured from saliva. Memory B cells are a type of memory cell with the capacity to remember previous exposure to an antigen and, thus, to hasten the immune response upon a subsequent encounter. Both memory B cells and memory T cells are efficient immune response cells. The cells are stored in the lymphatic tissue, waiting for a returning invader. Vaccines permit an initial, relatively mild exposure to an antigen, but they result in storage of the memory cells that can later prevent the illness.

ESSENTIAL POINTS

- Recognition, recruitment, response, and attenuation are the basis of all immune responses.
- Monocytes and macrophages are cells important to both the innate and acquired immune systems. They are phagocytes and an important first line of defense. They also prepare antigens for destruction by both B and T lymphocytes.
- Natural killer cells are important for locating and destroying viruses and cells that spontaneously become malignant.
- Memory B and T cells provide a qualitatively and quantitatively superior secondary immune response.

REFERENCES

Ader, R., Felten, D.L., and Cohen, N., Eds., *Psychoneuroimmunology*, 2nd ed., Academic Press, New York, 1991.

Adolphs, R., Tranel, D., Damasio, H., and Damasio, A., Impaired recognition of emotion in facial expressions following bilateral damage to the human amygdala, *Nature*, 372, 669–672, 1994.

Allman, J., and Brothers, L., Faces, fear and the amygdala, *Nature*, 372, 613–614, 1994.

Baker, D.G., Mendenhall, C.L., Simbartl, L.A., Magan, L.K., and Steinberg, J.L., Relationship between posttraumatic stress disorder and self-reported physical symptoms in Persian Gulf War veterans, *Arch. Intern. Med.*, 157 (18), 2076–2078, 1997.

Beckwith, B.E., Petros, T.V., Bergloff, P.J., and Staebler, R.J., Vasopressin analogue (DDAVP) facilitates recall of narrative prose, *Behavioral Neurosci.*, 101 (3), 429–432, 1987.

Beckwith, B.E., Till, R.E., and Schneider, V., Vasopressin analog (DDAVP) improves memory in human males, *Peptides*, 5 (4), 819–822, 1984.

Bellinger, D.L., Madden, K.S., Lorton, D., Thyagarajan, S., and Felten, D.L., Age-related alterations in neural–immune interactions and neural strategies in immunosenescence, in *Psychoneuroimmunology*, 3rd ed., Ader, R., Felten, D.L., and Cohen, N., Eds., Academic Press, New York, 2001, pp. 241–286.

Bernton, E.W., Beach, J.E., Holaday, J.W., Smallridge, R.C., and Fein, H.G., Release of multiple hormones by a direct action of interleukin-1 on pituitary cells, *Science*, 238 (4826), 519–521, 1987.

Cannon, W.B., Emergency function of the adrenal medulla in pain and major emotions, *Am. J. Physiol.*, 3, 356–372, 1914.

Davidson, R.J. and Irwin, W., The functional neuroanatomy of emotion and affective styles, *Trends Cognitive Sci.*, 3 (1), 11–21, 1999.

Davidson, R.J. and Slagter, H.A., Probing emotion in the developing brain: functional neuroimaging in the assessment of the neural substrates of emotion in normal and disordered children and adolescents, *Ment. Retard. Developmental Disabil. Res. Rev.*, 6 (3), 166–170, 2000.

Davidson, R.J., Coe, C.C., Dolski, I., and Donzella, B., Individual differences in prefrontal activation asymmetry predict natural killer cell activity at rest and in response to challenge, *Brain Behav. Immunity*, 13 (2), 93–108, 1999.

Delves, P.J. and Roitt, I.M., Review article: advances in immunology (first of two parts), *New England J. Med.*, 343 (1), 108–117, 2000.

Delves, P.J. and Roitt, I.M., Review article: advances in immunology (second of two parts), *New England J. Med.*, 343 (2), 37–49, 2000a.

Dossey, L., Prayer and medical science: a commentary on the prayer study by Harris et al. and a response to critics, *Arch. Intern. Med.*, 160 (12), 1735–1738, 2000b.

Eriksson, P.S., Perfilieva, E., Björk-Eriksson, T., Alborn, A.-M., Nordborg, C., Peterson, D.A., and Gage, F.H., Neurogenesis in the adult human hippocampus, *Nat. Med.*, 4 (11), 1313–1317, 1998.

Fágáráṣan, M.O. and Axelrod, J., Interleukin-1 amplifies the action of pituitary secretagogues via protein kinases, *Int. J. Neurosci.*, 51 (3–4), 311–313, 1990.

Gershon, M.D., *The Second Brain*, HarperCollins, New York, 1998.

Goetz, C.G. and Pappert, E.J., Eds., *Textbook of Clinical Neurology*, 1st ed., W.B. Saunders, Philadelphia, 1999.

Goyal, R.K. and Hirano, I., The enteric nervous system, *New England J. Med.*, 334 (17), 1106–1115, 1996.

Gruber, B.L., Hersh, S.P., Hall, N.R., Waletzky, L.R., Kunz, J.F., Carpenter, J.K., Kverno, K.S., and Weiss, S.M., Immunological responses of breast cancer patients to behavioral interventions, *Biofeedback Self Regul.*, 18 (1), 1–22, 1993.

Hastings, M., The brain, circadian rhythms, and clock genes, *Br. Medical J.*, 317 (7174), 1704–1707, 1998.

Huston, D.P., The biology of the immune system, *J. Am. Medical Assoc.*, 278 (2), 1804–1814, 1997.

Kalu, D.N., Comparison of the effects of DHEA and food restriction on serum calcitonin, *Experimental Aging Res.*, 10 (1), 3–5, 1984.

Kavelaars, A., Ballieux, R.E., and Cobi, J.H., β-endorphin secretion by human peripheral blood mononuclear cells: regulation by glucocorticoids, *Life Sci.*, 46 (17), 1233–1240, 1990.

Kiecolt-Glaser, J.K., Garner, W., Speicher, C.E., Penn, G.M., Holliday, J.E., and Glasser, R., Psychosocial modifiers of immunocompetence in medical students, *Psychosomatic Med.*, 46 (1), 7–14, 1984.

Krueger, J.M., Dinarello, C.A., Shoham, S., Davenne, D., Walter, J., and Kubillus, S., Interferon alpha-2 enhances slow-wave sleep in rabbits, *Int. J. Immunopharmacol.*, 9 (1), 23–30, 1987.

Lotze, M.T., Frana, L.W., Sharrow, S.O., Robb, R.J., and Rosenberg, S.A., *In vivo* administration of purified human interleukin 2, *J. Immunol.*, 134, 157–166, 1985.

MacLean, P.D., Brain evolution relating to family, play, and the separation call, *Arch. Gen. Psychiatry*, 42 (4), 405–417, 1985.

Ormazabal, M.J., Goicoechea, C., Sanchez, E., and Martin, M.I., Salmon calcitonin potentiates the analgesia induced by antidepressants, *Pharmacol., Biochem., Behav.*, 68 (1), 125–133, 2001.

Pauwells, P.J., Diverse signalling by 5-hydroxytryptamine (5-HT) receptors, *Biochemical Pharmacol.*, 60 (12), 1743–1750, 2000.

Peredery, O., Persinger, M.A., Blomme, C., and Parker, G., Absence of maternal behavior in rats with lithium/pilocarpine seizure-induced brain damage: support of MacLean's triune brain theory, *Physiol. Behav.*, 52 (4), 665–671, 1992.

Rizzo, A.J. and Goltzman, D., Calcitonin receptors in the central nervous system of the rat, *Endocrinology*, 108 (5), 1672–1677, 1981.

Robbins, J., Wired for sadness, *Discover*, April 21(4), 74–81, 2000.

Rothwell, N.J., CRF is involved in the pyrogenic and thermogenic effects of interleukin 1 beta in the rat, *Am. J. Physiol.*, 256 (1), E111–E115, 1989.

Rothwell, N.J., Functions and mechanisms of interleukin 1 in the brain, *Trends Pharmacological Sci.*, 12 (11), 430–436, 1991.

Streit, W.J. and Kincaid-Colton, C.A., The brain's immune system, *Sci. Am.*, 273 (5), 54–61, 1995.

Till, R.E. and Beckwith, B.E., Sentence memory affected by vasopressin analog (DDAVP) in cross-over experiment, *Peptides*, 6 (3), 397–402, 1985.

Travis, J., More than the brain's drain. Does cerebrospinal fluid help the brain convey messages? *Science News*, 155, 58–59, 1999.

Vacchio, M.S., Ashwell, J.D., and King, L.B., A positive role for thymus-derived steroids in formation of the T-cell repertoire, in Neuroimmunomodulation Molecular Aspects, Integrative Systems, and Clinical Advances, *Annals of the New York Academy of Sciences*, Vol. 840, McCann, S.M., Sternberg, E.M., Lipton, J.M., Chrousos, G.P., Gold, P.W., and Smith, C.G., Eds., New York Academy of Sciences, New York, 1998, pp. 317–327.

van Houten, M., Rizzo, A.J., Goltzman, D., and Posner, B.I., Brain receptors for blood-borne calcitonin in rats: circumventricular localization and vasopressin-resistant deficiency in hereditary diabetes insipidus, *Endocrinology*, 111 (5), 1704–1710, 1982.

Williamson, S.A., Knight, R.A., Lightman, S.L., and Hobbs, J.R., Effects of beta endorphin on specific immune responses in man, *Immunology*, 65 (1), 47–51, 1988.

Xu, S., Lundeberg, T., and Yu, L., Antinociceptive effects of calcitonin gene-related peptide injected into periaqueductal grey of rats with mononeuropathy, *Brain Res.*, 859 (2), 358–360, 2000.

Yamaga, N., Kawasaki, H., Inaizumi, K., Shimizu, M., Nakamura, A., and Kurosaki, Y., Age-related decrease in calcitonin gene-related peptide mRNA in the dorsal root ganglia of spontaneously hypertensive rats, *Japanese J. Pharmacol.*, 86 (4), 448–450, 2001.

Yamazaki, N., Umeno, H., and Kuraishi, Y., Involvement of brain serotonergic terminals in the antinociceptive action of peripherally applied calcitonin, *Japanese J. Pharmacol.*, 81 (4), 367–374, 1999.

Yehuda, R., Biology of posttraumatic stress disorder, *J. Clinical Psychiatry*, 61 (suppl. 7), 14–21, 2000.

ADDITIONAL RESOURCES

Beckwith, B.E., Petros, T.V., Bergloff, P.J., Swenson, R.R., and Paulson, R., Failure of posttrial administration of vasopressin analogue (DDAVP) to influence memory in healthy, young, male volunteers, *Peptides*, 16 (8), 1327–1328, 1995.

Beckwith, B.E., Till, R.E., Reno, C.R., and Poland, R.E., Dose-dependent effects of DDAVP on memory in healthy young adult males: a preliminary study, *Peptides*, 11 (3), 473–476, 1990.

Fleisher, T.A. and Tomar, R.H., Introduction to diagnostic laboratory immunology, *J. Am. Medical Assoc.*, 278 (22), 1823–1834, 1997.

Reichlin, S., Neuroendocrine-immune interactions, *New Engl. J. Med.*, 329 (17), 1246–1253, 1993.

2 Systems Integration: Psychoneuroimmunology

Even the ignorant know that man has a heart and lungs, brain and stomach; but he thinks that each of these organs are separate and independent things that have nothing to do with each other.

Paracelsus, 1493–1541
Swiss physician

It has become abundantly clear that there are probably no organ systems or homeostatic defense mechanisms that are not, in vivo, subject to the influence of interactions between behavioral and physiological events.

Ader, Felten, Cohen, 1990
Pioneers in the field of PNI

CONTENTS

It was only in the latter half of the 20th century that researchers teased apart the molecular and cellular basis of the immune system, began to understand the genetics of immunity, and elucidated patterns of interaction with antigen-presenting cells. All the material that we presented to you in the last chapter regarding the immune system took much research to amass. Currently, the frontier in medical scientific exploration involves the interface between such detailed understanding of cells and the examination of how one body system interacts with others to communicate vital information. This is the field of psychoneuroimmunology (PNI). Researchers study- ing cells of the immune system, for example, are finding that they have receptors for hormones of the endocrine system and neuropeptides of the nervous system (e.g., there are receptors in the lymphocyte for β-endorphins, enkephalins, somatostatin, and adrenocorticotropic hormone [ACTH], among others). These are the ground- breaking findings of the last 20 years, giving medical research a wholly new per- spective. And it quickly gets more complicated than that: the endocrine hormones actually modulate the response of the immune cells, for example, ACTH depresses the immune response and insulin stimulates it (Besedovsky and del Rey, 1996). Moreover, an antigen must stimulate a lymphocyte before the resting lymphocyte evidences a detectable receptor for insulin (Helderman and Strom, 1978). In other words, the lymphocyte does not even reveal that it has a receptor for insulin until it is faced with an antigen. Such results provide a glimpse of the complexity of systems integration.

Some investigators and scientists who write about the immune system are still resistant to incorporating discussion of systems interaction, which is evidenced by the fact that recently written, standard medical textbooks describe the immune system as an autonomous entity, entirely ignoring information about systems inte- gration. In looking at the history of medicine, there has been a propensity among the medical community to separate and simplify everything in the body. Yet, research has shown that neither cellular functions nor body systems are pristinely discrete units, as previously taught. Rather, they are intricately woven and cannot be sepa- rated. Upon close examination, a picture of the physiological systems as a harmo- nious network arises, and a clear, seminal pattern of the scientific bases of the mind–body connection becomes evident.

In spite of considerable capacity for self-regulation, the immune system can be modulated by endocrine and neural activity, and it can just as easily influence endocrine, neural, stress, and other behavioral functions (Ader et al., 1990). We will begin by reviewing numerous studies of functional and cellular interactions among the body systems. There are interactions between each of the classic body systems and the stress system as well. However, we will cover these issues in the chapter on stress (Chapter 3) and not here. The implications of systems integration for human disease will then be discussed and sometimes speculated upon. This chapter is not designed to be a comprehensive overview of the field of PNI. In fact, there are important areas of research, such as gene expression, cancer, and human immuno- deficiency virus (HIV), which we have consciously chosen not to include. The extensive bibliography will help you to explore further on your own. Our intention is to give the reader a sense of the sheer wonder of the body's intricate ability for systems interaction and to illustrate that this ubiquitous design reinforces the body's primary objective of maintaining homeostasis, which promotes self-regulation and, thus, self-healing.

DEFINITIONS

As we investigate systems integration, we will learn that immune cells secrete and have receptors for molecules that, up to now, exclusively have been called *hormones*, neurotransmitters, or neuropeptides. The researchers who many years ago designated what was and was not a hormone never imagined that an immune cell could secrete a "hormone." What do we call a substance that is secreted by an immune cell but is classically thought of as a hormone? It is important to recognize that we are now faced with terms whose meanings no longer fit their designated definition. In Chapter 1, we made every effort to define these terms by their classic or traditional terminology. It is beyond our interest and scope in this book to attempt to create new definitions (although it is our contention that they are needed), so we have chosen to use these words in their classic descriptive sense as we peruse the frontiers of medicine.

The following is a list of chemicals of communication:

• Hormones	• Neuropeptides
• Neurotransmitters	• Protein ligands
• Growth factors	• Cytokines

NEUROPEPTIDES: WHEN IMMUNE CELLS SECRETE HORMONES

Research concerning the interface between the nervous and endocrine systems falls largely into two categories. First, studies show that various neurons can have receptors for both hormones and neurotransmitters (i.e., both types of messengers can connect to a receptor site on the exact same neuron). This is a radical change in the understanding of transmitters. Second, investigations have revealed that many classic hormones behave like a neurotransmitter, that is, they are not only released from endocrine tissue, but from nerve cells as well. We call these neuropeptides to create a distinction. Therefore, hormones can be found in the brain of humans and various other mammals, functioning both as hormonal and electrical transmitters.

Neuropeptides and classic neurotransmitters can coexist in the same neuron. It seems that this coexistence promotes discrete behavioral effects. For example, the functional interactions between a neuropeptide, called *galanin*, and the classic neurotransmitter, acetylcholine, appear to be related to memory inhibition, and there is some suggestion that the mitigation of this interaction may benefit those suffering from various types of dementia (Crawley, 1990).

Table 2.1 lists the numerous hormones (neuropeptides) that are found in the brain. Some have been discovered by chemical means, others by immunological studies. Most of these neuropeptides previously were thought to be localized only in discrete areas of one of the three classically defined body systems and not in the brain. The list of neuropeptides is so numerous that there are undoubtedly some that

TABLE 2.1
Neuropeptides Found in the Brain

Hypothalamic-Releasing Hormones
Corticotropin-releasing hormone (CRH)
Thyroid-releasing hormone (TRH)
Growth-hormone-releasing hormone (GRH)
Somatostatin
Gonadotropin-releasing hormone (GnRH)
Prolactin-inhibiting hormone (dopamine)
Beacon[a]

Gastrointestinal Hormones
Gastrin
VIP
CCK
Substance P
Insulin
Glucagon
Motilin
Pancreatic polypeptide

Anterior Pituitary Hormones
Luteinizing hormone (LH)
α-melanocyte-stimulating hormone (α-MSH)
Thyroid-stimulating hormone (TSH)
Follicle-stimulating hormone(FSH)
Growth hormone (GH)
Prolactin (PRL)
Adrenocorticotropic hormone (ACTH)

Growth Factors
Insulin-like growth factor II (IGF II)
Fibroblast growth factor (FGF)
Endothelial cell growth factor

Posterior Pituitary Hormones
Vasopressin (also called *antidiuretic hormone* [ADH])
Oxytocin
Neurophasin(s)

Others
Carosine
Sleep peptide (S)
Calcitonin gene-related peptide (CGRP)
Neuropeptide Y
Thymosin
Cardionatriuretic peptide (also called *atrial natriuretic peptide*)
Angiotensin II
Bombesin
Bradykinin

Opioid Hormones
Dynorphin
β-endorphin
Met-enkephalin
Leu-enkephalin

[a] A recently discovered neuropeptide involved in the control of energy balance in the hypothalamus (Collier et al., 2000).

we have left out, and with equal assuredness, there are others that will be discovered in the near future. I reiterate; it is my contention that the brain is capable of secreting any hormone produced by the body, as needed, and that it is only a matter of time before this is determined scientifically.

The implications of the nervous and endocrine systems sharing transmitters is enormous and sets the stage for significant interactions with the immune and stress systems. Think about it. The body houses an efficient organization not only for the nervous system to communicate with the hormones of the endocrine system, or vice versa, but also, as we shall review, for the immune and stress systems to influence and be influenced by the nervous and endocrine systems.

CONDITIONED IMMUNE RESPONSES

Research elucidating the interactions between the nervous and immune systems began with studies on conditioned responses of the immune system. As mentioned in the "Introduction," in 1975, Robert Ader and his colleagues published research on the conditioned immune response in a rat population. If you recall, the rats in the experimental group were injected with cyclophosphamide (an immunosuppressive agent) and given drinking water flavored with saccharin. Rats later given only the saccharin-flavored water nevertheless continued to evidence reduced immune responses. Similarly, over a hundred years ago, Sir William Osler, the notable physician from Johns Hopkins, describes a patient having an asthma attack after smelling an artificial rose. Although the effects of such conditioning were experientially familiar to physicians, Ader's experiment was the first scientific proof of pavlovian conditioning of the immune response (see Cohen et al., 1994, for a review).

Ader's research opened the way to a plethora of studies that illustrate the conditioning of immune suppression and to some that define immune enhancement as well. Conditioned immune enhancement, like suppression, has now been illustrated with the use of the same chemical, cyclophosphamide, as well as by a variety of other stimuli, including taste and smell (Bovbjerg et al., 1987). However, much of the earlier research on conditioning involved studies of immune suppression. Many of these studies showed that an aversive stimulus can induce glucocorticoid elevation and immune suppression. It is clear is that the hypothalamic–pituitary–adrenal (HPA) axis is a predominant pathway for neuromodulation of the immune system, which will be elaborated later in this chapter. Ader's work also revealed that antibodies can increase simply by using an antigen as the unconditioned stimulus, postulating that it is the interaction between the immune and neuroendocrine systems that mediates the conditioned response (Ader et al., 1993). All of this research suggests that behavior itself is the regulator of immune function (Ader, 1990; Reichlin, 1993).

Figure 2.1 summarizes some of the systems interaction that you will read about throughout this chapter.

THE IMMUNE SYSTEM AS A SENSORY ORGAN

INTRODUCTION

Many neurotransmitters and their receptors, previously thought to be located only in the brain, have been found in the immune system (Reichlin, 1993). Conversely, accumulated research shows that any immune function can occur in the brain. Think about how amazing that statement is; our immune system is fully expressed in the home of our thoughts and emotions. When the central nervous system (CNS) receives cognitive stimuli that are relevant to the immune system, it conveys that information by hormonal pathways to receptors on immune cells, causing immunological changes. For example, γ-aminobutyric acid (GABA) receptors (GABA being the primary inhibitory neurotransmitter) and benzodiazepine receptors (benzodiazepines being powerful anti-anxiety molecules), typically thought of as being housed in the brain, have been discovered on immune cells and actually modulate the actions of

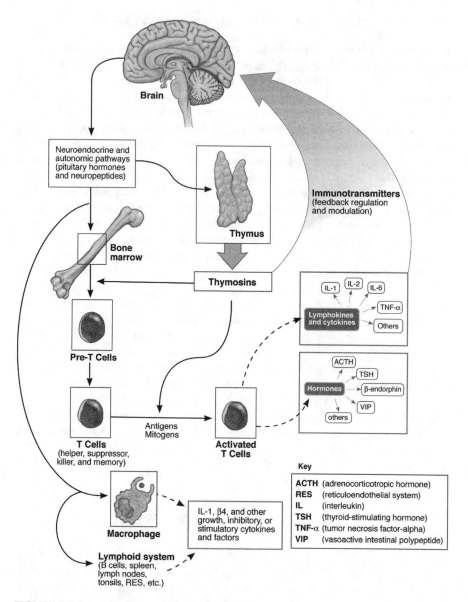

FIGURE 2.1 Interactions among the three classic body systems.

the immune system (Song and Leonard, 2000). This is the physical basis for the mind's impact on the development of disease—a primary example of the mind–body connection.

The nervous system communicates with the immune system via sympathetic fibers coming from and going to the brain. The fibers innervate the primary (i.e., bone marrow, thymus) and secondary (i.e., spleen, lymph nodes) immune organs and include noradrenergic (i.e., bearing receptors for norepinephrine), cholinergic (i.e., bearing receptors for acetylcholine), and peptidergic (i.e., bearing receptors for neuropeptides) nerve fibers (Ackerman et al., 1991; Bellinger et al., 1990; Felten, S.Y. and Felten, D.L., 1991). Neurotransmitters typically must be activated by the immune system before passing on their message.

So, how does the brain receive and respond to chemical and electrical information from the immune system? The CNS is capable of modulating the immune system from within the CNS itself (e.g., microglia have phagocytic functions in the brain). However, modulation predominantly occurs via peripheral immune stimuli affecting the autonomic nervous system (ANS). The information received involves messages about the general type and level of intensity of the intruder, not information about the specific antigen. In other words, the immune system alone detects an antigen, virus, or bacteria. It then lets the central and peripheral nervous systems in on the news, by way of its own mediators as well as via neuroendocrine mediators. The immune system's activation of the CNS most likely involves the older brain structures, such as the limbic system, and follows discrete neuronal pathways (Besedovsky and del Rey, 1991).

Interestingly, the immune stimulus (e.g., virus, bacteria, etc.) must reach an, as yet, undetermined but apparent threshold before it is capable of activating the CNS. The CNS then can generate neuroendocrine peripheral effects. There is, in fact, an interactional and functional relationship between the two systems. For example, when secreted from the sympathetic nerves, epinephrine and norepinephrine generally *suppress* the immune system, but both have distinct immune *enhancing* effects in the CNS, potentiated by the immune system's own cytokines, interleuken (IL)-1 and -2 (Zalcman et al., 1994). Based on these findings, researchers have designated the immune system a *sensory organ* for its ability to obtain, process, and then dispatch information to the CNS (Besedovsky et al., 1983a; Blalock, 1984, 1988).

One of the greatest examples of the interdependency of the nervous and immune systems came out of pioneering work begun in the late 1970s, which was performed by Hugo Besedovsky and his colleagues in Germany. They determined that neuronal firing rates increased in the hypothalamus during peak antibody response to an immunization, with a corresponding decrease of norepinephrine content in the hypothalamus. Norepinephrine also showed a time-dependent decrease in the spleens of mice following immunization as well as after antigen challenge (Besedovsky et al., 1977, 1979, 1983, 1985). Ten years later, a pattern of increased firing rate corresponding to antibody production was ascertained by another investigator as well (Saphier et al., 1987).

Any alteration in neuroendocrine factors, whether local or systemic, can markedly alter the immune activity (Felten et al., 1991, 1993; Madden et al., 1994, 1995; Stanisz et al., 1986; Strom et al., 1972; and many more). Given the mobile nature of immune cells, messages can reach the immune system by nerves in the vicinity of the target immune cells or via the circulation (i.e., local or systemic influences) (Felten, S.Y. and Felten, D.L., 1991). The first evidence that immune/brain communication causes a peripheral response was the observation that glucocorticoid levels increase when the HPA axis is activated (Besedovsky et al., 1975). This systemic change results in immune system adjustments, which we will discuss in detail in the chapter on stress (Chapter 3). Likewise, local synthesis and secretion of neuropeptides by immune cells are important for subtler adjustments in the maintenance of immune homeostasis (see a full discussion on pituitary-like hormones later in this chapter).

Research eventually focused on the precise modulating activities of the neuropeptides as they affect immune cell function and of the immune cells on neuroendocrine tissue and organs. Bear in mind that the body systems are sharing receptors for multiple possible combinations of immune, endocrine, stress, and/or nervous system factors that can be elaborated either within or between one another. We will now take a look at a few of these modulating molecules.

CYTOKINES AS IMMUNOLOGICAL MESSENGERS

Cytokines are non-antibody proteins that function like hormones and can trigger further cytokine and hormonal secretions. Cytokines are the immune system's own mediators and are capable of modulating the immune system in a localized manner. For example, IL-1 stimulates itself as well as tumor necrosis factor (TNF), IL-2, and IL-6 and results in immune modulation (Dinarello et al., 1987, 1989; Le and Vilcek, 1987). In addition, cytokines are the principal mediators of communication between the immune and neuroendocrine systems, which also results in immune system modulation, particularly regarding inflammation and infection. The immune system has receptors for foreign stimuli, such as antigen, virus, or bacteria, which, as mentioned, the CNS is incapable of recognizing on its own. However, the immune system can communicate the presence of such stimuli through cytokine immunological messengers (Bulloch, 1985). Upon CNS recognition of the cytokine, the information is converted to neuroendocrine signals, resulting in chemical messages being sent back to the immune system, with ensuing physiological changes.

By and large, the cytokines (and their receptors) that are found in the nervous system are localized to the brain. While most research has been performed on rodents, TNF and interferon-γ (INF-γ) have been found in human brain tissue and IL-1 in human hypothalamus, human thyroid, and ovary tissue as well (Breder et al., 1988; Hurwitz et al., 1992; Svenson et al., 1991; Tada et al., 1994). Detailed analysis shows that different cytokines have discrete portions of the brain that they are capable of stimulating: dopamine in the striatum, prefrontal cortex, and hippocampus; serotonin predominantly in the hippocampus; and tryptophan accumulating in a more diffuse fashion in the CNS (Besedovsky and del Rey, 1996, 2001). The effect of having cytokines localized in the brain is that they are capable of influencing neuroendocrine production. Among the first cytokines found to have hormonal function were INF, which increases glucocorticoid production, and IL-1, which increases hypothalamic secretion of corticotropin-releasing hormone (CRH) (Blalock and Harp, 1981; Tsagarakis et al., 1989). However, now we know that cytokines are responsible for numerous neuroendocrine alterations (see partial list in Table 2.2).

The activated immune system sends both humoral and neural messages to the brain that there is some type of intruder (antigen, virus, or bacteria) present in the body (Besedovsky and del Rey, 2001). Upon CNS recognition of the cytokine, the brain converts the information to neuroendocrine signals, resulting in chemical messages being sent back to the immune system. The CNS response to the cytokine

TABLE 2.2
Effects of Various Cytokines on the Body

Cytokine	Species	Effect
		Thyroid (*in vivo*)
IL-1β	Rat	Decrease free T4 (first 2–4 days); decrease plasma total T4 and T4 binding the whole week; depending on dose, decrease plasma TSH and impaired TSH responsiveness to TRH
IL-1α	Mouse	Decrease serum T4 due to inhibition of release; thyroid *in vitro* unresponsive to TSH; increase pituitary TSH 22 and 31 days after treatment
TNF-α	Rat	Decrease T4; decrease binding of T4 in plasma caused by reduction of T4 binding pre-albumin; no effect on basal or TRH-stimulated TSH levels
TNF-α	Mouse	Decrease rT3; increase T3 T4 ratio; decrease T3 and T4 responses to TSH
TNF-α	Human	Decrease T3 and TSH; increase rT3; no effect on T4 and free T4
		Hypothalamus–Pituitary Axis (*in vivo*)
IL-1β	Mouse	Increase ACTH
IL-1α	Mouse	Increase ACTH
IL-1α	Rat	Increase ACTH
IL-1β	Rat	Increase ACTH; increase vasopressin
IL-6	Mouse	Increase ACTH
IL-6	Rat	Increase ACTH; increase CRH
TNF-α	Rat	Increase ACTH
TNF-α	Human	Increase LH; no change in FSH
		Adrenal Gland (*in vitro*)
IL-1	Human	Increase cortisol (more effect with monocyte supernatant)
IL-1	Bovine	Increase cortisol (mediated by PG)
IL-1	Rat	Increase corticosterone (mediated by PG)
IL-2	Rat	Increase corticosterone (mediated by PG) (effect only with rat IL-2, not with human IL-2)
IL-6	Rat	Increase corticosterone (mediated by PG)
TNF-α	Human, fetal	Decrease cortisol; shift to androgen production
INF-γ	Human, fetal	Increase mRNA insulin-like growth factor II
		CNS (*in vivo*)
IL-1α,β	Mouse	Increase cerebral concentration MHPG (largest in hypothalamus, medial division); increase Trp throughout the brain
IL-2	Mouse	Increase NE turnover in hypothalamus and DA turnover in prefrontal cortex, but not 5-HT

Note: IL = interleukin; TNF = tumor necrosis factor; INF = interferon; TSH = thyroid-stimulating hormone; TRH = thyroid-releasing hormone; ACTH = adrenocorticotropic hormone; CRH = corticotropin-releasing hormone; LH = luteinizing hormone; FSH = follicle-stimulating hormone; PG = prostaglandin; MHPG = 3-methoxy 4-hydroxy-phenylglycol; Trp = tryptophan; NE = norepinephrine; DA = dopamine; 5-HT = 5-hydroxytryptamine.

Source: Besedovsky, H.O. and del Rey, A., *Endocrine Rev.*, 17 (1), 64–102, 1996.

message either affects distinct neuroendocrine functions that are under the control of the CNS (e.g., stimulating the HPA axis), or it promotes behavioral properties of peripheral cytokines (e.g., fever) (Brown et al., 1991; Dantzer et al., 1998; Linthorst et al., 1995). The hypothalamus, hippocampus, and the pituitary of the CNS as well as the sympathetic nerve terminals of the peripheral nervous system are the primary sites at which communication occurs (Scarborough, 1990).

Another route for cytokine modulation in the CNS is via immune cells themselves (Fontana et al., 1982; Frei et al., 1989, 1992). Activated immune cells are capable of permeating the blood–brain barrier and secreting cytokine mediators. This interaction is distinct from the cytokines independently traveling to the CNS. Studies show that these brain-born cytokines can influence peripheral neuroendocrine functions and influence behavioral effects, particularly those associated with the hypothalamus and hippocampus (Kent et al., 1992; Pitossi et al., 1997). These actions probably help maintain homeostasis by modulating the interaction of the systems during antigen challenge.

Moreover, fascinating research shows that IL-1, IL-2, IL-6, TNF-α, and INF-γ all cause pituitary-like hormones to be secreted by immune cells in a localized autocrine- and paracrine-type manner (Carr and Blalock, 1991). This news is astounding, and the implications for modulation and integration of systems are profound. These lymphocyte-derived, pituitary-like hormones actually modulate subtle adjustments in pituitary hormone secretions (Schwartz, 2000). For example, IL-1 regulates anterior pituitary cell growth, while IL-2 and IL-6 inhibit normal growth yet encourage tumor growth (Arzt et al., 1998). As in the other aspects of the immune–neuroendocrine bidirectional communication, we see that cytokines play an enormously important role in system homeostasis during immune challenges.

NEUROENDOCRINE HORMONES AS IMMUNOLOGICAL MESSENGERS

There are numerous neuroendocrine hormones that have receptors on and that are produced by immune cells (Reichlin, 1993). In other words, stimulated lymphocytes produce neuropeptides to modulate their own immunity (Smith and Blalock, 1981). In fact, lymphocytes secrete numerous types of hormones, including ACTH and endorphins (Blalock and Smith, 1980); substance P (Weinstock et al., 1988); vasoactive intestinal polypeptide (VIP) (Cutz et al., 1978); thyroid-stimulating hormone (TSH) (Smith et al., 1983); prolactin (Hiestand et al., 1986); growth hormone (GH) (Weigent et al., 1988); and others (Bost, 1988). This was one of the first major findings in immune/neuroendocrine research: that lymphocytes secrete and have receptors for hormones. That is pretty dramatic information. Table 2.3 is a chart of some of the neuropeptides that are produced in the immune system.

We will next briefly review the ways in which some of the neuroendocrine hormones can affect immune function.

PRO-OPIOMELANOCORTIN (POMC) MOLECULES

You will recall from the endocrine section in Chapter 1 that the POMC molecule is made in a variety of tissues, including the lymphocytes, the brain, and the anterior and posterior pituitary. Studies in the area of immune–neuroendocrine interactions

---

TABLE 2.3
Neuropeptide Receptors on Cells

Neuropeptide	Immune Cell Carrying the Receptor
β-Endorphin	B and T lymphocytes, natural killer cell (NK)
Enkephalin	B lymphocytes
Somatostatin	Mononuclear lymphocyte, mast cell, neutrophil
VIP	Mononuclear lymphocyte, mast cell

Source: Adapted from Blalock, J.E., *Physiolog. Rev.*, 69 (1), 1–32, 1989.

---

began with the POMC-derived peptides. Enormously significant were the findings that leukocytes (after antigen stimulation) secreted ACTH and endorphins that were identical to pituitary ACTH and endorphin (Blalock and Smith, 1980; Smith and Blalock, 1981). CRH actually encourages leukocytes to secrete ACTH and endorphins—molecules that are typically secreted during a stress response. In addition to β-endorphins and ACTH, lipoproteins and melanocyte-stimulating hormone (MSH) have receptors on and are secreted by lymphocytes.

ACTH

ACTH is capable of several types of immunomodulatory activities, and there is much evidence for bidirectional communication of this hormone. It decreases antibody production by B lymphocytes and INF-γ synthesis by T lymphocytes (Weigent et al., 1990). Its ability to suppress immune function via glucocorticoid stimulation will be discussed later in this chapter.

Enkephalins and Endorphins

Enkephalins and endorphins help regulate the immune system. In 1979, T lymphocytes were shown to have receptors for enkephalins (Wybran et al., 1979). This was astounding news. Enkephalins are now known to increase NK cell activity levels and IL-2 production in humans, which stimulates T-lymphocyte proliferation and B-cell production of immunoglobulins for a specific antigen (Faith et al., 1987; Weigent et al., 1990; Wybran et al., 1987). Receptors for endorphins were first located on virus-infected leukocytes (Blalock and Smith, 1980). Endorphins can either potentiate or inhibit lymphocyte proliferation. Both opioids increase NK cell activity levels, suppress antibody production, and stimulate cytotoxic T lymphocytes (Weigent et al., 1990). Furthermore, both endorphin and enkephalin secretion during stress contribute to an immunomodulating function, inhibiting ACTH (which attenuates the stress response) and, thus, stimulating the immune system (Morgan et al., 1990).

Generally, α-endorphin and the enkephalins (to a lesser extent) inhibit antibody production, and β- and γ-endorphins increase antibody production. Some of the opioid–lymphocyte interaction occurs in a localized manner within lymphoid tissues. Therefore, it is probable that the endogenous opioids complete a circuit, linking the immune with the nervous and endocrine systems as well as acting independently within each system (Smith et al., 1987).

α-MSH

α-MSH has complex behavioral and immune effects. It is associated with control of food intake, the regulation of skin pigmentation, protection against microbes, and the modulation of inflammation. It is secreted from the pituitary gland and from human immune cells. α-MSH is a powerful anti-inflammatory agent. It acts both by modulating inflammatory mediators, such as cytokines, and at peripheral inflammatory receptors. α-MSH increases during an immune response, but generally decreases with age. Individuals capable of producing greater amounts of α-MSH will have significantly less disease progression. It may be that pharmacological use of α-MSH can help alleviate inflammatory diseases in the future (Catania et al., 2000a, 2000b; Ichiyama et al., 1999; Lipton and Catania, 1998).

OTHER IMMUNE MESSENGER MOLECULES

- GH stimulates NK cell activity levels, augments antibody synthesis, and increases the proliferation of cytotoxic T lymphocytes, generally enhancing immune responses (Kelley, 1989, 1990). Curiously, it may also be involved with aging (Kelley, 1991; Pierpaoli et al., 1969).
- VIP inhibits T-cell proliferation and migration, alters antibody production, and reduces NK cell activity levels (Bellinger et al., 1990; Stanisz et al., 1986).
- Nerve growth factor (NGF), required for the maintenance of sensory and sympathetic neurons, enhances the secretion of IL-2, thus promoting T-lymphocyte proliferation and B-cell production of immunoglobulins for a specific antigen (Thorpe et al., 1990).
- Substance P stimulates T-cell and antibody proliferation as well as stimulating mast cells and basophils to release histamine.
- TSH enhances antibody production (Bellinger et al., 1990; Weigen et al., 1990).
- Somatostatin inhibits T-cell formation (Bellinger et al., 1990; Weigent et al., 1990).
- Prolactin appears to inhibit NK activity (Matera et al., 1990).
- Insulin enhances the proliferation and differentiation of antigen-stimulated T cells (DeBenedette and Snow, 1990).

Table 2.4 summarizes this information.

THYMUS AND PINEAL GLANDS: FACILITATORS OF BIDIRECTIONAL COMMUNICATION

So, the immune and neuroendocrine systems share signaling molecules, primarily neuropeptides and cytokines, which promote communication within and between systems. We will now take a look at the thymus and pineal glands as organs that have major roles as facilitators of immune and neuroendocrine communication.

TABLE 2.4
Messenger Molecules and Their Immune Actions

Hormone	Immune Action
Growth hormone	↑ NK cell activity and cytotoxic T lymphocytes
Vasoactive intestinal polypeptide	↓ NK cell activity and T-cell proliferation
Nerve growth factor	↑ IL-2 and thus ↑ B and T lymphocytes
Substance P	↑ B- and T-lymphocyte proliferation
Thyroid-stimulating hormone	↑ Antibody production
Somatostatin	↓ T-cell formation
Prolactin	↓ NK cell activity
Insulin	↑ Antigen-stimulated, T-lymphocyte proliferation

THYMUS GLAND

In addition to its role as the master trainer of the immune system, the thymus is also a very active endocrine gland. It is capable of secreting various hormones and is influenced by neurotransmitter secretions, resulting in actions that both regulate the immune system and impact on other body systems. Incorporated on this gland there is actually an integration of all three classic systems.

Thymic hormones regulate IL-2 production, which then aids in the maturation of thymocytes and the presence of IL-2 receptors on mature T cells. This effect appears to be synergistic with IL-1 (Hadden et al., 1991). In addition, numerous hormones produced within the thymus are classically thought of as pituitary hormones (e.g., GH, prolactin, ACTH, luteinizing hormone [LH], and others). I cannot emphasize enough the importance of such findings. It has forced us to alter our whole concept of how the body functions. These thymic hormones have paracrine–autocrine actions, which serve to regulate immune action and influence neuroendocrine functions that affect the regulation of the HPA axis (Savino et al., 1998). Glucocorticoids play a particularly interesting role in T-lymphocyte development. At high concentrations, they induce thymocyte apoptosis, but at lower concentrations, they actually potentiate thymocyte maturation (Vacchio et al., 1998). We will come back to this point when we look at the role that glucocorticoids play in stress (see Chapter 3, which covers the stress system).

Sympathetic noradrenergic innervation of the thymus is well established both from animal and human studies, and norepinephrine is the primary hormone affecting the thymus (Ackerman et al., 1991; Bellinger et al., 1988, 2001a; Bulloch and Pomerantz, 1984). There is evidence that norepinephrine regulates lymphocyte entry and exit of immune organs in general and with the thymus in particular (Madden, 2001; Wiedmeier et al., 1987). Moreover, changes in noradrenergic innervation occur with aging (Madden, 2001). As the thymic cortex progressively alters in composition with age, noradrenergic innervation becomes denser and norepinephrine increases, possibly playing a role in immune regulation (Bellinger et al., 2001b). An aging thymus contributes to decreased efficacy of the immune system because of a reduction in secretion of thymic hormones and fewer T lymphocytes capable of functioning at full competency. It also affects B-cell efficacy, possibly because there are fewer helper T cells to prepare the antigen for the B cells. Both decreased T- and B-lymphocyte function subsequently result in fewer cytokines, such as IL-1, which in turn, is important for inducing T-cell proliferation—a web of interacting molecules.

PINEAL GLAND

The pineal gland is eminently important to systems integration; in fact, it is my contention that the pineal gland, *not* the pituitary, is the master gland (see Chapter 6 on the pineal gland). The pineal gland is to the endocrine system what the cerebellum is to the nervous system—the root of orchestration and modulation. Its hormonal products affect all of the classic body systems. It is the primary neuroendocrine energy transducer, which means that its sensory receptors are capable of receiving environmental stimuli and converting them into action potentials capable of communicating with the brain. In short, the pineal can take one form of energy and transform it into another. The most well-studied environmental energy transduction involving the pineal gland is the transformation of light–dark sensory information into the modulation that we call the circadian rhythm and into the production of the hormone, melatonin. This one hormone is capable of regulating myriad endocrine and immune functions.

Pineal innervation is supplied by the sympathetic nervous system as well as by fibers coming directly from the brain. Nerve endings typically are found in proximity to the specialized secretory cells of the pineal gland, called *pinealocytes*, which are the cells that elaborate melatonin. The primary neurotransmitter is norepinephrine, which acts on β-adrenergic receptors on the pinealocyte membrane. However, some researchers describe the pineal gland as having numerous types of receptors (Ebadi, 1986). The neuronal pathways are connected to the hypothalamus and, in particular, its suprachiasmatic nucleus (the home of our biological clock). This ebb and flow of melatonin provides us with the circadian rhythm governing our daily sleep cycles and the seasonal cycles of many animals.

Melatonin has been shown to stimulate immune function and reduce the deleterious effects of stress. It fits into its own receptor but also into the benzodiazepine receptor. Notably, the immune-boosting effects of melatonin appear to be mediated by opioid agonists. These opioid agonists arise when melatonin stimulates T-lymphocyte helper cells that have already been stimulated by an antigen (Maestroni and Conti, 1991). And with sheer wonder at the complexity of it all, this is what we call systems integration.

EXAMPLES OF SYSTEMS INTEGRATION

One of the best ways to understand systems integration is to take a couple of examples and play it out, uncovering the network of connections and interweavings. We have chosen the stress–immune system and the neural, immune, and endocrine factors that contribute to intercellular communication in the anterior pituitary as two examples to bring alive for you the countless ways in which the systems interact.

First Example: HPA Axis and the Immune System

It was Hans Selye, in 1936, who first showed that adverse stimuli (e.g., stress, fear) activate the HPA axis. Selye was the first to recognize the common, nonspecific aspects of disease. At the time, pathologists were concerned with defining the discrete components of each disease (e.g., what bacteria or virus caused the disease). Selye observed that no matter what the specific disease, there is a collective set of signs and symptoms affecting patients and lowering their immunity. Today researchers continue to uncover the neuroendocrine actions that Selye observed.

In 1977, Hugo Besedovsky, a researcher in the field of neuroendocrine and immune system interactions, hypothesized that in order for neuroendocrine cells to modulate immune cells, the immune cells must be capable of informing neuroendocrine structures about their functional state. Besedovsky believed that an immune–neuroendocrine network existed, which he postulated was based on the existence of a bidirectional, afferent–efferent pathway between the immune and neuroendocrine structures (Besedovsky and Sorkin, 1977). Besedovsky proposed that glucocorticoids are responsible for preserving the specificity of immune reactions because they prevented immune overactivity, that is, autoimmunity or an allergic response. Scientific evidence supports Besedovsky's theory, and the interactions between the HPA axis and the immune system now have been elucidated.

As we have already discussed, the immune system is a sensory receptor organ that sends information to CNS-controlled structures, via the cytokines, and that the information received by the brain is not antigen-specific but rather involves messages about the general type and level of intensity of the intruder (Besedovsky et al., 1983a; Blalock, 1984). Activated CNS structures, such as the hippocampus and hypothalamus, then cause neuroendocrine immune peripheral effects, attesting to the fact that either direct or indirect brain stimulation has occurred (Besedovsky and del Rey, 1991).

Prior to the discovery that lymphocytes can secrete and have receptors for POMC peptides, there were already studies showing that the immune system stimulates the HPA axis. As mentioned, most illuminating was the finding that when the immune system reaches a given threshold in response to an antigen, it causes the HPA axis to stimulate the adrenal cortex to release glucocorticoids (Besedovsky et al., 1975). However, some researchers feel that the lymphocyte-derived ACTH is not the same as that secreted by the pituitary. Studies show that lymphocyte-derived ACTH is incapable of increasing the secretion of corticosterone from the adrenal cortex of animals (Dunn et al., 1987; Olsen et al., 1992). However, both these studies were performed on hypophysectomized (i.e., the pituitary gland is removed) rats or mice, possibly rendering their adrenal glands powerless to make such a response. Many other experiments, both *in vitro* and *in vivo*, demonstrate that antigen-stimulated lymphocytes do indeed increase either or both ACTH and glucocorticoid levels, sometimes mediated by cytokines (Besedovsky et al., 1981; del Rey et al., 1998). Further research showed that the lymphocyte-derived ACTH and endorphins are virtually identical in both composition and function to the same pituitary hormones (Blalock et al., 1985; Blalock and Smith, 1985). The increased glucocorticoid levels may serve the purpose of increasing glucose levels and allowing the individual to have sufficient energy to respond to the antigenic insult, but, as we will see, it is also integrally involved in an immune–neuroendocrine network, subtly tuning the body's homeostasis.

As previously reviewed, research on the immune system has revealed that cytokines stimulate the pituitary to release the POMC-derived peptides (ACTH) and β-endorphin, which means that the immune system has the ability to directly stimulate the HPA response (Bernton et al., 1991; del Rey et al., 1987). There is still controversy as to whether CRH is an obligatory precursor or whether cytokines can directly affect ACTH and glucocorticoid secretion (Besedovsky et al., 1986; Kehrer et al., 1988; Milenković et al., 1989; Naitoh et al., 1988; Uehara et al., 1987). Nevertheless, current thinking is that the cytokine, IL-1, is the primary mediator of increased glucocorticoid levels induced by virus, although IL-1 does not modify the activity of other stress hormones to nearly the same extent (Berkenbosch et al., 1989; Besedovsky et al., 1986). Other cytokines (e.g., IL-1, IL-2, IL-6, INF, and TNF-α) also are capable of initiating secretion of CRH, ACTH, or glucocorticoids and causing HPA axis activation (Karanth and McCann, 1991 [IL-2]); (Naitoh et al., 1988; Späth-Schwalbe et al., 1994 [IL-6]); (Holsboer et al., 1988 [INF]); (Milenković et al., 1989; Sharp et al., 1989 [TNF]). However, IL-1 appears to be a more potent stimulator of glucocorticoids (Besedovsky and del Rey, 1991). It is my contention that further research will reveal increasingly more information on the effects of the other cytokines and their role in immune system homeostasis. For example, IL-6 is stimulated by IL-1 and subsequently inhibited by glucocorticoids (Schöbitz et al., 1993; Spangelo et al., 1991a, 1991b). Undoubtedly, there is much ahead of us to learn in this field of investigation.

One important feature of neuroendocrine–immune research is the finding that a threshold in immune response had to be met before the HPA was activated. Below this threshold, the immune system appears to work somewhat autonomously. At the time of peak immune response, the HPA axis is initiated, and activated leukocytes and cytokines increase the level of glucocorticoids circulating in the blood, which subsequently initiates an immunosuppressive effect (Besedovsky et al., 1975, 1985). So, the instigation of the HPA axis response occurs only when its immunomodulating effect is necessary. Cytokines provide a feedback circuit that ameliorates over-responsiveness (which can cause autoimmunity) because virtually all aspects of the immune system are inhibited by cortisol (Besedovsky and del Rey, 2001; Sternberg et al., 1989). A feedback loop that has the net result of bolstering the immune system occurs when cortisol reaches levels that cause ACTH to decrease (and eventually lower cortisol levels). For instance, immunoglobulins (Ig) M, IgG, and IgA are increased in the spleen of mice when glucocorticoids are decreased (del Rey et al., 1984). It appears that both glucocorticoids and cytokines are active modulators of the immune system.

Furthermore, little-known studies reveal intricate and discrete modulating capacities for glucocorticoids and cytokines. For example, lymphocytes with lower antigen affinity are more likely to be destroyed by glucocorticoids, possibly a mechanism to control over-responsiveness (Besedovsky et al., 1981). In contrast, glucocorticoids in initial stages of the immune response actually enhance antibody production, contrary to its typical immune-suppressing actions (Besedovsky et al., 1979b).

Finally, as mentioned, cytokine stimulation causes immune cells to produce pituitary-like peptides. Each of these actions are examples of the immune system fine-tuning itself for optimal operation.

Activation of the stress response during injury or illness, paradoxically, causes immune suppression and is an effective way to control its overexpression. When glucocorticoids cannot ameliorate the immune response, the result may be autoimmune disease (Reichlin, 1993). Conversely, if the immune mediators are unchecked, perpetual glucocorticoid secretion would result in serious if not catastrophic immune suppression. The bidirectional communication between the immune and neuroendocrine systems is undoubtedly one of the most crucial to the body's homeostasis and self-regulation. Researchers Carr and Blalock call integration of the immune and neuroendocrine systems a "bidirectional pathway of intersystem communication" (Carr and Blalock, 1991). Immune organs are innervated; cytokines and other immune neuropeptides send messages to the brain; the messages are heard by both the neuroendocrine and immune systems ... this is systems integration.

Second Example: Intercellular Communication in the Anterior Pituitary

As we have already reviewed, IL-1, IL-2, IL-6, TNF-α, and INF-γ directly affect the pituitary gland, and immune cells secrete pituitary-like hormones following cytokine stimulation. These cytokines influence cell function (i.e., regulate the secretion of pituitary hormones) and cell growth via autocrine and paracrine actions (Arzt and Stalla, 1996; Arzt et al., 1999; Carr and Blalock, 1991). Recent studies, which are not only engaging but are undoubtedly pioneering a new field of integral medicine, reveal a variety of pituitary factors (other than the classic hormones) that act as messengers with distinct paracrine- and autocrine-type actions within the pituitary gland. Autocrine or paracrine actions occur at high concentrations or in a persistent fashion, chronically exposing the target cell. There is substantial evidence that these novel pituitary-like hormones subtly adjust and modulate the classic pituitary gland hormones, thus affecting both function and cell growth (Renner et al., 1996; Schwartz, 2000). While any one of these various modulators would have an insignificant impact on pituitary secretions, unbelievably, their overall influence is significant to an integrated hormonal response and affects pituitary homeostasis. The impact of these subtle adjustments is still not entirely understood. A survey of all known anterior pituitary communicators is available (see Schwartz, 2000) as well as reviews of various specific messengers (Arzt et al., 1998, 1999; Denef and Van Bael, 1998; Ganong, 1993; Houben and Denef, 1994; Ray and Melmed, 1997). Therefore, to demonstrate the theory, we have chosen to review two of these locally acting messengers (i.e., factors that act as an intrapituitary signal)—galanin and α-MSH.

Galanin

One of the most interesting anterior pituitary paracrine messengers is galanin, classically thought of as a polypeptide neurotransmitter in the hypothalamus and pituitary and as a hormone that influences smooth-muscle contraction in the gut (not exactly your most frequently discussed hormone). Galanin is synthesized and secreted in the anterior pituitary and influences intrapituitary hormonal activity, particularly of prolactin, which stimulates lymphocytes to secrete cytokines (Schwartz, 2000). Recent research indicates that it mediates the paracrine-induced effect of estrogen secretion by cells that secrete prolactin (Wynick et al., 1993). Estrogens, in turn, modulate galanin, with estradiol significantly increasing its secretion (Hammond et al., 1997; Wynick et al., 1993). Galanin decreases prolactin and GH levels, while estrogen increases galanin secretion (Cai et al., 1998 [prolactin]; Schwartz and Cherney, 1992 [GH]; Wynick et al., 1993 [estrogen]). Both galanin and estradiol decrease ACTH secretion, possibly modulating the HPA response (Cimini, 1996). Finally, galanin is implicated in the stimulation of LH secretion that is induced by GnRH—both related to sexual function (Todd et al., 1998). Sufficiently confused? The idea here is that a little-known hormone significantly influences pituitary secretions, which affect sexual and growth functions as well as modulating the stress and immune responses. We have to begin to let go of our ideas that the major hormones are the only ones that have a notable impact on systems regulation.

α-MSH

Our second example of a paracrine messenger that affects the pituitary in a totally novel manner is α-MSH. The classic hormone α-MSH is synthesized and secreted by anterior pituitary cells. The actions of the novel immune-cell–secreted, pituitary-derived α-MSH are different and distinct from the well-known classic endocrine effects. The pituitary-derived α-MSH hormone stimulates secretion of prolactin (which is also synthesized in the anterior pituitary) by paracrine action. The secretion of the prolactin is significant enough to then elevate thyrotropin-releasing hormone (TRH) and adenosine triphosphate (ATP) (Schwartz, 2000). TRH stimulates the release of thyrotropin (which helps stimulate and sustain hormonal secretions from the thyroid) from the anterior pituitary. ATP is an enzyme that is capable of producing high amounts of chemical energy for the body and, thus, is crucial as the source of energy for many physiological functions, from muscle contraction to metabolism. Just to add one more layer of interaction, recall that we just learned that immune-cell–secreted, pituitary-derived galanin decreases prolactin and, here, that α-MSH increases it. The intricacy of interaction is staggering.

Perhaps these paracrine pituitary-like messengers can be seen as the archetypal "feminine" aspect of the body system, or as Eastern philosophers would call it, the yin. Historically discovered first were the powerful, strong system modulators, such as the hypothalamic hormones that inhibit or potentiate the systemically influential hormones of the pituitary. These may be thought of as representing the archetypal "male" energy, or yang. Currently, the subtle modulators, such as those acting as intrapituitary signals, are beginning to be discovered and acknowledged for their importance to overall body functioning. Their physiological significance and power is in the ability to interact and integrate. It is an accumulation of subtle effects, rather than the more expressive impact of the strong system modulators. Both are fundamentally important to system homeostasis.

INTEGRATION: THE POTENTIAL FOR HARMONY

We are just beginning to understand systems integration. Chemical and electrical transmitters, once thought to have limited and discrete functions, are found to have significant impacts on one another, often interchanging functional roles. Although studies bringing to light specifics such as the fact that lymphocytes have receptors for and secrete neuropeptides are of enormous significance to medical science, I speculate that the intricacy in systems interaction that will be revealed in the coming decade will be far more astounding. Now that scientists have discovered the functional modulators that have the most dynamic influence on the body, increasingly subtler ones are being detected. We have approached this stranger from a distance but are now beginning to draw nearer and get an impression of some of the detailed features.

In Chapter 1, we learned that the HPA axis is connected to a memory system for stress and trauma. We can now begin to speculate that the immune system too has a memory beyond that specific to antigen memory. In this chapter, we have seen that the same sites (e.g., the hippocampus and hypothalamus) that are recognized as crucial for memory functions for stress are also fundamentally important in the immune–neuroendocrine bidirectional communication pathway. These sites are both important transfer stations for cytokines, the all-important interceding messengers. The ubiquitous and intricate array of electrical and chemical routes of communication that are already known to make up the immune response is a compelling indication that there could be a memory for the emotional or behavioral components of illness. It is my contention that we will eventually learn that there is consciousness, therefore the potential for memory, in every living cell—in the nucleus and chromatin of every living cell.

What are some of the practical implications of understanding that our bodies are integrated networks? We know that illness and psychosocial factors, such as stress, bereavement, or divorce, can change or deplete immune performance and alter neuroendocrine function. In the next chapter on stress, we will review diverse situations in which people are at significantly greater risk for illness (e.g., relatives of Alzheimer's patients; medical students taking exams; individuals experiencing bereavement, especially men). The impact of these events on one's health is more fully understood from the perspective of systems integration, as discussed in this chapter.

An analogy can be made between the body and a transportation department. There are passengers traveling from one destination to another. There are managers concerned with tracking the arrival and departure of these passengers and their luggage. There are separate discrete events transpiring, yet there is also an interconnectedness that ideally allows for an overall efficient management. Our bodies have the capacity to function in a similar manner, with separate, yet fully interactive, parts maintaining homeostasis. There is a harmony whose sum is greater than the parts—in other words, there is integral physiology. This statement reflects the ancient concept of Taoism: "If you want to be whole, let yourself be partial.... If you want to become full, let yourself be empty. If you want to be reborn, let yourself die. If you want to be given everything, give everything up." We are approaching a time when the scientific knowledge of the intricate interrelationships of every cell as well as the integration of the classic body systems will come to be seen as the most profound reflection of the subtle energies that interconnect all beings.

The practice of medicine they split up into separate parts, each doctor being responsible for the treatment of only one disease. There are, in consequence, innumerable doctors, some specializing in diseases of the eyes, others of the head, others of the teeth, others of the stomach, and so on; while others, again, deal with the troubles which cannot be exactly localized.

Herodotus, 484–424 B.C., *Histories*
Greek historian, considered "The Father of History"

ESSENTIAL POINTS

- We are now faced with terms whose meanings no longer fit their designated definitions.
- The nervous and endocrine systems share neurotransmitters.
- The brain is capable of both receiving and responding to chemical and electrical information from the immune system.
- The immune system is called a *sensory organ* because it can obtain, process, and then dispatch information to the CNS.
- Cytokines are the principal mediators of communication between the immune and neuroendocrine systems.
- Receptors have been located in the lymphocyte for β-endorphin, the enkephalins, somatostatin, substance P, VIP, GH, TSH, ACTH, and others.
- Lymphocytes secrete neuropeptides.
- Thymic hormones can influence neuroendocrine functions in ways that affect the regulation of the HPA axis.
- The pineal gland is the master gland. Its hormonal products affect all of the classic body systems.
- There is a bidirectional, afferent–efferent pathway between the immune and neuroendocrine systems, promoting homeostasis.
- Cytokines stimulate the pituitary to release the POMC-derived peptides, ACTH and β-endorphin, making the immune system capable of directly affecting the stimulation of the HPA response.
- At high concentrations, glucocorticoids induce thymocyte apoptosis, but at lower concentrations, they actually potentiate thymocyte maturation.
- Integral physiology is a seamless integration of the classic body systems, which now must incorporate the impact of thoughts, emotions, and beliefs on the nervous system.

REFERENCES

Ackerman, K.D., Bellinger, D.L., Felten, S.Y., and Felten, D.L., Ontogeny and senescence of noradrenergic innervation of the rodent thymus and spleen, in *Psychoneuroimmunology*, 2nd ed., Ader, R., Felten, D.L., and Cohen, N., Eds., Academic Press, New York, 1991, pp. 71–125.

Ader, R., Immune-derived modulation of behavior, in *Annals of the New York Academy of Sciences*, Vol. 594, Neuropeptides and Immunopeptides: Messengers in a Neuroimmune Axis, O'Dorisio, M.S. and Panerai, A., Eds., New York Academy of Sciences, New York, 1990, pp. 280–288.

Ader, R., Felten, D.L., and Cohen, N., Interactions between the brain and the immune system, *Ann. Rev. Pharmacol. Toxicol.*, 30, 561–602, 1990.

Ader, R., Kelly, K., Moynihan, J.A., Grota, L.J., and Cohen, N., Conditioned enhancement of antibody production using antigen as the unconditioned stimulus, *Brain, Behav., Immunol.*, 7 (4), 334–343, 1993.

Arzt, E. and Stalla, G.K., Cytokines: autocrine and paracrine roles in the anterior pituitary, *Neuroimmunomodulation*, 3 (1), 28–34, 1996.

Arzt, E. et al., Cytokine expression and molecular mechanisms of their auto/paracrine regulation of anterior pituitary function and growth, in Neuroimmunomodulation Molecular Aspects, Integrative Systems, and Clinical Advances, *Annals of the New York Academy of Sciences*, Vol. 840, McCann, S.M., Sternberg, E.M., Lipton, J.M., Chrousos, G.P., Gold, P.W., and Smith, C.G., Eds., New York Academy of Sciences, New York, 1998, pp. 525–531.

Arzt, E., Pereda, M.P., Castro, C.P., Pagotto, U., Renner, U., and Stalla, G.K., Pathophysiological role of the cytokine network in the anterior pituitary gland, *Frontiers Neuroendocrinology*, 20 (1), 79–95, 1999.

Bellinger, D.L., Felten, S.Y., and Felten, D.L., Maintenance of noradrenergic sympathetic innervation in the involuted thymus of the aged Fischer 344 rat, *Brain, Behavior Immunity*, 2 (2), 133–150, 1988.

Bellinger, D.L., Lorton, D., Lubahn, C., and Felten, D.L., Innervation of lymphoid organs— association of nerves with cells of the immune system and their implications in disease, in *Psychoneuroimmunology*, 3rd ed., Ader, R., Felten, D.L., and Cohen, N., Eds., Academic Press, New York, 2001a, pp. 55–111.

Bellinger, D.L., Lorton, D., Romano, T.D., Olschowka, J.A., Felten, S.Y., and Felten, D.L., Neuropeptide innervation of lymphoid organs, in Neuropeptides and Immunopeptides: Messengers in a Neuroimmune Axis, *Annals of the New York Academy of Sciences*, Vol. 594, O'Dorisio, M.S. and Panerai, A., Eds., New York Academy of Sciences, New York, 1990, pp. 17–33.

Bellinger, D.L., Madden, K.S., Lorton, D., Thyagarajan, S., and Felten, D.L., Age-related alterations in neural–immune interactions and neural strategies in immunosenescence, in *Psychoneuroimmunology*, 3rd ed., Ader, R., Felten, D.L., and Cohen, N., Eds., Academic Press, New York, 2001b, pp. 241–286.

Berkenbosch, F., de Goeji, D.E., del Rey, A., and Besedovsky, H.O., Neuroendocrine, sympathetic and metabolic responses induced by interleukin-1, *Neuroendocrinology*, 50 (5), 570–576, 1989.

Bernton, E.W., Bryant, H.U., and Holaday, J.W., Prolactin and immune function, in *Psychoneuroimmunology*, 2nd ed., Ader, R., Felten, D.L., and Cohen, N., Eds., Academic Press, New York, 1991, pp. 403–428.

Besedovsky, H.O. and del Rey, A., Physiological implications of the immune-neuro-endocrine network, in *Psychoneuroimmunology*, 2nd ed., Ader, R., Felten, D.L., and Cohen, N., Eds., Academic Press, New York, 1991, pp. 589–608.

Besedovsky, H.O. and Sorkin, E., Network of immune-neuroendocrine interactions, *Clinical Experimental Immunol.*, 27 (1), 1–12, 1977.

Besedovsky, H.O. and del Rey, A., Immune-neuro-endocrine interactions: facts and hypotheses, *Endocrine Rev.*, 17 (1), 64–102, 1996.

Besedovsky, H.O. and del Rey, A., Cytokines as mediators of central and peripheral immune–neuroendocrine interactions, in *Psychoneuroimmunology*, 3rd ed., Ader, R., Felten, D.L., and Cohen, N., Eds., Academic Press, New York, 2001, pp. 1–17.

Besedovsky, H.O., del Rey, A., and Sorkin, E., Antigenic competition between horse and sheep red blood cells as a hormone-dependent phenomenon, *Clinical Experimental Immunol.*, 37 (1), 106–113, 1979a.

Besedovsky, H.O., del Rey, A., and Sorkin, E., Lymphokine-containing supernatants from con A-stimulated cells increase corticosterone blood levels, *J. Immunol.*, 126 (1), 385–387, 1981.

Besedovsky, H.O., del Rey, A., and Sorkin, E., What do the immune system and the brain know about each other? *Immunol. Today*, 4, 342–346, 1983a.

Besedovsky, H.O., del Rey, A., Sorkin, E., Da Prada, M., Burri, R., and Honegger, C., The immune response evokes changes in brain noradrenergic neurons, *Science*, 221 (4610), 564–566, 1983b.

Besedovsky, H.O., del Rey, A., Sorkin, E., Lotz, W., and Schwulera, U., Lymphoid cells produce an immunoregulatory glucocorticoid increasing factor (GIF) acting through the pituitary gland, *Clinical Experimental Immunol.*, 59 (3), 622–628, 1985.

Besedovsky, H.O., del Rey, A., Sorkin, E., Da Prada, M., and Keller, H.H., Immunoregulation mediated by the sympathetic nervous system, *Cell. Immunol.*, 48 (2), 346–355, 1979b.

Besedovsky, H.O., del Rey, A., Sorkin, E., and Dinarello, C.A., Immunoregulatory feedback between interleukin-1 and glucocorticoid hormones, *Science*, 233 (4764), 652–654, 1986.

Besedovsky, H.O., Sorkin, E., Felix, D., and Haas, H., Hypothalamic changes during the immune response, *Eur. J. Immunol.*, 7 (5), 323–325, 1977.

Besedovsky, H.O., Sorkin, E., Keller, M., and Müller, J., Changes in blood hormone levels during the immune response, *Proc. Soc. Experimental Biol. Med.*, 150 (2), 466–470, 1975.

Blalock, J.E., The immune system as a sensory organ, *J. Immunol.*, 132 (3), 1067–1070, 1984.

Blalock, J.E., Production of neuroendocrine hormones by the immune system, in *Neuroimmunoendocrinology*, Blalock, J.E. and Bost, K.L., Eds., Karger, Basel, Switzerland, 1988, pp. 1–13.

Blalock, J.E., A molecular basis for bidirectional communication between the immune and neuroendocrine systems, *Physiolog. Rev.*, 69 (1), 1–32, 1989.

Blalock, J.E. and Smith, E.M., A complete regulatory loop between the immune and neuroendocrine systems, *Fed. Proc., Fed. Am. Soc. Experimental Biol.*, 44 (1), 108–111, 1985.

Blalock, J.E. and Harp, C., Interferon and adrenocorticotropic hormone induction of steroidgenesis, melanogenesis and antiviral activity, *Arch. Virol.*, 67 (1), 45–49, 1981.

Blalock, J.E. and Smith, E.M., Human leukocyte interferon: structural and biological relatedness to adrenocorticotropic hormone and endorphins, *Proc. Natl. Acad. Sci. U.S.A.*, 77 (10), 5972–5974, 1980.

Blalock, J.E., Harbour-McMenamin, D., and Smith, E.M., Peptide hormones shared by the neuroendocrine and immunologic systems, *J. Immunol.*, 135 (2 suppl.), 858–861, 1985.

Bost, K.L., Hormone and neuropeptide receptors on mononuclear leukocytes, *Prog. Allergy*, 43, 68–83, 1988.

Bovbjerg, D., Cohen, N., and Ader, R., Behaviorally conditioned enhancement of delayed-type hypersensitivity in the mouse, *Brain, Behav. Immunity*, 1 (1), 64–71, 1987.

Breder, C.D., Dinarello, C.A., and Saper, C.B., Interleukin-1 immunoreactive innervation of the human hypothalamus, *Science*, 240 (4850), 321–324, 1988.

Brown, R. et al., Suppression of splenic macrophage interleukin-1 secretion following intracerebroventricular injection of interleukin-1 beta: evidence for pituitary–adrenal and sympathetic control, *Cell. Immunol.*, 132 (1), 84–93, 1991.

Bulloch, K., Neuroanatomy of lymphoid tissue: a review, in *Neural Modulation of Immunity*, Guillemin, R., Cohn, M., and Melnechuk, T., Eds., Raven, New York, 1985, pp. 111–141.

Bulloch, K. and Pomerantz, W., Autonomic nervous system innervation of thymic-related lymphoid tissue in wildtype and nude mice, *J. Comp. Neurol.*, 228 (1), 57–68, 1984.

Cai, A., Bowers, R.C., Moore, J.P., and Hyde, J.F., Function of galanin in the anterior pituitary of estrogen-treated Fischer 344 rats: autocrine and paracrine regulation of prolactin secretion, *Endocrinology*, 139 (5), 2452–2458, 1998.

Carr, D.J. and Blalock, J.E., Neuropeptide hormones and receptors common to the immune and neuroendocrine systems: bidirectional pathway of intersystem communication, in *Psychoneuroimmunology*, 2nd ed., Ader, R., Felten, D.L., and Cohen, N., Eds., Academic Press, New York, 1991, pp. 573–588.

Catania, A., Airaghi, L., Colombo, G., and Lipton, J.M., Alpha-melanocyte-stimulating hormone in normal human physiology and disease states, *Trends in Endocrinology and Metabolism*, 11 (8), 304–308, 2000a.

Catania, A., Cutuli, M., Garofalo, L., Airaghi, L., Valenza, F., Lipton, J.M., et al., Plasma concentrations and anti-L-cytokine effects of alpha-melanocyte stimulating hormone in septic patients, *Crit. Care Med.*, 28 (5), 1403–1407, 2000b.

Cimini, V., Galanin inhibits ACTH release *in vitro* and can be demonstrated immunocytochemically in dispersed corticotrophs, *Experimental Cell Res.*, 228 (2), 212–215, 1996.

Cohen, N., Moynihan, J.A., and Ader, R., Pavlovian conditioning of the immune system, *Int. Arch. Allergy Immunol.*, 105 (2), 101–106, 1994.

Collier, G.R. et al., Beacon: a novel gene involved in the regulation of energy balance, *Diabetes*, 49 (11), 1766–1771, 2000.

Crawley, J.N., Coexistence of neuropeptides and "classical" neurotransmitters: functional interactions between galanin and acetylcholine, in A Decade of Neuropeptides: Past Present, and Future, *Annals of the New York Academy of Sciences*, Vol. 579, Koob, G.F., Sandman, C.A., and Fleur, L.S., Eds., New York Academy of Sciences, New York, 1990, pp. 233–245.

Cutz, E., Chan, W., Track, N.S., Goth, A., and Said, S., Release of vasoactive intestinal polypeptide in mast cells by histamine liberators, *Nature (London)*, 275 (5681), 661–662, 1978.

Dantzer, R., Bluthé, R.M., Layé, S., Bret-Dibat, J., Parnet, P., and Kelley, K.W., Cytokines and sickness behavior, in Neuroimmunomodulation: Molecular Aspects, Integrative Systems, and Clinical Advances, *Annals of the New York Academy of Sciences*, Vol. 840, McCann, S.M., Lipton, J.M., Sternberg, E.M., Chrousos, G.P., Gold, P.W., and Smith, C.C., Eds., New York Academy of Sciences, New York, 1998, pp. 586–590.

DeBenedette, M. and Snow, E.C., Insulin modulates the interleukin-2 responsiveness of T lymphocytes, *Reg. Immunol.*, 3 (2), 82–87, 1990.

del Rey, A., Besedovsky, H., and Sorkin, E., Endogenous blood levels of corticosterone control the immunologic cell mass and B cell activity in mice, *J. Immunol.*, 133 (2), 572–575, 1984.

del Rey, A., Besedovsky, H.O., Sorkin, E., and Dinarello, C.A., Interleukin-1 and glucocorticoid hormones integrate an immunoregulatory feedback circuit, in Neuroimmune Reactions: Proceedings of the Second International Workshop on Neuroimmunomodulation, *Annals of The New York Academy of Sciences*, Vol. 496, Janković, B.D., Marković, M., and Spector, N.H., Eds., New York Academy of Sciences, New York, 1987, pp. 85–90.

del Rey, A., Klusman, I., and Besedovsky, H.O., Cytokines mediate protective stimulation of glucocorticoid output during autoimmunity: involvement of IL-1, *Am. J. Physiol.*, 275 (4), R1146–R1151, 1998.

Denef, C. and Van Bael, A., A new family of growth and differentiation factors derived from the N-terminal domain of proopiomelanocortin (N-POMC), *Comp. Biochem. Physiol. Part C, Pharmacol. Toxicol. Endocrinol.*, 119 (3), 317–324, 1998.

Dinarello, C.A., Interleukin-1 and its biologically related cytokines, *Adv. Immunol.*, 44, 153–205, 1989.

Dinarello, C.A. et al., Interleukin 1 induces interleukin 1: I, Induction of circulating interleukin 1 in rabbits *in vivo* and in human mononuclear cells *in vitro*, *J. Immunol.*, 139 (6), 1902–1910, 1987.

Dunn, A.J., Powell, M.L., and Gaskin, J.M., Virus-induced increases in plasma corticosterone, *Science*, 238 (4832), 1423–1425, 1987.

Ebadi, M. and Govitrapong, P., Orphan transmitters and their receptor sites in the pineal gland, in *Pineal Research Reviews*, Vol. 4, Reiter, R.J., Ed., Alan R. Liss, New York, 1986, pp. 1–54.

Faith, R.E., Murgo, A.J., Clinkscales and Plotnikoff, N.P., Enhancement of host resistance to viral and tumor challenge by treatment with methionine-enkephalin, in Neuroimmune Reactions: Proceedings of the Second International Workshop on Neuroimmunomodulation, *Annals of The New York Academy of Sciences*, Vol. 496, Janković, B.D., Marković, M., and Spector, N.H., Eds., New York Academy of Sciences, New York, 1987, pp. 137–145.

Felten, D.L., Cohen, N., Ader, R., Felten, S.Y., and Carlson, S.L., Central neural circuits involved in neural-immune interactions, in *Psychoneuroimmunology*, 2nd ed., Ader, R., Felten, D.L., and Cohen, N., Eds., Academic Press, New York, 1991, pp. 1–25.

Felten, D.L., Felten, S.Y., and Madden, K.S., Fundamental aspects of neural-immune signaling, *Psychotherapy Psychosomatics*, 60 (1), 46–56, 1993.

Felten, S.Y. and Felten, D.L., Innervation of lymphoid tissue, in *Psychoneuroimmunology*, 2nd ed., Ader, R., Felten, D.L., and Cohen, N., Eds., Academic Press, New York, 1991, pp. 27–61.

Fontana, A., Kristensen, F., Dubs, R., Gemsa, D., and Weber, E., Production of prostaglandin E and interleukin-1 like factors by cultures astrocytes and C6 glioma cells, *J. Immunol.*, 129 (6), 2413–2419, 1982.

Frei, K., Malipiero, U.V., Leist, T.P., Zinkernagel, R.M., Schwab, M.E., and Fontana, A., On the cellular source and function of interleukin 6 produced in the central nervous system in viral diseases, *Eur. J. Immunol.*, 19 (4), 689–694, 1989.

Frei, K., Nohava, K., Malipiero, U.V., Schwerdel, C., and Fontana, A., Production of macrophage colony-stimulating factor by astrocytes and brain macrophages, *J. Neuroimmunology*, 40 (2–3), 189–195, 1992.

Ganong, W.F., Blood, pituitary, and brain renin-angiotensin systems and regulation of secretion of anterior pituitary gland, *Frontiers Neuroendocrinology*, 14 (3), 233–249, 1993.

Hadden, J.W., Hadden, E.M., and Coffey, R.G., First and second messengers in the development and function of thymus-dependent lymphocytes, in *Psychoneuroimmunology*, 2nd ed., Ader, R., Felten, D.L., and Cohen, N., Eds., Academic Press, New York, 1991, pp. 529–560.

Hammond, P.J., Khandan-Nia, N., Withers, D.J., Jones, P.M., Ghatei, M.A., and Bloom, S.R., Regulation of anterior pituitary galanin and vasoactive intestinal peptide by oestrogen and prolactin status, *J. Endocrinol.*, 152 (2), 211–219, 1997.

Helderman, J.H. and Strom, T.B., Specific binding site on T and B lymphocytes as a marker of cell activation, *Nature*, 274 (5666), 62–63, 1978.

Hiestand, P.C., Mekler, P., Nordmann, R., Grieder, A., and Permmongkol, C., Prolactin as a modulator of lymphocyte responsiveness provides a possible mechanism of action for cyclosporine, *Proc. Natl. Acad. Sci. U.S.A.*, 83 (8), 2599–2603, 1986.

Holsboer, F., Stalla, G.K., von Bardeleben, U., Hammann, K., Muller, H., and Muller, O.A., Acute adrenocortical stimulation by recombinant gamma interferon in human controls, *Life Sci.*, 42 (1), 1–5, 1988.

Houben, H. and Denef, C., Bioactive peptides in the anterior pituitary cells, *Peptides*, 15 (3), 547–582, 1994.

Hurwitz, A. et al., Human intraovarian interleukin-1 (IL-1) system: highly compartmentalized and hormonally dependent regulation of the genes encoding IL-1, its receptor, and its receptor antagonist, *J. Clinical Invest.*, 89 (6), 1746–1754, 1992.

Ichiyama, T., Sakai, T., Catania, A., Barsh, G.S., Furukawa, S., Lipton, J.M., Inhibition of peripheral NF-kappaB activation by central action of α-melanocyte-stimulating hormone, *J. Immunol.*, 99 (2), 211–217, 1999.

Karanth, S. and McCann, S.M., Anterior pituitary hormone control by interleukin-2, *Proc. Natl. Acad. Sci. U.S.A.*, 88 (7), 2961–2965, 1991.

Kehrer, P., Turnill, D., Dayer, J.M., Muller, A.F., and Gaillard, R.C., Human recombinant interleukin-1 beta and alpha, but not recombinant tumor necrosis factor alpha stimulate ACTH release from rat anterior pituitary cells *in vitro* in a prostaglandin E_2 and cAMP independent manner, *Neuroendocrinology*, 48 (2), 160–166, 1988.

Kelley, K.W., Growth hormone, lymphocytes and macrophages, *Biochemical Pharmacol.*, 38 (5), 705–713, 1989.

Kelley, K.W., The role of growth hormone in modulation of the immune response, in Neuropeptides and Immunopeptides: Messengers in a Neuroimmune Axis, *Annals of the New York Academy of Sciences*, Vol. 594, O'Dorisio, M.S. and Panerai, A., Eds., New York Academy of Sciences, New York, 1990, pp. 95–103.

Kelley, K.W., Growth hormone in immunobiology, in *Psychoneuroimmunology*, 2nd ed., Ader, R., Felten, D.L., and Cohen, N., Eds., Academic Press, New York, 1991, pp. 377–402.

Kent, S. et al., Different receptor mechanisms mediate the pyrogenic and behavioral effects of interleukin 1, *Proc. Natl. Acad. Sci. U.S.A.*, 89 (19), 9117–9120, 1992.

Le, J. and Vilcek, J., Tumor necrosis factor and interleukin 1: cytokines with multiple overlapping biological activities, *Lab. Invest.*, 56 (3), 234–248, 1987.

Linthorst, A.C., Flachskamm, C., Muller-Preuss, P., Holsboer, F., and Reul, J.M., Effect of bacterial endotoxin and interleukin-1 beta on hippocampal serotonergic neurotransmission, behavioral activity, and free corticosterone levels: an *in vivo* microdialysis study, *J. Neurosci.*, 15 (4), 2920–2934, 1995.

Lipton, J.M. and Catania, A., Mechanisms of antiinflammatory action of the neuroimmuno-modulatory peptide alpha-MSH, in Neuroimmunomodulation Molecular Aspects, Integrative Systems, and Clinical Advances, *Annals of the New York Academy of Sciences*, Vol. 840, McCann, S.M., Sternberg, E.M., Lipton, J.M., Chrousos, G.P., Gold, P.W., and Smith, C.G., Eds., New York Academy of Sciences, New York, 1998, pp. 373–380.

Madden, K.S., Catecholamines, sympathetic nerves, and immunity, in *Psychoneuroimmunology*, 3rd ed., Ader, R., Felten, D.L., and Cohen, N., Eds., Academic Press, New York, 2001, pp. 197–216.

Madden, K.S., Felten, S.Y., Felten, D.L., Hardy, C.A., and Livnat, S., Sympathetic nervous system modulation of the immune system; II: Induction of lymphocyte proliferation and migration *in vivo* by chemical sympathectomy, *J. Neuroimmunology*, 49 (1–2), 67–75, 1994.

Madden, K.S., Sanders, V.M., and Felten, D.L., Catecholamine influences and sympathetic neural modulation of immune responsiveness, *Ann. Rev. Pharmacol. Toxicol.*, 35, 417–448, 1995.

Maestroni, G.J.M. and Conti, A., Role of the pineal neurohormone melatonin in the psy-cho–neuroendocrine–immune network, in *Psychoneuroimmunology*, 2nd ed., Ader, R., Ed., Academic Press, New York, 1991, pp. 495–513.

Matera, L., Cesano, A., Veglia, F., and Muccioli, G., Effect of prolactin on natural killer activity, in Neuropeptides and Immunopeptides: Messengers in a Neuroimmune Axis, *Annals of the New York Academy of Sciences*, Vol. 594, O'Dorisio, M.S. and Panerai, A., Eds., New York Academy of Sciences, New York, 1990, pp. 396–398.

Milenković, L., Rettori, V., Snyder, G.D., Beutler, B., and McCann, S.M., Cachectin alters anterior pituitary hormone release by a direct action *in vitro*, *Proc. Nat. Acad. Sci. U.S.A.*, 86 (7), 2418–2422, 1989.

Morgan, E.L., Janda, J.A., McClurg, M.R., and Buchner, R.R., Neuroendocrine hormone-mediated suppression of human B cell activation, in Neuropeptides and Immunopep-tides: Messengers in a Neuroimmune Axis, *Annals of the New York Academy of Sciences*, Vol. 594, O'Dorisio, M.S. and Panerai, A., Eds., New York Academy of Sciences, New York, 1990, pp. 482–484.

Naitoh, Y. et al., Interleukin-6 stimulates the secretion of adrenocorticotropic hormone in conscious, freely moving rats, *Biochemical Biophysical Res. Commun.*, 155 (3), 1459–1463, 1988.

Olsen, N.J., Nicholson, W.E., DeBold, C.R., and Orth, D.N., Lymphocyte-derived adrenocor-ticotropin is insufficient to stimulate adrenal steroidgenesis in hypophysectomized rats, *Endocrinology*, 130 (4), 2113–2119, 1992.

Pierpaoli, W., Baroni, C., Fabris, N., and Sorkin, E., Hormones and immunological capacity; II: Reconstruction of antibody production in hormonally deficient mice by somato-tropic hormone, thyrotropic hormone, and thyroxin, *Immunology*, 16 (2), 217–230, 1969.

Pitossi, F., del Rey, A., Kabiersch, A., and Besedovsky, H.O., Induction of cytokine transcripts in the central nervous system and pituitary following peripheral administration of endotoxin to mice, *J. Neurosci. Res.*, 48 (4), 287–298, 1997.

Ray, D. and Melmed, S., Pituitary cytokine and growth factor expression and action, *Endocrine Rev.*, 18 (2), 206–228, 1997.

Reichlin, S., Neuroendocrine-immune interactions, *New England J. Med.*, 329 (17), 1246–1253, 1993.

Renner, U., Pagotto, U., and Stalla, G.K., Autocrine and paracrine roles of polypeptide growth factors, cytokines and vasogenic substances in normal and tumorous pituitary function and growth: a review, *Eur. J. Endocrinol.*, 135 (5), 515–532, 1996.

Saphier, D., Abramsky, O., Mor, G., and Ovadia, H., Multiunit electrical activity in conscious rats during an immune response, *Brain, Behav., Immunity*, 1 (1), 40–51, 1987.

Savino, W., Villa-Verde, D.M.S., Alves, L.A., and Dardenne, M., Neuroendocrine control of the thymus, in Neuroimmunomodulation Molecular Aspects, Integrative Systems, and Clinical Advances, *Annals of the New York Academy of Sciences*, Vol. 840, McCann, S.M., Sternberg, E.M., Lipton, J.M., Chrousos, G.P., Gold, P.W., and Smith, C.G., Eds., New York Academy of Sciences, New York, 1998, pp. 470–477.

Scarborough, D.E., Cytokine modulation of pituitary hormone secretion, in Neuropeptides and Immunopeptides: Messengers in a Neuroimmune Axis, *Annals of the New York Academy of Sciences*, Vol. 594, O'Dorisio, M.S. and Panerai, A., Eds., New York Academy of Sciences, New York, 1990, pp. 169–187.

Schöbitz, B., Van Den Dobbelsteen, M., Holsboer, F., Sutano, W., and De Kloet, E.R., Regulation of interleukin 6 gene expression in rat, *Endocrinology*, 132 (4), 1569–1576, 1993.

Schwartz, J., Intercellular communication in the anterior pituitary, *Endocrine Rev.*, 21 (5), 488–513, 2000.

Schwartz, J. and Cherny, R., Intercellular communication within the anterior pituitary influencing the secretion of hypophysial hormones, *Endocrine Rev.*, 13 (3), 453–475, 1992.

Sharp, B.M., Matta, S.G., Peterson, P.K., Newton, R., Chao, C., and Mcallen, K., Tumor necrosis factor-alpha is a potent ACTH secretagogue: comparison to interleukin-1 beta, *Endocrinology*, 124 (6), 3131–3133, 1989.

Smith, E.M. and Blalock, J.E., Human lymphocyte production of corticotropin and endorphin-like substances: association with leukocyte interferon, *Proc. Nat. Acad. Sci. U.S.A.*, 78 (12), 7530–7534, 1981.

Smith, E.M., Phan, M., Kruger, T.E., Coppenhaver, D.H., and Blalock, J.E., Human lymphocyte production of immunoreactive thyrotropin, *Proc. Nat. Acad. Sci. U.S.A.*, 80 (19), 6010–6013, 1983.

Smith, E.M., Harbour, D.V., and Blalock, J.E., Leukocyte production of endorphins, in Neuroimmune Reactions: Proceedings of the Second International Workshop on Neuroimmunomodulation, *Annals of The New York Academy of Sciences*, Vol. 496, Janković, B.D., Marković, M., and Spector, N.H., Eds., New York Academy of Sciences, New York, 1987, pp. 192–195.

Song, C. and Leonard, B.E., *Fundamentals of Psychoneuroimmunology*, John Wiley & Sons, Chichester, U.K., 2000.

Spangelo, B.L., Jarvis, W.D., Judd, A.M., and MacLeod, R.M., Induction of interleukin-6 release by interleukin-1 in rat anterior pituitary cells *in vitro*: evidence for an eicosanoid-dependent mechanism, *Endocrinology*, 129 (6), 2886–2894, 1991a.

Spangelo, B.L., Judd, A.M., Isakson, P.C., and MacLeod, R.M., Interleukin-1 stimulates interleukin-6 release from rat anterior pituitary cells *in vitro*, *Endocrinology*, 128 (6), 2685–2692, 1991b.

Späth-Schwalbe, E. et al., Interleukin-6 stimulates the hypothalamus-pituitary-adrenocortical axis in man, *J. Clinical Endocrinol. Metab.*, 79 (4), 1212–1214, 1994.

Stanisz, A.M., Befus, D., and Bienenstock, J., Differential effects of vasoactive intestinal peptide, substance P, and somatostatin on immunoglobulin synthesis and proliferations by lymphocytes from Peyer's patches, mesenteric lymph nodes, and spleen, *J. Immunol.*, 136 (1), 152–156, 1986.

Sternberg, E.M. et al., Inflammatory mediator-induced hypothalmic–pituitary–adrenal axis activation is defective in streptococcal cell wall arthritis-susceptible Lewis rats, *Proc. Nat. Acad. Sci. U.S.A.*, 86 (7), 2374–2378, 1989.

Strom, T.B., Deisseroth, A., Morganroth, J., Carpenter, C.B., and Merrill, J.P., Alteration of the cytotoxic action of sensitized lymphocytes by cholinergic agents and activators of adenylate cyclase, *Proc. Nat. Acad. Sci. U.S.A.*, 69 (10), 2995–2999, 1972.

Svenson, M., Kayser, L., Hansen, M.B., Rasmussen, A.K., and Bendtzen, K., Interleukin-1 receptors on human thyroid cell line FRTL-5, *Cytokines*, 3 (2), 125–130, 1991.

Tada, M., Diserens, A.C., Desbaillets, I., and de Tribolet, N., Analysis of cytokine receptor messenger RNA expression in human glioblastoma cells and normal astrocytes by reverse-transcription polymerase chain reaction, *J. Neurosurgery*, 80 (6), 1063–1073, 1994.

Thorpe, L.W., Jerrells, T.R., and Perez-Polo, J.R., Mechanisms of lymphocyte activation by nerve growth factor, in Neuropeptides and Immunopeptides: Messengers in a Neuroimmune Axis, *Annals of the New York Academy of Sciences*, Vol. 594, O'Dorisio, M.S. and Panerai, A., Eds., New York Academy of Sciences, New York, 1990, pp. 78–84.

Todd, J.F., Small, C.J., Akinsanya, K.O., Stanley, S.A., Smith, D.M., and Bloom, S.R., Galanin is a paracrine inhibitor of gonadatroph function in the female rat, *Endocrinology*, 139 (10), 4222–4229, 1998.

Tsagarakis, S., Gillies, G., Rees, L.H., Besser, M., and Grossman, A., Interleukin-1 directly stimulates the release of corticotropin releasing factor from rat hypothalamus, *Neuroendocrinology*, 49 (1), 98–101, 1989.

Uehara, A., Gottschall, P.E., Dahl, R.R., and Arimura, A., Interleukin-1 stimulates ACTH release by an indirect action which requires endogenous corticotropin releasing factor, *Endocrinology*, 121 (4), 1580–1582, 1987.

Vacchio, M.S., Ashwell, J.D., and King, L.B., A positive role for thymus-derived steroids in formation of the T-cell repertoire, in Neuroimmunomodulation Molecular Aspects, Integrative Systems, and Clinical Advances, *Annals of the New York Academy of Sciences*, Vol. 840, McCann, S.M., Sternberg, E.M., Lipton, J.M., Chrousos, G.P., Gold, P.W., and Smith, C.G., Eds., New York Academy of Sciences, New York, 1998, pp. 317–327.

Weigent, D.A., Baxter, J.B., Wear, W.E., Smith, L.R., Bost, K.L., and Blalock, J.E., Production of immunoreactive growth hormone by mononuclear leukocytes, *FASEB J.*, 2 (12), 2812–2818, 1988.

Weigent, D.A., Carr, D.J.J., and Blalock, J.E., Bidirectional communication between the neuroendocrine and immune systems, in A Decade of Neuropeptides: Past, Present, and Future, *Annals of the New York Academy of Sciences*, Vol. 579, Koob, G.F., Sandman, C.A., and Fleur, L.S., Eds., New York Academy of Sciences, New York, 1990, pp. 17–27.

Weinstock, J.V., Blum, A., Walder, J., and Walder, R., Eosinophils from granulomas in murine *Schistosomiasis mansoni* produce substance P, *J. Immunol.*, 141 (3), 961–966, 1988.

Wiedmeier, S.E., Burnham, D.K., Singh, U., and Daynes, R.A., Implantation of thymic epithelial grafts into the anterior chamber of the murine eye: an experimental model for analyzing T-cell ontogeny, *Thymus*, 9 (1), 25–44, 1987.

Wybran, J., Appleboom, T., Famaey, J.P., and Govaerts, A., Suggestive evidence for receptors for morphine and methionine-enkephalin receptors on normal blood T lymphocytes, *J. Immunol.*, 123 (3), 1068–1070, 1979.

Wybran, J. et al., Immunologic properties of methionine-enkephalin, and therapeutic impli-
cations in AIDS, ARC, and cancer, in Neuroimmune Reactions: Proceedings of the
Second International Workshop on Neuroimmunomodulation, *Annals of the New York
Academy of Sciences*, Vol. 496, Janković, B.D., Marković, M., and Spector, N.H.,
Eds., New York Academy of Sciences, New York, 1987, pp. 108–114.

Wynick, D., Hammond, P.J., Akinsanya, K.O., and Bloom, S.R., Galanin regulates basal and
oestrogen-stimulated lactotroph function, *Nature*, 364 (6437), 529–532, 1993.

Zalcman, S. et al., Cytokine-specific central monoamine alterations induced by interleukin-
1, -2, and -6, *Brain Res.*, 643 (1–2), 40–49, 1994.

ADDITIONAL RESOURCES

Angeletti, R.H. and Hickey, W.F., Neuroendocrine cells within immune tissues, in Neuroimmune Reactions: Proceedings of the Second International Workshop on Neuroimmunomodulation, *Annals of the New York Academy of Sciences*, Vol. 496, Janković, B.D.,
Marković, M., and Spector, N.H., Eds., New York Academy of Sciences, New York,
1987, pp. 78–84.

Besedovsky, H.O., del Rey, A.E., and Sorkin, INITIALS, Immune-neuroendocrine interactions, *J. Immunol.*, 135 (2 suppl.), 750–754, 1985.

Blalock, J.E., The syntax of immune-neuroendocrine communication, *Immunology Today*, 15
(11), 504–511, 1994.

Blalock, J.E. and Bost, K.L., Eds., *Neuroimmunoendocrinology*, Karger, Basel, Switzerland,
1988.

Janković, B.D., Marković, M., and Spector, N.H., Eds., Neuroimmune Reactions: Proceed-
ings of the Second International Workshop on Neuroimmunomodulation, *Annals of
The New York Academy of Sciences*, Vol. 496, New York Academy of Sciences, New
York, 1987.

Marić, D. and Janković, B.D., Enkephalins and immunity I: *in vivo* modulation of cell-
mediated immunity, in Neuroimmune Reactions: Proceedings of the Second International Workshop on Neuroimmunomodulation, *Annals of the New York Academy of
Sciences*, Vol. 496, Janković, B.D., Marković, M., and Spector, N.H., Eds., New York
Academy of Sciences, New York, 1987, pp. 126–136.

Plotnikoff, N.P., Faith, R.E., Murgo, A.J., and Good, R.A., Eds., *Enkephalins and Endorphins,
Stress and the Immune System*, Plenum Press, New York, 1986.

Polan, M.L., Loukides, J.A., and Honig, J., Interleukin-1 in human ovarian cells and in
peripheral blood monocytes increases during the luteal phase: evidence for a midcycle
surge in the human, *Am. J. Obstet. Gynecol.*, 170 (4), 1000–1006, 1994.

Turnbull, A.V. et al., Inhibition of tumor necrosis factor-alpha action within the CNS markedly
reduces the plasma adrenocorticotropin response to peripheral local inflammation in
rats, *J. Neurosci.*, 17 (9), 3262–3273, 1997.

Zalcman, S., Green-Johnson, J.M., Murray, L., Wan, W., Nance, D.M., and Greenberg, A.H.,
Interleukin-2-induced enhancement of an antigen-specific IgM plaque-forming cell
response is mediated by the sympathetic nervous system, *J. Pharmacol. Experimental
Ther.*, 271 (2), 977–982, 1994.

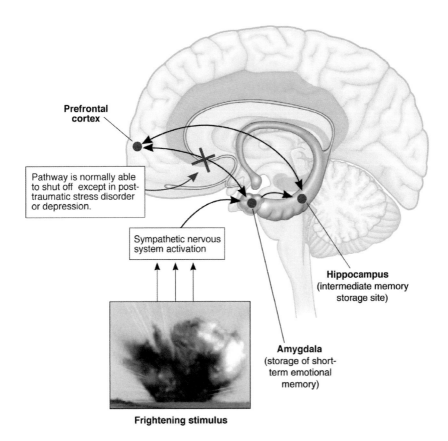

Prefrontal cortex

Pathway is normally able to shut off except in post-traumatic stress disorder or depression.

Sympathetic nervous system activation

Hippocampus (intermediate memory storage site)

Amygdala (storage of short-term emotional memory)

Frightening stimulus

FIGURE 3.6 Diagram of the fear response.

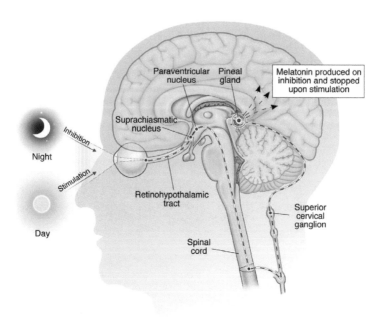

FIGURE 6.1 Neural pathway from the eye to the pineal.

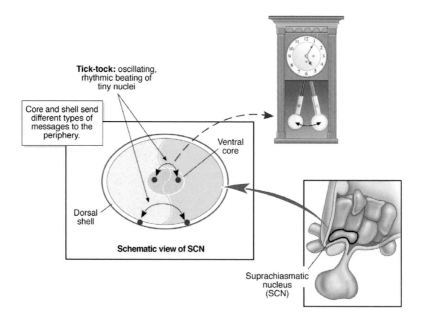

FIGURE 6.4 Oscillating patterns within the SCN.

3 The Stress System

A merry heart doeth a man good, while a broken spirit drieth the bones.

King Solomon
Proverbs

CONTENTS

A BRIEF HISTORY

We begin the chapter on stress by returning to the work of Hans Selye, who is rightly known as the "father of stress." The story begins when, as a medical student in Czechoslovakia in the 1920s, Selye observed that patients at the hospital in which he worked appeared to have a fairly common set of symptoms, regardless of their specific diagnosis. This was a significant deviation from the thinking of the time, which postulated that discrete agents caused disease and that symptoms are restricted to that specific disease. Selye, knowing that there would be no support for his theory, did not pursue it, but neither did he forget it.

Then, in 1936 at McGill University in Montréal, where Selye was working as a research physician, he conducted an experiment that would forever change our understanding of medicine. The experiment involved frequently injecting rats with a putative placental hormone (which he never succeeded in purifying). After days of constant abuse from repeated injections, the rats developed gastric ulcers, enlarged adrenals, and involuted thymuses—all the signs that we now associate with a stress reaction. However, much to Selye's astonishment, the rats that had been subjected to the same protocol, but were injected with saline instead of the putative hormone, had the identical set of symptoms. Experiments using other types of stressors yielded the same results, giving Selye the explanation for the common symptoms he had seen in the patients at the hospital in Czechoslovakia. Selye called this nonspecific reaction to disease the *stress response*, and he expanded this concept to include a response to all types of stress, whether or not the stress was of a physiological or psychological origin.

In the subsequent 10 years, Selye developed his ideas on stress and eventually published a paper delineating his comprehensive theory of stress, called the *general adaptation syndrome* (see Figure 3.1) (Selye, 1949). Selye understood that this nonspecific response was hormonally triggered and involved the hypothalamic–pituitary–adrenal (HPA) axis. As his work proceeded, he unraveled the relationship between glucocorticoids and the inflammatory response and was the first to recognize the importance of glucocorticoids in the stress response. Selye then outlined the relationship between stress and disease, expounding on the various potential malfunctions of the general adaptation syndrome. He determined that adrenocorticotropic hormone (ACTH) and cortisol were related to the suppression of inflammation and determined that either an excess or deficiency of these and other hormones could cause a "derailment" in the adaptation response (Selye, 1949; Selye; 1955). Far more is now known about the cellular and systems interactions involved in the stress response. Nonetheless, as one peruses the literature, it is always Selye's work against which theory or accuracy is measured. Selye's discovery that the neuroendocrine and immune systems interact during stress, disease, and injury arguably makes him the father of the field of psychoneuroimmunology (PNI) as well.

Prior to Selye's work, the physiologist Walter Cannon was the person to actually introduce the use of the word *stress*. Cannon borrowed the term *de facto* from physics and applied it to the phenomenon of the organism reaching a breaking point in which homeostasis cannot be maintained. He also adopted use of the word *strain* from physics, which is intended to include the concept of elasticity. Strain is an important

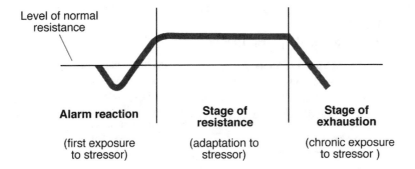

FIGURE 3.1 Selye's general adaptation syndrome.

concept, and later in this chapter, we will discuss the differences between stress and strain as they apply to our daily lives. Cannon also coined the term *homeostasis*, which is the harmonious equilibrium of myriad factors that permit the body to maintain a steady state of health. He pioneered the roles of epinephrine/norepinephrine and the sympathetic nervous system in the stress response and described an adaptive stress reaction that he called "fight or flight," which we now know as the stress response (Cannon, 1914). Given that researchers only recently have unequivocally agreed that stress is a contributing factor to disease, it seems amazing that it has been almost a century since Cannon recognized that both physical and emotional factors can disrupt the body's homeostasis (Cannon, 1914; Chrousos and Gold, 1992).

Against this backdrop, Selye began his pioneering work, confronted by a skeptical medical community that largely relegated his findings to the psychological professionals. Emotional issues had no place in medicine. After all, physicians were beginning to find cures to discrete diseases and to tease apart the molecular underpinnings of the immune system.

WHAT IS STRESS?

Selye's research gave us information about the chemical pathway, and Cannon's work gave us the outline of the electrical pathway of the stress response. Each investigator recognized that stress is a departure from homeostasis. Selye's concept of the adaptation response, which now is referred to as a *stress response*, is the body's constant effort to right any physical or mental stressor, maintaining physiological, mental, and emotional harmony or homeostasis (see Table 3.1). Stress, therefore, is the absence of homeostasis or an imbalance in the harmonious workings of the organism, which results in the body's concerted effort to reestablish that balance. If the organism is incapable of reestablishing the homeostasis, typically the consequence is disease. In humans, activation of the chemical stress pathway (glucocorticoids) tends to be associated with depression, whereas activation of the electrical stress pathway (epinephrine) more frequently is correlated with anxiety (Sapolsky, 1994).

TABLE 3.1
Selye's Stress Response Theory

Selye's Signs of Stress	The Stress Response
Adrenal hypertrophy	Increased blood pressure
Thymus involution	Increased pulse rate
Spleen involution	Elaboration of stress hormones
Lymph node involution	Increased muscle tension
Reduced lymphocyte count	Rapid, shallow respiration

With illness comes symptoms that are both specific to the disease but also those that are the nonspecific symptoms that Selye first observed in the 1920s. Selye labeled protracted or chronic stress, such as that seen in seriously ill patients, the *stress syndrome*. Recall the discussion in Chapter 2 regarding the immune system reaching a given threshold in response to an antigen before it stimulates the HPA axis (Besedovsky et al., 1975). Similarly, an individual's level of stress must qualitatively and quantitatively reach a given (but as yet undetermined) threshold before the stress syndrome develops. Today it is recognized that the stress syndrome is not limited to the physically ill but occurs as well in chronically emotionally stressed individuals, such as caregivers of Alzheimer's patients, as well as numerous people affected by the stress of work, financial concern, divorce, or bereavement.

Selye believed that some types of stress actually could be advantageous and pleasantly stimulating. This theory has been affirmed by numerous studies in the subsequent 60 years. Interestingly, the physiological basis for this beneficial low-grade stress has now been established. While studies show that glucocorticoids that are secreted in a prolonged manner, as a result of chronic stress, induce apoptosis of thymocytes during the maturation process, recent research indicates that there is actually immune enhancement, via the promotion of T-cell development, when glucocorticoids are secreted in small amounts (Munck and Guyre, 1991; Vacchio et al., 1998). Once again, there is an undetermined setpoint at which glucocorticoids become detrimental to the body's homeostasis.

Several studies have established this setpoint in number of days for a given protocol (McEwen, 1998; Munck and Guyre, 1991). The conversion to a harmful response after that given number of days is quite consistent. In this chapter, we will discuss the physiological underpinnings of chronic stress in order to understand why it can be so destructive and then review the patterns of behavior that can induce such a response. Memory, which plays a significant role in the perpetuation of stress, will also be discussed. We humans are capable of worrying ourselves sick, and as we will see, we actually are capable of worrying ourselves to death.

THE STRESS RESPONSE

Underlying the stress syndrome are changes that are associated with both the electrical and chemical stress response. The stress response is designed to empower the gazelle fleeing the lion on the savanna; in other words, it is the fight-or-flight response (see Figure 3.2). Let us quickly review what was covered in Chapters 1 and 2. The

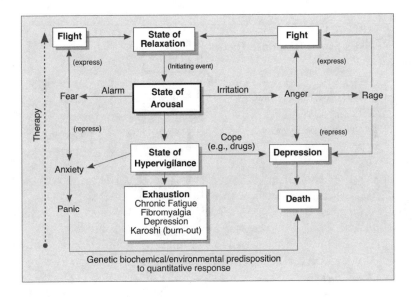

FIGURE 3.2 Clinical stress response.

stressful stimulus causes the hypothalamus to secrete corticotropin-releasing hormone (CRH) and antidiuretic hormone (ADH). CRH stimulates the release of ACTH from the pituitary, which in turn causes the adrenal cortex to release corticosteroids, primarily the glucocorticoid, cortisol. Meanwhile, the autonomic nervous system (ANS) stimulates the adrenal medulla to release epinephrine (adrenaline), which initiates all the classic sympathetic nervous system responses, such as increased heart rate, blood pressure, and respiratory rates. Release of these adrenal medulla hormones also results in increased arousal and anxiety (see Figure 3.3).

The glucocorticoids, epinephrine, and norepinephrine all can inhibit insulin secretion, which results in the conversion of stored protein and fat to useable energy for exertion (the hormone glucagon also helps do this). So, when stress occurs, the stored energy becomes usable glucose and free fatty acids that enter the blood stream for quick energy use. The energy conversion is complemented by increased depth of respiration in the wings, which increases the available oxygen supply. The circulating blood directs the oxygen and glucose to the specific organs and muscles essential for physical exertion and avoids those that are not absolutely necessary for survival. This is how the 110-pound woman is able to lift the family van off of her husband trapped beneath. Hormones related to functions that are nonessential to goals of acute stress, such as reproduction (prolactin, luteinizing hormone, follicle-stimulating hormone), appetite (insulin), and vigilant immune system function, are inhibited. Simultaneously, endorphins, which are strong analgesics, are released.

Keep in mind that the electrical pathway (which also includes hormones) responds to a stressor immediately, whereas the hormonal response is slower but more sustained. While glucocorticoids and epinephrine are the dynamos of the stress response, in this chapter we will cover other molecules that influence or sustain the stress response in subtler ways. Having now learned so much about systems inter-

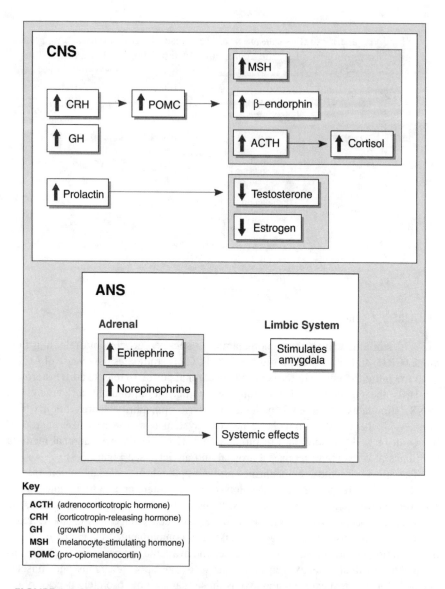

FIGURE 3.3 Endocrine stress response.

action, you will not be surprised to hear that the lines between what we called the chemical (CRH/ACTH/cortisol) and electrical (ANS/epinephrine) pathways are not pristinely separated. For example, norepinephrine stimulates the hypothalamus to secrete CRH, which helps to instigate the stress response of the sympathetic nervous system, stimulating the secretions of both epinephrine and norepinephrine (Cunningham et al., 1990; Dunn and Berridge, 1990). Furthermore, ADH, which works synergistically with CRH to stimulate ACTH, also appears to work synergistically to promote behavioral effects (e.g., memory enhancement) of the stress response (Elkabir et al., 1990; Rittmaster et al., 1987).

I will tell you a story to illustrate the stress response. Several summers ago, I was heading down the Snake River in Wyoming and saw a herd of buffalo. I had my corncob pipe and my hat, but I did not have a gun because I do not hunt. However, I did have my camera. I figured that it would be fun to go up close to the bison. So, I did. I heard a snort. What happened next was that my body experienced a great deal of sensory input. There was rapid input into my amygdala—the fear center. It took about a half a millisecond for my amygdala to say to itself, "Connect, danger, danger!" The hormonal cascade of the stress response was initiated—first the ANS, adrenal medulla, and epinephrine, then CRH, ACTH, and the glucocorticoids. My sympathetic nervous system threw out all sorts of signals, and right after I snapped the picture that you see in Figure 3.4, I ran for my life! Never have I run that fast! I am a big guy, and I could never run a marathon. But, I ran my own marathon in Yellowstone Park that day. I got back to the car (which was across the river) in about 20 seconds, no kidding!

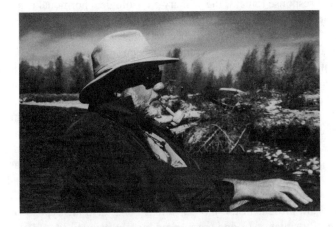

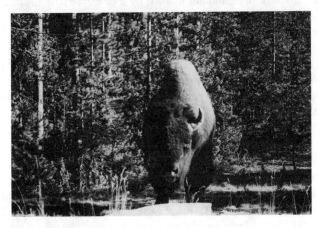

FIGURE 3.4 The buffalo story.

This is an example of the fight-or-flight HPA stress response in its classic sense. The response was clearly designed to give the body immediate energy. My endocrine system was just surging. Adrenaline (i.e., epinephrine), cortisol, and other hormones were secreted. The stored sugar and fats were flowing in my bloodstream, providing fuel for my Yellowstone Park marathon. Likewise, more blood was directed to my large muscles to enable the exertion. My respiratory rate increased, providing more oxygen for the run. My heartbeat was soaring. My blood pressure shot up. In other words, I became a temporary Superman. It didn't last, the Superman part that is. What typically follows an acute stress is sheer exhaustion.

DO WOMEN HAVE THEIR OWN DISCRETE STRESS RESPONSE?

In a well-publicized paper, Shelly Taylor and colleagues at the University of California in Los Angeles discuss their theory of a markedly different pattern of response to stress in women than in men (Taylor et al., 2000). While acknowledging that the fight-or-flight response remains the primary physiological hormonal response in both sexes, they tease out a pattern of stress response that is unique to women. They call this pattern "tend-and-befriend" and speculate that it is the female's counterpart to the infant's attachment mechanism, which has been so thoroughly examined by child development professionals. Based on both human and animal studies, Taylor et al. hypothesize that the "tend-and-befriend" pattern is mediated by a stress regulatory system composed of female reproductive hormones and endogenous opioids but primarily involving the secretion of oxytocin. Taylor and colleagues cite numerous studies that demonstrate the anxiolytic properties of oxytocin, including mild sedation, decreased blood pressure, lower sensitivity to pain, and decreased glucocorticoid secretion. Furthermore, they point out that oxytocin levels increase as a response to massage and decrease with sadness. The researchers then go on to make the case that the same properties, which cause the "tend-and-befriend" pattern in response to stress and are present in the mother–infant bond, also are typical of women in various stressful situations—and are marked by a propensity to affiliate. One study that Taylor et al. cite on coping behavior found that women seek and use social support more than men—the combined significance was beyond the $P < .0000001$ level! What is so remarkable about this theory is that the physiological response results in a hormonal cascade as well as social/emotional behavior that is a healthy response to stress. Oxytocin is essentially a relaxation hormone, which is now known to be secreted in women during stress. In the next chapter, other hormones that produce a relaxation response will be reviewed.

ALLOSTATIC LOAD

CRH is supposed to stop being secreted when the glucocorticoids reach a theoretical setpoint, at which time the negative feedback loop ought to do its job and shut down the secretion of glucocorticoids. While glucocorticoid suppression of the immune system is helpful, if not lifesaving in short-term situations, chronic stress can alter the feedback regulation and cause prolonged glucocorticoid secretion, which can be profoundly detrimental. The stress response was not designed to be a prolonged physiological event, but rather a relatively short sprint away from the buffalo or other ominous critter (angry humans not excluded). The symptoms that occur from chronic stress, of any etiology, correlate to those physiological changes that are induced by and supportive of the fight-or-flight response. The symptoms (e.g., weight loss, loss of sexual drive, peptic ulcers, and of course immune suppression, which can lead to serious illness) have become exaggerated versions of an initially adaptive response.

In 1993, researcher Bruce McEwen published his views of the complex process of the body's effort to maintain homeostasis (McEwen and Stellar, 1993). McEwen realized that the concept of a static internal system maintaining a constant homeostatic steady state was entirely unrealistic. He recognized that the body is constantly fluctuating in its effort to maintain homeostasis. McEwen used the concept of *allostasis*, coined by researchers Sterling and Eyer in the 1980s, to express his premise. Allostasis is defined as the "operating range" of the body or the body's ability to adjust various vital functions (e.g., HPA axis, cardiovascular, metabolic, endocrine, nervous, or immune systems) in order to reset itself to a steady state (i.e., a state of relative homeostasis) following stress of any sort. It is the ability of the body to "achieve stability through change" (McEwen, 1998). McEwen took this concept one step further and coined the term *allostatic load* (graphically depicted in Figure 3.5). He defined allostatic load as the state of an organism in which "the strain on the body produced by repeated ups and downs of physiological response, as well as by the elevated activity of physiological systems under challenge, and the changes in metabolism and the impact of wear and tear on a number of organs and tissues, can predispose the organism to disease" (McEwen and Stellar, 1993). In other words, there comes a point at which the strain of accommodating the stress becomes too much, and the body can no longer handle the load. At that point, the person enters a state of chronic stress, with all the accompanying physiological breakdown.

According to Larry Dossey, M.D., there is something akin to allostatic load, which he calls time sickness or hurry sickness. We are victims of time sickness syndrome. Many of us are always feeling rushed, and it is a major cause of stress in our culture. It is similar to a sensory overload syndrome. You are handling all of the stress, and then there is just one more thing that happens, but it happens at the wrong time. You just crash, and your sympathetic nervous system flares. You may subsequently do or say something you might not normally do or say. Or, if you are capable of being calmer in the face of such overload, you are undoubtedly thinking thoughts that you would rather not think.

What glucocorticoids can do! Selye gave us the basics: thymic involution (reduction in size and function of the thymus), lymphopenia (decrease in proportion of blood lymphocytes), eosinopenia (decrease in eosinophils in blood), and decreased lymph node size. We now know that glucocorticoids inhibit cytokine release (essential to both T- and B-cell maturation), suppress natural killer (NK) cell activity, and promote lymphocyte apoptosis, which is programmed cellular death (Hetts, 1998; Munck and Guyre, 1991). Yet, in contrast, the acute stress response has been shown to strengthen the immune system and provide an immunological memory (McEwen,

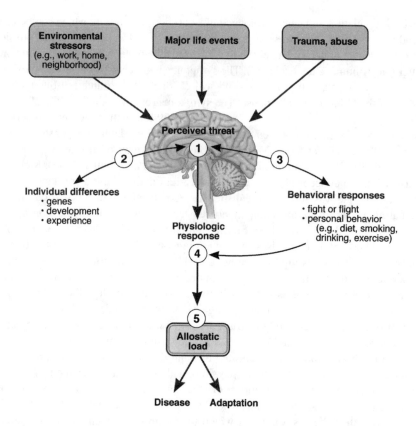

FIGURE 3.5 McEwen's allostatic load.

1998). Sometimes I think of acute stress as the body's way of staying in shape, of exercising the stress factor. If we never experienced stress, we would lose our vitality and vigor for life. A muscle never used becomes useless. Recent studies, however, have provided more understanding of the extensive implications of allostatic load (McEwen, 1998, 2000c, 2000d). This basic concept of allostatic load is an important one to keep in mind as we proceed to examine different factors that may be supportive during acute stress but maladaptive during chronic stress.

HORMONAL AND NEUROTRANSMITTER INFLUENCES ON STRESS

The major hormones and neurotransmitters of the stress system are beneficial modulators, but these same elements cause its malfunction, potentially leading to serious illness. There actually are numerous other factors that contribute to the stress–immune homeostasis, but for the most part, discussion in this section will be limited to what happens physiologically during chronic stress (see Khansari et al., 1990, for a review). Further, we will look at the role of opioids in HPA–immune interactions, determining their modulating role in both systems.

Glucocorticoids

Well over 100 years ago, the physician Thomas Addison identified a condition (that later came to be known as Addison's disease) in which the adrenals secrete insufficient amounts of cortisol and the patient evidences abnormally high levels of white blood cells (leukocytosis). Based on this finding, physicians decided that glucocorticoids were immune enhancing. That concept should have been dispelled in the mid-20th century, when glucocorticoids were shown to have anti-inflammatory properties (Hench et al., 1949). Yet, the idea that glucocorticoids stimulate the immune response persisted. Research in the latter part of the 20th century fully established the correlation between high doses of glucocorticoids (e.g., prednisone) and suppression of the immune response, even when administered to healthy adults (Rinehart et al., 1975).

On the heels of these studies came the work of researchers, such as Hugo Besedovsky, who looked at the actions of the glucocorticoids from a systems interaction perspective and surmised that the net effect of glucocorticoids was modulatory. Besedovsky felt that the glucocorticoids prevent immune overactivity and permit specificity (e.g., magnitude, duration) of immune reactions (Besedovsky et al., 1975; Besedovsky and Sorkin, 1977; Munck et al., 1984). They are a little like the foot controlling the gas pedal. He showed that lymphocytes with lower antigen affinity are more sensitive to the effects of glucocorticoids, once again, possibly a means for controlling overresponsiveness of the immune system (Besedovsky et al., 1981).

Glucocorticoids suppress the immune system by decreasing the production of many factors that facilitate B- and T-cell proliferation, including the cytokines, β-endorphin, and insulin. Inhibition of these mediators reduces proper functioning of monocytes and macrophages (Guyre et al., 1988; Moynihan and Stevens, 2001; Munck and Guyre, 1991). High levels of glucocorticoids also reduce NK cell activity levels in mice and humans (Cox et al., 1983; Holbrook et al., 1983; Keller et al., 1991; Oya et al., 2000; Shavit, 1991). Curiously, one experiment showed that rats, who were administered corticosterone in amounts equal to those induced by inescapable tail shock, did not have antibody suppression like the shocked animals (Fleshner et al., 1998). This finding supports the argument that there is a combination of factors that contribute to the immune-suppressing effects of glucocorticoids and that we do not yet fully understand these factors.

Many physicians today are not aware that brief exposure to glucocorticoids actually enhances the immune response, but there are many studies illustrating this point. In one experiment, γ-interferon was shown to completely abolish the immune suppressive actions of glucocorticoids (Girard et al., 1987; Morganelli and Guyre, 1988). Furthermore, Allen Munck and Paul Guyre, at Dartmouth Medical School, concluded from analysis of various studies that steroids must saturate at least 50% of the glucocorticoid receptors for a minimum of 24 hours before monocyte or macrophage inhibition occurs (Munck and Guyre, 1991). The research supports Selye's premise that some stress is important. The role of glucocorticoids, both in controlling overresponsiveness of the immune system and in enhancing the immune system at low levels, are illustrations of the body seeking homeostasis. Both responses are adjustments to help lower the allostatic load, anticipative of maintaining or regaining health.

ADRENOCORTICOTROPIC HORMONE (ACTH)

Recall that the secretion of ACTH from the pituitary, prompted by CRH from the hypothalamus, stimulates the adrenals to secrete glucocorticoids. Fascinating research shows that during chronic stress, glucocorticoid levels remain high, while ACTH returns to normal or slightly below normal levels. In other words, the ACTH levels no longer correlate to those of the glucocorticoids (Bornstein and Chrousos, 1999). Curious! So, researchers began to try to figure out why this happens. It is well known that the adrenals atrophy if the pituitary is removed and that exogenous ACTH can reinstate normal glucocorticoid secretion. So, how can the adrenals continue to secrete high levels of cortisol during chronic stress if ACTH has all but shut down?

Well, a few creative individuals, from several different countries, broke from the conventional thinking that the adrenal medulla and the adrenal cortex are two proximate glands that lack any pathway for communication. For the reader who is new to the topic, this theory might seem like the obvious. Although it is known that fetal and neonatal adrenal function occurs independently of pituitary ACTH, medical students today are still being taught that the two segments of the adrenals have nothing to do with one another. (McDonald and Nathanielsz, 1998, includes a review of adrenal innervation.) The finding that the adrenal medulla and cortex communicate introduced a potentially new route for mechanisms of hormonal action during chronic stress. The observations opened the way to a whole new field of research, called *non-ACTH* or *ACTH-independent regulation of the adrenal cortex*.

Chromaffin cells of the adrenal medulla extensively communicate with the steroid-producing cells of the adrenal cortex (also called *adrenocortical cells*) in such a manner as to elevate cortisol (Bornstein et al., 1997; Haidan et al., 1998). *In vitro* studies show that when adrenocortical cells are mixed with medulla chromaffin cells, they produce ten times the amount of glucocorticoids as adrenocortical cells alone (Bornstein and Ehrhart-Bornstein, 2000). This means that we probably do not need ACTH to keep the cortisol pumping during stress. Several mechanisms of paracrine bidirectional communication have been proposed. First, neuropeptides and small amounts of CRH and ACTH from the adrenal medulla may influence cortisol secretion, although the effect is probably minor (Bornstein and Chrousos, 1999; Ehrhart-Bornstein et al., 1998). Second, and probably more importantly, various immune cytokines are secreted by the adrenal cortex and may play a role in immune–adrenal regulation, which could theoretically stimulate cortisol (Bornstein and Chrousos, 1999; Bornstein and Ehrhart-Bornstein, 2000). For example, IL-6, during chronic but not acute stress, increases steroid production (Päth et al., 1997). And, when pituitary ACTH shuts down during chronic stress, it appears that the chromaffin cells of the medulla become potent stimulators of adrenocortical steroidogenesis via a paracrine mechanism. Recent research suggests the activation of the sympathetic nervous system and the secretion of epinephrine from chromaffin cells of the medulla as a route by which cortisol is stimulated (Haidan et al., 2000; Pignatelli et al., 1998).

Speculatively, it could be the collaboration of all three of the mechanisms mentioned that produces the effects of non-ACTH–mediated cortisol during chronic stress—or that the most salient factor has not yet been discovered. Recall from Chapter 2 that, historically speaking, the major systemically influential hormones, such as the hypothalamic and pituitary hormones, were first discovered. In recent years, subtler modulators, such as those involving paracrine and autocrine interactions, have been acknowledged for their importance to overall physiologic functioning. The significance resides in their ability to interact and integrate. It appears that research on stress has now entered a phase in which the subtler interactions of the adrenals are being elucidated as significant to prolonged stress.

Corticotropin-Releasing Hormone (CRH)

CRH, isolated from the hypothalamus in 1955, is best known for its role as the hormone released from the hypothalamus to stimulate the secretion of ACTH (see Saffran and Schaly, 1955; Taylor and Fishman, 1988; Vale et al., 1981, for a review). CRH is a very powerful hormone that is capable of affecting multiple human functions, including mood, growth, and reproduction (Chrousos, 1999; Ghizzoni et al., 1996; Gold et al., 1987; Habib et al., 2000). CRH stimulates the secretion of epinephrine from the adrenal medulla and is stimulated by norepinephrine (Pacak et al., 1995; Pacak, 2000). In fact, norepinephrine and CRH are capable of stimulating one another and appear to operate differently during acute stress than during chronic stress (Calogero et al., 1988; Kiss and Auguilera, 1992, 2000).

Intriguing research on adult male rhesus macaques using a CRH antagonist confirms just how germane CRH is to the malfunction of the HPA response. Researchers synthesized a CRH antagonist and determined the dose at which it reduced ACTH blood levels. They administered it to the monkeys who, 90 minutes later, were exposed to the acute psychosocial stress of being placed in a cage with two unfamiliar monkeys in adjacent cages, separated only by Plexiglas. The exposure lasted for 30 minutes, and behaviors were recorded. The episode elicited symptoms of acute stress in the controls, including hitting the Plexiglas, audible teeth grinding, body tremors, grimacing, urination, and defecation. However, the rhesus macaques that were given the CRH antagonist exhibited significantly less anxiety and aggression. Blood tests showed that the monkeys given the CRH antagonist had significantly lower ACTH, cortisol, norepinephrine, and epinephrine (Habib et al., 2000).

The findings of CRH antagonist-related stress levels in macaques confirmed previous studies on rats (Webster et al., 1998). Researchers speculate that a CRH antagonist could have therapeutic potential for inflammatory conditions, sexual disorders, growth retardation, and gastrointestinal disorders. Additional research revealed that administration of the CRH antagonist did not result in adrenal atrophy—an enormously important finding if it were ever to be used as a therapeutic agent (Bornstein et al., 1998).

OPIOIDS AND STRESS

Numerous studies link opioids, particularly the endorphins, to HPA stimulation of the immune system. Opioids appear to have immune-modulating characteristics, variously increasing or decreasing the immune response (see Moynihan and Stevens, 2001, for a review.) Endorphins are secreted by the adrenal medulla during the stress response and are primarily associated with the reduction of pain. Leukocytes have opioid receptors specific to the opioid type. For instance, NK cell activity levels are enhanced by β-endorphin, γ-endorphin, and met-enkephalin, but not by α-endorphin or leu-enkephalin.

Endorphins have neurotransmitter properties as well as CNS involvement and, therefore, communicate back and forth between the HPA axis and the immune system about both cognitive and noncognitive stimuli (Smith et al., 1985). β-endorphin stimulation of NK cell activity can be reversed by naloxone, an opioid antagonist, which means that increased NK activity is opioid-mediated. CRH indirectly modulates the immune system by augmenting the production of β-endorphins by leukocytes and by inducing monocytes to secrete IL-1 (Carr and Blalock, 1990). IL-1 causes B cells, but not T cells, to secrete β-endorphin, which in turn enhances the immune response (Kavelaars et al., 1990). Thus, we have another great example of systems interaction and integration.

In the 1980s, researchers made a distinction between opioid and non-opioid forms of stress. Yehuda Shavit, who began this work as a graduate student in psychology at UCLA, showed that, depending on the length and intensity of the stressor, the body responds with either an opioid-mediated or a nonopioid–mediated form of analgesia. Rats exposed to prolonged intermittent foot shock (inescapable shock) demonstrated an opioid-mediated route of analgesia (ascertained by its ability to be blocked by the opioid antagonist, naloxone). These experiments caused an "escape or avoidance learning deficit" or "learned helplessness" (Shavit, 1991). However, rats exposed to brief but continuous foot shock, given for the same cumulative amount of time, elicited a non-opioid analgesic response to a degree comparable with that of the opioid-mediated analgesia.

So, why are the two different routes of analgesia significant? Research shows a correlation between opioid-mediated analgesia and depressed NK activity levels as well as decreased tumor median survival time with tumor (Shavit et al., 1985). Similar research shows a depressed mitogen (i.e., a substance that aids lymphocyte proliferation) response can result from just one instance of intermittent foot shock. When the protocol was changed to continuous foot shock, the mitogen suppression was correlated to β-endorphin stimulation (Panerai et al., 1997). Additional research showed that learned helplessness correlates to decreased norepinephrine and to depression (Weiss and Simson, 1988).

Although opioids, such as β-endorphin, help limit the stress response via their analgesic effects, the analgesic effect can fail when stress causes chronic activation of the HPA axis (Chrousos, 1998). One study on the effects of exercise-induced stress showed that mild excercise enhances immunity, while continuous excercise that exhausts the opioid system can result in immunosuppression (Ilyinsky et al., 1990). The fact that different stress parameters variously evoke opioid or non-opioid forms of analgesia may be one factor behind the inconsistent results found in studies on stress.

THE IMMUNE SYSTEM PREPARES FOR ACTION

During an acute stress response, the HPA stimulates the immune response and arouses immunological memory for invaders (Dhabhar and McEwen, 1996). The stress stimulus instigates a process by which leukocytes (particularly T cells and monocytes) move from the blood stream to the walls of blood vessels, lymph nodes, or bone marrow, in preparation to mount an immune response, if there is a need to do so (Dhabhar et al., 1996). This phenomenon is evidenced by a reduction of blood leukocytes (over 50%), an increase in neutrophils (over 80%), and an increase in the number of leukocytes in other areas, particularly the skin (Dhabhar and McEwen, 1996; Dhabhar et al., 1996). Following acute stress, it appears that some of these leukocytes are retained in certain areas of the skin and that γ-interferon, as a local mediator of this enhanced skin immunity, fosters immunological memory (Dhabhar et al., 2000). However, research shows that glucocorticoids are the primary mediators of the leukocyte shift. So, in spite of overall statistics indicating the destructive aspects of glucocorticoids, again we see that they enhance the immune response in the initial stages.

The researchers describe the leukocyte migration as "battle or communication stations" for the enhancement of cell-mediated immunity, that is, T cell immunity (Dhabhar et al., 1996). This seems to be an appropriate function from the evolutionary perspective—an individual in a fight-or-flight scenario would need to mount a rapid immune response if injury occurred during conflict. It also makes logical sense that this immune readiness would be beneficial to immune challenges, such as wounds, but would most likely exacerbate immune challenges in systemic disorders (Dhabhar and McEwen, 1996). A contrasting profile emerges of the immune response during acute versus chronic stress, as chronic stress not only causes leukocyte function to be inhibited, but also induces a decrease in the redistribution of lymphocytes from the blood to the immune compartments (Dhabhar and McEwen, 1997, 1999). Typically, an immune-enhancing effect will endure for 3 to 5 days, after which time the allostatic load becomes too great, and features of chronic stress emerge (McEwen, 1998).

THE DISEASES WE GET FROM PROLONGED STRESS

CASE STUDY: ROSETO, PENNSYLVANIA

Dr. Stewart Wolf studied the town of Roseto, Pennsylvania, for 28 years. There was a group of Italian immigrants from a small town in southern Italy that had moved to Roseto, and basically, they were in each other's kitchens. They were in each other's pasta and tomato sauce—butter, pasta, wine, and a lot of love. There were intermarriages among the family members, a true modern-day tribe.

They lived with the feeling of being more than themselves, a feeling of being connected, a feeling of identity, and with the security that they had a place, an inherent place in life. What Wolf found in Roseto was that the incidence of heart disease and mortality was lower when compared with neighboring towns. But, unfortunately, the Roseto story has a sad ending. During the last 10 years of the study, the young people began moving out. They wanted more in life. They felt there was more out there that they did not have. Technology crept in. Some of the people did well with their lives, and instead of living on Gabriel Avenue in the center of town, they moved to a big house on top of the hill. Soon, the woman who lived in the nice house on top of the hill started complaining that nobody comes around to visit anymore. Feelings of isolation and loneliness crept in. And, with all these changes, the incidence of heart disease rose significantly. But, for so many years, these people had dietary habits that were absolutely horrific by most conventional standards, yet the incidence of myocardial infarction and cardiovascular disease was incredibly low (Wolf, 1992).

AN EASTERN PERSECTIVE OF STRESS

The emotions we feel, we feel in our bodies. We burn with anger, tremble with fear, and are choked up with sadness. Our stomachs turn with revulsion. Humans experience unpleasant emotions as unpleasant bodily sensations, and thus they feel physically distressed when emotionally distressed. According to Chinese medicine, there is a particular type of energy called *shen*, which is one's spiritual vitality. It may be recognized by a brilliant glow in the eyes, even of a dying person. It may be absent in a person with a relatively minor illness and is an indication of the patient's will.

Shen resides in various organs, correlating to the primary emotion that one is experiencing. For example, burning with anger is manifested by burning in the liver. When you are feeling grief, you feel it in the lungs, and sadness is felt in the heart. When you are feeling fear, you feel it in the kidneys. So, for example, when someone is very fearful for a long period of time, often that person may go to the doctor complaining of low back pain, prostate, or menstrual disorders. If you are a physician or healthcare practitioner of any sort, you might want to pick up a book on the five Chinese elements and learn how emotions affect the different organ systems. You can watch for the clinical correlation in your practice. In 6 months, I think you will be surprised by what you have observed. I should not have been surprised, but I was, which was my scientific skepticism showing.

The effects of stress are numerous: physical, emotional, behavioral, and cognitive. It has become the mode in which a lot of us function. Most of the patients I see, to one degree or another, suffer from stress. It is the sign of an exhausted, unhealthy culture. Repressed emotions are a significant factor in the cause of disease. It is my feeling that we are taught to repress powerful emotions in our culture. Repression of anger, fear, and grief may lead to chronic disease, helplessness, depression, and alexithymia (i.e., the inability to verbalize one's emotions). In the next section, we will discuss memory and trauma, and the engrams that crystallize in our personalities. These engrams are repressed emotions that can cause disease. According to Chinese tradition, when you repress an emotion, it creates an energetic imbalance. This imbalance, over a long period of time, will be translated into functional pathology, like back pain.

A CLINICAL PERSPECTIVE OF STRESS

A fascinating study was published in *Science* in 1983 (Ekman et al., 1983). An actor was instructed to depict various emotions through facial distortions and to poignantly express an emotion: anger, fear, sadness, happiness, surprise, and disgust. He was connected to monitors that measured several physiological parameters. The technician in the other room could guess what emotion he was showing by the physiological response seen on the monitors. For example, if he had a high skin temperature and pulse rate, the technician knew that he was angry. If his skin temperature went up but his pulse rate was low, he was either fearful or sad, and so on. This landmark study showed a direct physiological correlation to an emotion simply *performed* by an actor. Recall that magnetic resonance imaging (MRI) of the brain shows that the right prefrontal cortex governs negative feelings (which would manifest on the left side of the face) and that the left prefrontal cortex governs positive emotions (manifesting on the right side of the face) (Jackson et al., 2000). Just as with our actor, something so simple as contracting a few muscles may actually alter your mood.

There are various captivating studies showing how different types of stress can be detrimental to the body and how certain personalities are more vulnerable to particular types of stress than others. First, I want briefly to share with you an example of this in the animal world. It comes from the work of Robert Sapolsky, a neuroendocrinologist who is in Kenya researching baboons when he is not teaching at Stanford University (Sapolsky, 1990, 1994). In his study of baboons, Sapolsky initially determined that the dominant male baboon had a resting cortisol that was significantly lower than the subordinate males. Predictably, when the pecking order changed, so did the cortisol levels of the respective baboons.

Continuing his research, Sapolsky uncovered the intriguing fact that there were actually larger discrepancies in the cortisol levels between dominant males with different personality traits than there were between dominants and subordinates. Among the personality traits that kept dominant males with a healthier cortisol profile were the ability to discriminate between a neutral and threatening action of another baboon and, in the latter situation, to be the one to control the situation by initiating a fight. Dominant baboons that lose a fight and control the situation by displacing their aggression (and perhaps frustration) on to another baboon also have relatively lower cortisol levels. As you may have guessed, the issue of control is the salient one, but it also correlates to issues of security and predictability and, in humans, to social support as well.

A researcher, Eileen Kobasa, studied corporate mentality at a large company that was undergoing a merger and cutback of employees. (Is this not somewhat akin to a group of baboons changing their pecking order?) She looked at stress patterns and found something she called *hardiness* (Kobasa, 1979, 1983). Similarly, I was the corporate medical director of Marriott International, Inc. for 20 years, and there were people in the corporation who we called *shock absorbers*. We'd say: "Joe can handle that. Give him more work. Pete left? Give it to Joe. George left? Give it to Joe. He can handle it." Joe was our number-one shock absorber. Kobasa wanted to know what makes a shock absorber a true shock absorber, not just someone who is repressing his or her feelings. She found that the common factors were the three Cs: commitment, challenge, and control (that is control of oneself, not control of the outside environment). Kobasa writes that "high stress/low illness executives show, by comparison with high stress/high illness executives, more hardiness, that is, [they] have a stronger commitment to self, an attitude of vigorousness toward the environment, a sense of meaningfulness, and an internal locus of control" (Kobasa, 1985). These individuals manifested coherence between their internal and external environments. Remember the phrase "coherence of the internal and external environment," as it will be revisited.

A chronic state of high anxiety and vigilance is destructive to health, in part, as a result of chronic suppression of the immune system. HPA hyperfunction is corre-lated to heart disease, osteoporosis, depression, and age-related diseases, to name a few (Chrousos, 2000). The work of researchers, such as Soloman, Cohen, Felten, and Ader, described in previous chapters, paved the way for recognition of the interface between disease and various behavioral factors that provoke an altered immune response. In short, the immune system is depressed when one has a pro-longed stress response. There are many human studies on bereavement, depression, stress of exams, space flight, sleep deprivation, loneliness, divorce, cancer, the heartbreak of herpes, helplessness, and loneliness all showing the same thing—that each type of stress leaves us more vulnerable to illness (see Biondi, 2001; Calabrese et al., 1987; Friedman et al., 1996; Glaser and Kiecolt-Glaser, 1994; Kiecolt-Glaser et al., 1987, 1988; Kiecolt-Glaser and Glaser, 1991, for reviews). The next section will review a few of these illnesses and their known correlation to stress.

ILLNESS AND STRESS

HEART

There is an increased risk of myocardial ischemia for individuals enduring either acute or chronic stress (Jiang et al., 1996; Krantz et al., 1999; Krantz et al., 2000; O'Connor et al., 2000). Over 20 years ago, researchers showed that acute mental stress in patients with coronary artery disease causes ischemia; the startling part was that it was symptomatically silent in 83% of their subjects (Rozanski et al., 1988). More recently published studies are detailing stress-induced abnormalities, such as abnormal vasomotor response and blood flow velocity, occurring with patients suf-fering from coronary artery disease (Kop et al., 2001; Yeung et al., 1991). Stress has also been shown to increase platelet activation, increasing susceptibility to heart attack (Markovitz and Mathews, 1991).

The heart is affected both by stress and by depression (Januzzi et al., 2000). An article in the *Journal of the American Medical Association* (*JAMA*) showed that depression correlates to an independent and higher mortality rate. In a prospective study performed at a cardiac care unit of a university-affiliated hospital, researchers amazingly found that major depression is as much a risk factor for cardia-related mortality as a previous myocardial infarction (MI) (Frasure-Smith et al., 1993). A similar study published in *Lancet* shows that patients with post-infarction depression are at high risk for incomplete recovery in the 6-month period following an acute MI compared with those patients who are not suffering from depression (Ladwig et al., 1994). More recently, research confirmed earlier findings of increased risk of mortality for those with post-infarction depression (O'Connor et al., 2000).

As mentioned in our story about the baboons, social stresses contribute to a measurable increase in stress hormones, which are damaging to the cardiovascular system. It is clear that there is a strong correlation between social stresses of various sorts and heart disease in humans. The years of studies and debate (beginning in the 1960s) about type-A personalities and myocardial infarction ended up ferreting out anger and hostility as the two most salient qualities correlated to heart disease. Researchers are indeed still finding solid correlation between anger and heart disease (Moller et al., 1999). However, Levin points out that any personality characteristic may or may not have a detrimental effect, depending upon whether it is adaptive. For example, he and his colleagues found a protective effect for type-A individuals who were *not* religious (Levin, 2001).

Marital status also has correlates to cardiac events. Women (but not men) in stressful marriages as well as unmarried men both are at greater risk for heart disease (Kumlin et al., 2001; Orth-Gomer et al., 2000). For the first time, hopelessness has been identified as a risk factor for hypertension in men, which we had already gleaned from our rodent studies (Everson et al., 2000).

A physician, Robert Eliot, did some very interesting research on personality and stress. He identified the common, but previously unknown, phenomenon by which individuals have normal blood pressure during an office visit but highly elevated blood pressure when confronted with normal daily challenges. He calls these people *hot reactors* (Eliot and Breo, 1989). Eliot, a driven cardiologist until he suffered his own heart attack at the age of 44 years, asked himself, "Is any of this worth dying for?" His resounding "no!" compelled him to find ways to help others reduce stress and the risk of heart disease. Amazingly, one in five of us seemingly healthy individuals is a *hot reactor*.

In the late 1960s, Eliot was asked to go to NASA to determine why so many NASA employees were dying suddenly from cardiac arrest. Autopsies showed mysterious microscopic lesions, called *contraction band lesions*. These lesions are difficult to observe with current heart imaging techniques. Contraction band lesions are tiny ruptures in muscle fibers of the heart that cause microscopic electrical short circuits, which can lead to ventricular fibrillation and sudden death because the heart muscle is so extensively damaged that it literally dissolves. It took Eliot and his colleagues 16 years to determine that the cause of the contraction band lesions are dose-related, continuously high levels of the catecholamine stress hormones. Contraction band lesions can, in fact, cause death in people whose arteries are patent and healthy looking. Sociologically, Eliot learned that the NASA scientists who died of sudden myocardial infarcts were frequently the highly educated astrophysicists or jet propulsion experts, whose jobs were highly specialized and not transferable to employment anywhere else in the country. Once a rocket program was completed, they were laid off and often forced to take menial jobs, such as pumping gas, in order to help feed their families. The stress was literally fatal (Eliot, 1994). Eliot devoted himself to educating people on how to prevent the development of contraction band lesions.

A phenomenon called *karoshi*, literally death (*shi*) from overwork (*karo*), is the second leading cause of death (after cancer) in Japan, according to the Japanese Ministry of Health. Karoshi affects managers and supervisors, primarily in their 30s and 40s. These men (it seems it is exclusively men) suddenly die from stroke or heart attack—perhaps from contraction band lesions. They are forced to work 70-hour weeks, week after week, month after month. In addition, they tend to use cigarettes and alcohol to reduce their stress. The labor ministry is now granting compensation to widows of these men, while still denying the existence of karoshi. Sadly, these men simply lose their ability to function, sometimes while at work. If they are lucky enough to survive, they are taken to a specialized medical facility, called a *karoshi unit*, for physical and emotional rehabilitation, where they learn relaxation techniques and self-management skills (see Neunan and Hubbard, 1998, for a review of workplace stress).

The Common Cold

Researchers have confirmed age-old anecdotal reports that increased stress is related to catching the common cold (Cohen and Miller, 2001). One landmark study concludes that "psychological stress was associated in a dose-response manner with an increased risk of acute infectious respiratory illness" (Cohen et al., 1991).

Wound Healing

In a much-publicized study involving caretaker relatives of Alzheimer's patients, it was found that healing from a punch-biopsy wound took significantly longer—an average of 9 days longer—than that of matched controls (Kiecolt-Glaser et al., 1995). Caregivers reported greater levels of perceived stress and were producing lower levels of a cytokine known to be important in wound healing than the controls. Subsequent examinations of the topic have sought to understand more fully the neuroendocrine regulation of wound healing and its clinical implications (Marucha et al., 2001).

Exam Stress

Several studies show that examination stress affects students' immune systems, resulting in increased morbidity. Students tend to get upper respiratory tract infections and bronchitis following the stress of the exam. An important study, which occurred in 1984, involved 75 first-year medical students at The Ohio State University College of Medicine. Blood samples drawn on the first day of final examinations, compared with blood drawn a month prior, revealed declines in NK cell activity levels. Students with higher stress and loneliness scores had statistically significantly lower NK cell activity between blood samples (Kiecolt-Glaser et al., 1984). Other research shows increases in plasma cortisol and salivary norepinephrine as well as elevated antibody titers to various latent herpes viruses (Kiecolt-Glaser and Glaser, 1991; Lacey et al., 2000; McClelland et al., 1985).

CANCER

Research shows a correlation between stress and cancer incidence. There is also an association between factors such as social support, lack of control, and suppression of emotion with cancer progression and possibly survival (see Rosch, 1996; Spiegel, 2000; Turner-Cobb et al., 2001, for reviews). There are various studies on personality characteristics that are predictive of cancer. Among the earliest and better known of these studies is the work of Carolyn Biddell Thomas, at Johns Hopkins University. She followed several graduating classes of medical students for up to a 30-year period. Thomas found that those students who later were diagnosed with cancer had reported (at the time of graduation) feeling a lack of a close relationship to parents (especially fathers with sons). This effect persisted even when various known risk factors, such as smoking and drinking, were controlled (Schaffer et al., 1982a; Thomas et al., 1979). Students who scored higher on a test designed to elicit levels of nervous tension and those who had fewer intellectual interests in life also were at a statistically significant greater risk of developing cancer (Schaffer et al., 1982b; Thomas and McCabe, 1980).

Another prospective study showed that women with breast cancer, who had relapses, had a 5.67-fold higher incidence of bereavement or job loss compared with controls who remained in remission (Ramirez et al., 1989). Similarly, a joint study between researchers in Sweden and UCLA's School of Public Health revealed a 5.5-fold increase in colorectal disease for individuals with severe stress in the workplace in the prior 10 years (Courtney et al., 1993). Researchers speculate that the constant stress may lead to changes in lifestyle that increase a variety of risk factors for disease.

In contrast, there are various studies showing that social support improves outlook and health of cancer patients (Bloom and Spiegel, 1984; Butler et al., 1999; Koopman et al. 1998; Schrock et al., 1999; Spiegel, 1999a; Spiegel et al., 1999). One study revealed that metastatic breast cancer patients who scored higher on subscales of belonging and tangible social support on a personality inventory had lower salivary cortisol levels, which correlates to greater immune function (Turner-Cobb et al., 2000).

David Spiegel, who is at Stanford University School of Medicine, was the pioneer in finding a link between group therapy for breast cancer patients and stress reduction, improved quality of life, and possibly prolonged survival. His first published piece of research revealed that breast cancer patients who participated in a weekly support group and used self-hypnosis for pain had a mean survival time of 36.6 months compared with 18.9 months for the control group (Spiegel et al., 1989). His later work delineates factors that undermine a patient's sense of support, which if inadequate, can have both adverse medical and emotional consequences (Spiegel, 1997, 1999; Spiegel et al., 1999). He designed a 12-week, supportive–expressive group for breast cancer patients that could be implemented effectively in community settings. Group participation reduced patients' distress by 40%, as measured by a mood disturbance scale taken before and after the 12-week session (Spiegel et al., 1999). Other studies have supported his results (Blake-Mortimer et al., 1999; Kogon et al., 1997). Similarly, researchers also have found that psychological therapy, relaxation, guided imagery, and biofeedback are correlated with both reduction of anxiety and improved immune parameters (Gruber et al., 1993; Watson et al., 1999).

BEREAVEMENT

There are numerous studies that illustrate the correlation between bereavement and a depressed immune system. Many studies show that the bereaved have a poorer lymphocyte response to an immune challenge (Bartrop et al., 1977; Schleifer et al., 1983). Epidemiological research and studies of select populations of bereaved individuals show that the alteration in immune competence actually corresponds to greater illness and even higher mortality rates. Risk of death for individuals with cancer who suffered the loss of a child is greatly increased, as is the death rate of bereaved spouses (bereaved men experience twice the incidence as bereaved women) in the 7- to 12-month period following the bereavement (Levav et al., 2000; Schaefer et al., 1995).

DIVORCE

The correlation between the stress of separation or divorce and immune suppression is quite well documented and results in even greater health risks than bereavement (see Kiecolt-Glaser and Glaser, 1991, for a review). Once again (like our baboons), the salient issue appears to be one of control. Individuals who initiate the separation or who do not remain attached to their ex-spouse fare better both psychologically and in regard to immune function than those who do not sever attachments (Kiecolt-Glaser et al., 1987; Kiecolt-Glaser et al., 1988).

PHYSICIANS BE WARNED

Physicians are not immune to the devastating effects of stress. In 2001, *JAMA* published an article advising increased self-awareness of emotions related to the stresses of patient care (Meier et al., 2001). While couched in conservative language: "Our approach is based on the standard medical model of risk factors, signs and symptoms, differential diagnosis, and intervention," the report clearly expounds on issues that may increase "physician distress." Undoubtedly, it was an appropriate admonition. A prior survey on physician burnout indicated that 58% reported being "highly" emotionally exhausted (Deckard et al., 1994). Women physicians appear to be more at risk of burnout than men (McMurray et al., 2000). Compared with their male counterparts, female physicians reported being more satisfied with their specialty as well as with their patient and colleague relationships ($P < .05$); however, they reported significantly less work control and were paid a mean income about

$22,000 less than matched males. Once again, compared with male physicians, women physicians were 1.6 times more likely to state they had burnout ($P < .05$). Strikingly, after working an initial 40 hours, the odds of burnout increased 12 to 15% for each additional 5 hours worked per week ($P < .05$).

STRESS AND AGING

Not only can we acquire a variety of illnesses from stressing ourselves, we also can accelerate our aging process. Aging, by definition, includes decreased levels of circulating hormones and a decline in immune efficacy—all of which are exacerbated by stress (Friedman et al., 1996; Soloman and Benton, 1994; Soloman and Morley, 2001). One study showed that prolonged cortisol exposure in chronically stressed elderly subjects was correlated to hippocampus memory deficits (Lupien et al., 1998). Various studies support the theory that prolonged stress in the elderly, particularly when they become caregivers, carries with it an increased risk of mortality (Kiecolt-Glaser and Glaser, 1999).

Chronic stress and the overproduction of the inflammatory cytokine IL-6 have been strongly implicated in a host of age-related diseases and conditions. A summary of the conference held at the National Institutes of Health in 1998 and moderated by Dr. Dimitris Papanicolaou described IL-6 as "a potent stimulator of the hypothalamic–pituitary–adrenal axis" and stated that it is secreted during stress (Papanicolaou et al., 1998). A seminal study compared 119 men and women who were primary caregivers for a spouse who suffered dementia (included in the data were individuals who lost their spouse during the study) with 106 men and women who were noncaregivers (Kiecolt-Glaser et al., 2003). Caregivers had an increase in the average rate of IL-6 that was four times the rate of the noncaregivers. The effect persisted for years after the death of the spouse. Based on epidemiological studies on aging, the researchers predicted that the caregivers had a risk of death at around age 75 compared with age 90 for noncaregivers, the primary cause likely being the premature aging of the immune system.

SUMMARY

Stress reduces immune competence, leaving us more susceptible to a host of diseases. Stress accelerates the impact of discordant emotions, pollution, environmental factors (e.g., chemical, electromagnetic), and personal lifestyle factors (e.g., drugs, alcohol, smoking, poor nutritional habits) on our well-being. Response to stress depends on our psychological reaction to it. As with baboons, factors such as outlets for frustration, social support, predictability and warning, a sense of control, or a perception that things are improving all help to reduce stress (Weiss, 1972).

MEMORY AND STRESS

We, cave dwellers in three-piece suits, no longer need a buffalo chasing us (or anything else so dramatic) to activate the stress response. We are fully capable of sitting quietly and arousing a stress response simply with our thoughts and memories.

How can it happen that mere memories can arouse stress reactions? Negative emotional thoughts activate the stress system and interact with particular facets of the CNS that are involved in the storage of memories. These memory storage areas are significant to memory retrieval and emotional discernment of any given stress (Chrousos and Gold, 1992). To understand this phenomenon more fully we need to take a look at where and how memories are stored in our brains.

There are various sites in the brain in which short-term memories are stored. The amygdala is important because it is the short-term storage site at which contextual information acquires an emotional significance, such as fear (LeDoux, 1994, 1996). However, the cortex, particularly the prefrontal cortex, also is vital to short-term memory storage. Subjects who are depressed show deficits that include an inability of the brain to turn off the fear messages from the amygdala. This can develop into an inability to turn off the amygdala's fear response to just about anything and may be the physiological setup of the behavioral conditioning that occurs in posttraumatic stress disorder (Yehuda, 2000).

Long-term memory storage is largely the responsibility of the hippocampus. It is a center of learning as well as memory. The hippocampus stores memories that are associated with trauma and deeply imprints them in the memory. Information is moved from the various storage sites of short-term memories to the hippocampus for longer-term storage. Eventually, usually after about 3 years, the hippocampus relinquishes the storage of a memory to the neocortex (LeDoux, 1996). With Alzheimer's disease, patients preserve the oldest memories the longest because the disease is very advanced by the time it affects the neocortex.

A stressful thought is capable of causing the sympathetic nervous system to secrete norepinephrine, activating the amygdala, which in turn activates the stress response. Norepinephrine also can directly trigger the HPA axis and is an important factor in sustaining hypercortisolism during chronic stress (Wong et al., 2000). Furthermore, norepinephrine not only facilitates the movement of negatively charged memories from temporary storage in the amygdala to long-term storage in the hippocampus, but, as depicted in Figure 3.6, it *strengthens* the stressful memories, as they reside in the hippocampus (Habib et al., 2000). In other words, each time you have a negative experience that is similar to one that is already in storage, the traumatic aspects of the first experience will be reinforced by the subsequent stressful experience. The hippocampus even remembers relationships between stimuli (LeDoux, 1996). Norepinephrine also is the culprit in stress-related impairment of the prefrontal cortex and is associated with a decreased attention span, poor working memory, and a lack of inhibition in behavior (Birnbaum et al., 1999).

There is a particular part of the amygdala that has β-adrenergic receptors for epinephrine as well as receptors for glucocorticoids. The activation of the epinephrine receptors is crucial to the modulation of the glucocorticoids that infuse the amygdala during stress. It has been shown that blocking the β-adrenergic receptors largely blocks the ability of glucocorticoids to promote memory storage in the hippocampus (Ferry et al., 1999; Quirarte et al., 1997). A small amount of glucocorticoids enhance memory, which is important for recall of dangerous incidents, but too much stress impairs memory.

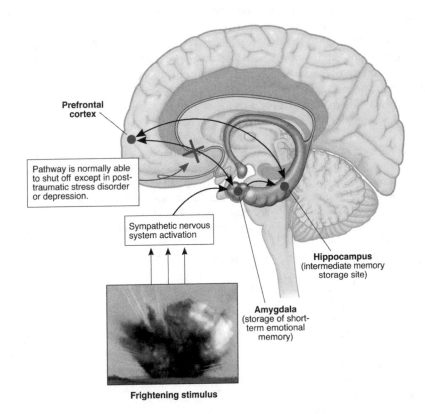

Prefrontal
cortex

Pathway is normally able
to shut off except in posttraumatic stress disorder
or depression.

Sympathetic nervous
system activation

Hippocampus
(intermediate memory
storage site)

Amygdala
(storage of short-
term emotional
memory)

Frightening stimulus

FIGURE 3.6 Diagram of the fear response. (See color insert following page 74.)

Chronic stress can be devastating to the brain. As the brain is continuously bathed in cortisol, the hippocampus begins to atrophy, causing plasticity (McEwen, 2000b). Dendrites, which increase the available area for a neuron to receive incoming information, shorten and lose their branches. In addition, neurons in a part of the hippocampus called the *dentate gyrus* have a suppressed neurogenesis (McEwen, 2000a; Ohl et al., 2000). This reduces the ability of the hippocampus to perform vital functions, including those involving declarative, spatial, and contextual memory. Neurons in the hippocampus actually die because of exposure to glucocorticoids, even in a petri dish (Sapolsky, 1994). The hippocampus is the first part of the brain to be affected by glucocorticoids, which is a staggering thought when you consider the level of lifetime exposure that many of us experience. Their insidious effects appear to increase with aging (Sapolsky et al., 1986). Estrogen, which ameliorates the deleterious effects of stress, decreases with age (particularly in women), which is of concern because aging brains of individuals who have endured chronic stress would be more affected by memory loss (McEwen, 2000c).

The destructive ramifications of glucocorticoids are reversible if the neurons are injured but not destroyed. As discussed in the first chapter, neurogenesis can occur in the hippocampus. Therefore, healing can occur. However, recent studies point to a decrease in the size of the hippocampus with chronic stress and a correlated inhibition of hippocampus-associated types of memory (Ohl et al., 2000). One experiment, using high-resolution techniques, showed that the number of days spent in depression corresponds to the amount of hippocampal atrophy. The study was done on formerly depressed individuals so that the affects of acute stress could be eliminated (Sheline et al., 1996). Similarly, possible links with chronic stress in certain forms of dementia, such as Alzheimer's disease, are being researched (Soloman and Morley, 2001).

> High levels of glucocorticoids from chronic stress desensitize the brain. Sometimes, especially when I am tired, I put on the news and, inevitably, hear about a disaster that is occurring. Instead of feelings of sorrow or compassion, I just feel numb. When you feel numb from hearing about devastation and you cannot respond, you are putting out a lot of cortisol. You are in a hypervigilant state. You can almost taste the anxiety. If you have experienced losing a loved one, you probably have experienced a feeling akin to having cotton wool in your head, you cannot put thoughts together, and feel dissociated from life event. That is the state that I believe corresponds to hypercortisolism.

Therefore, if you are experiencing stress, you are secreting norepinephrine, which alerts the hippocampus to be incredibly vigilant to stimuli and the recording of memories. The amygdala receives the incoming sensory information and checks in with the hippocampus to see if there is what I have termed an *engram*, that is, an engrained thought pattern, associated with a traumatic memory to which the hippocampus can respond. The amygdala is scouting around to see if there is a match. It is somewhat like doing an FBI computer search for a fingerprint. If the sensory data is close, you get a hit, and the sympathetic nervous system fastens onto the incoming information. The information locks into the amygdala and hippocampus in such a manner that you carry that engram with you until you find a way or receive help to erase it. Many individuals proceed through life accumulating engrams and, consequently, becoming generally more fearful as they age. It is my contention that engrams can be minimized, or even erased, through deep introspection or professional assistance.

When my first child was about to be born, I started acting, well, a little strange. I noticed that I was tightly gripping the car steering wheel as I drove the Washington, D.C., beltway, and I started getting feelings of impending doom. I said to myself, "I am an internal medicine resident. Hey, why am I afraid that I am going to die?" In those days, I saw myself as invincible and detached from the struggles of my patients, yet I was preoccupied with dying—from instant to instant. What was my amygdala honing in on? (Nobody knew what the amygdala did 20 years ago. Scientists thought it had something to do with angry animals because when their amygdala was taken out, they calmed down. You could even pet a lion. This is all we knew about the amygdala in those days.) What was going on? I finally broke down and spoke to a psychiatrist friend of mine: "So, Bruce, I have a young patient who is unreasonably apprehensive about dying." Knowing me well, Bruce responded, "So, what's really the matter, Lenny?" Bruce helped me into a state of deep relaxation. I recognized that my daughter's imminent birth had evoked in me a fear of fatherhood, because my father had died when I was young. I was actually programming myself to think that I was supposed to die now, because I was to become a father. With Bruce's help, I understood the connection, and it was a remarkable revelation. There was a complete erasure of that particular engram for me, and I felt calm and at peace, joyfully anticipating the birth of my daughter.

Encoded traumatic memories, or engrams, are hard to change. I see them as crystallizing, but not indelible. It is possible to erase traumatic memories or to override them with higher-ordered cognitive functions, closing the loop on the system of traumatic memory (LeDoux, 1996). Understanding how engrams form is key to resolving fears. Fear underlies a good deal of our physiological derailment. The fear may be associated with traumas that go back to a time prior to language acquisition, a time void of the ability to form contextual thoughts. Engrams frequently form during childhood. Regardless, with courage and conscious awareness, erasure of the engram and healing can occur. There are various strategies that aid this process, and they will be discussed thoroughly in the chapter on relaxation therapeutic modalities (Chapter 5). But we cannot emphasize strongly enough that each of us harbors the power and the ability to understand and dissolve our long-crystallized engrams.

APOPTOSIS

In 1972, Kerr and colleagues published the groundbreaking results of their work on a new type of cell death, which they called *apoptosis* from the Greek for "a falling off" (Kerr et al., 1972). Apoptosis is the end result of chronic stress. It is programmed cellular death, and it can be programmed death of the individual. Basically, there are two ways cells die. One is an inflammatory response, called *necrosis*, by which cells expand and essentially burst. The contents inside of the cell, such as the cytoplasm and nuclear particles, spill out into the intercellular spaces, causing inflammation. Various roving phagocytes surround the necrotic material and ingest the debris, effectively clearing it away. Although necrosis is the process of cellular death that typically occurs with injury and some inflammatory conditions, apoptosis is the most common mechanism of cell death overall.

During apoptosis, cells shrink because the chromatin condenses and fragments the cell's contents into membrane-bound particles. The nucleus involutes, and the cell implodes, instead of exploding. As with necrosis, the dead material is phagocytized. Because the cells shrink, there is no inflammation caused by intercellular deposits as occurs with necrosis. Much of what is known about apoptosis was gleaned from a nematode worm, the *Caenorhabditis elegans*, whose genetic model of apoptosis is remarkably similar to, although far less complex than, humans. The existence of apoptosis in the nematode indicates that the process has been conserved in evolution.

Apoptosis can be called a *programmed cellular death* because it is genetically determined (Hetts, 1998). Tissue-specific signals elicit protein products from a gene that researchers named the *CED-4* gene. *CED-4* activates the *CED-3* gene to instigate the process of apoptosis. Various commitment signals cause the process of apoptosis to begin, while other signals inhibit it. In other words, there are pro-death ligands, and there are anti-death ligands. Research is still being conducted on various commitment signals, but let us look at one death ligand, the Fas protein, to generally explain the process. When a cytotoxic T lymphocyte binds to an antigen, it causes the elaboration of the Fas ligand (FasL). The FasL easily binds to Fas, which is a cell-surface death receptor that is found on most cells. This interaction results in apoptosis, which in this instance would cause the death of the cell. The Fas receptor is like a smart bomb; it turns on the genetic material to initiate a cascade that commits the cell to destruction.

Glucocorticoids are known to induce apoptosis, particularly in thymocytes and activated T cells, but they also are able to rescue immune cells from apoptosis (Hetts, 1998; Planey and Litwack, 2000; Tolosa and Ashwell, 1999). Survival of activated T cells is mediated by glucocorticoid receptors, with signaling between the T cell antigen receptor and the glucocorticoid receptor (Jamieson and Yammoto, 2000). In addition, certain proteins (of the Bcl-2 family) may influence the lymphocytes to surrender to the apoptotic process or not (Huang and Cidlowski, 1999).

Importantly, apoptosis may be a crucial factor in the development of autoimmunity. If a cytotoxic T lymphocyte binds to a self-antigen, mistaking it for a foreign antigen, apoptosis ideally protects the body from such a defective T lymphocyte receptor (Hetts, 1998). However, when this process fails, autoimmunity occurs. For instance, if a viral antigen, whose DNA is similar to a normal cell, activates the Fas receptor, the normal cells then are marked for destruction. They are victims of friendly fire, which could be the basis of autoimmune thyroiditis or Hashimoto's thyroiditis.

As we have shown, there are pro-death ligands that trigger the apoptotic cascade in response to stress and other psychological factors. If someone went to a country abounding with occult rituals and had a curse placed on her or him, she or he might begin to believe that the ritualistic action could be fatal, and it might well be so. Death-ligand neuropeptides could cause the process of apoptosis to be instigated, and the individual, in a most extreme case, could die. Researchers continue to study the physiological basis of the apoptotic form of psychoneuroimmunology—or what might be called the *physiological basis of the voodoo response*. It is also called the *nocebo response* or the *negative response*.

I think that there is a physiological basis to the nocebo response that is very dramatic. I am no longer willing to try to withhold my passion regarding the way in which some doctors unwittingly program illness in their patients. I have seen it time and time again in my clinical practice. The physician says something akin to any of the following statements: "You have 6 months to live." "You have diabetes. If you don't control your blood sugar, in 2 years you're going to need an amputation." "Sorry, you have multiple sclerosis. That's a chronic disease; you're going to be in a wheelchair in about 3 months." I am concerned that some physicians do not grasp the powerful effect that their communication can have. This is an entire area of psychoneuroimmunology that warrants more study—how we communicate with our patients. Negative programming is much like implanting an emotionally destructive thought virus. I call the process "voodoo medicine." It is the antithesis of being a physician. Remember, above all, *do no harm*. Particularly with life-threatening diseases, the patients come in feeling vulnerable. In the office, they are literally physically naked, and they are emotionally naked, hanging on every word the physician says.

Are physicians doing an adequate job of helping the patient cope with the emotional aspects of their disease? This is not an issue of being willing to offer alternative or complementary medicine to a patient. It is about bringing the heart, the feeling, the caring, and the nurturing back to medicine. A physician's work ought to include trying to instill hope, while indicating that there is much that scientists just do not understand about the mystery of the healing process. Be artful, positive, a pillar of strength for your patients. Sometimes I feel like the most important thing I can do is to try to give the patient hope so that if bodily healing cannot occur, at least inner healing can.

Now, recall the story in the introduction about Steve, who got 10 years more to live. How do you explain it? It is the opposite of the nocebo response or of programmed cellular death. We can leave it to the Great Mystery. But, we also can see that this new science is beginning to explain some of these previously unknown phenomena that many physicians, if they are honest, will admit to having seen in their clinical practices. Unfortunately, because of the acculturation of physicians to be obligate scientists, we are loath to discuss these incredibly special, sanctified experiences we have with our patients. As integral medicine and the true art of healing—which is an approach to healing the whole person: the body, mind, emotions, and spirit—becomes commonly accepted, physicians will be joyfully swapping stories of patients like Steve.

LOOKING AHEAD

Stress management involves looking at our personal needs: support, intimacy, loving, caring, recreation, relaxation, joyful creativity, as well as spiritual concerns. There are many modalities that offer relaxation techniques to reduce the impact of stress. We will review some of these in Chapter 5. The topic of spiritual "needs" is very interesting because this is the latest area of research in psychoneuroimmunology. There are spiritual leaders, yogis, Tibetan monks, and such who are being studied physiologically. They are wonderful human beings, allowing themselves to be poked, probed, and measured to help us understand the physiological impact on the body of a person who lives a balanced existence. So, rather than calling these individuals the super-healthy, we might refer to them as the super-aware, evidencing the benefits of a tranquil lifestyle. We will closely examine the impact of spiritual awareness and development in the last chapters of the book. For now, we turn to learning about the relaxation system in Chapter 4.

REFERENCES

Bartrop, R.W., Luckhurst, E., Lazarus, L., Kiloh, L.G., and Penny, R., Depressed lymphocyte function after bereavement, *Lancet*, 1, 834–836, 1977.

Besedovsky, H.O. and Sorkin, E., Network of immune-neuroendocrine interactions, *Clinical Experimental Immunol.*, 27 (1), 1–12, 1977.

Besedovsky, H.O., Sorkin, E., Keller, M., and Müller, J., Changes in blood hormone levels during the immune response, *Proc. Soc. Experimental Biol. Med.*, 150 (2), 466–470, 1975.

Besedovsky, H.O., del Rey, A., and Sorkin, E., Lymphokine-containing supernatants from con A-stimulated cells increase corticosterone blood levels, *J. Immunol.*, 126 (1), 385–387, 1981.

Biondi, M., Effects of stress on immune functions: an overview, in *Psychoneuroimmunology*, 3rd ed., Ader, R., Felten, D.L., and Cohen, N., Eds., Academic Press, New York, 2001, pp. 189–226.

Birnbaum, S., Gobeske, K.T., Auerbach, J., Taylor, J.R., and Arnsten, A.F., A role for norepinephrine in stress-induced cognitive deficits: alpha-1-adrenoreceptor mediation in the prefrontal cortex, *Biological Psychiatry*, 46 (9), 1266–1274, 1999.

Blake-Mortimer, J., Gore-Felton, C., Kimmerling, J.M., Turner-Cobb, J.M., and Spiegel, D., Improving the quality and quantity of life among patients with cancer: a review of the effectiveness of group psychotherapy, *Eur. J. Cancer*, 35 (11), 1581–1586, 1999.

Bloom, J.R. and Spiegel, D., The relationship of two dimensions of social support to the psychological well-being and social functioning of women with advanced breast cancer, *Soc. Sci. Med.*, 19 (8), 831–837, 1984.

Bornstein, S.R. and Chrousos, G.P., Adrenocorticotropin (ACTH)- and non-ACTH-mediated regulation of the adrenal cortex: neural and immune inputs, *J. Clinical Endocrinol. Metab.*, 84 (5), 1729–1736, 1999.

Bornstein, S.R. and Ehrhart-Bornstein, M., Basic and clinical aspects of intraadrenal regulation of steroidogenesis, *Zeitschrift Rheumatologie*, 59 (2), 12–17, 2000.

Bornstein, S.R., Ehrhart-Bornstein, M., and Scherbaum, W.A., Morphological and functional studies of the paracrine interaction between cortex and medulla in the adrenal gland, *Microsc. Res. Tech.*, 36 (6), 520–533, 1997.

Bornstein, S.R. et al., Chronic effects of nonpeptide corticotropin-releasing hormone type I receptor antagonist on pituitary–adrenal function, body weight, and metabolic regulation, *Endocrinology*, 139 (4), 1546–1555, 1998.

Butler, L.D., Koopman, C., Classen, C., and Spiegel, D., Traumatic stress, life events, and emotional support in women with metastatic breast cancer: cancer-related traumatic stress symptoms associated with past and current stressors, *Health Psychol.: Off J. Div. Health Psychol., Am. Psychological Assoc.*, 18 (6), 555–560, 1999.

Calabrese, J.R., Kling, M.A., and Gold, P.W., Alterations in immunocompetence during stress, bereavement, and depression: focus on neuroendocrine regulation, *Am. J. Psychiatry*, 144 (9), 1123–1134, 1987.

Calogero, A.E., Gallucci, W.T., Gold, P.W., and Chrousos, G.P., Multiple feedback regulatory loops upon rat hypothalamic corticotropin-releasing hormone secretion, *J. Clinical Invest.*, 82 (3), 767–774, 1988.

Cannon, W.B., Emergency function of the adrenal medulla in pain and major emotions, *Am. J. Physiol.*, 3, 356–372, 1914.

Carr, D.J. and Blalock, J.E., Corticotropin-releasing hormone enhances murine natural killer cell activity through an opioid-mediated pathway, in Neuropeptides and Immunopeptides: Messengers in a Neuroimmune Axis, *Annals of the New York Academy of Sciences*, Vol. 594, O'Dorisio, M.S. and Panerai, A.E., Eds., New York Academy of Sciences, New York, 1990, pp. 371–373.

Chrousos, G.P., Stress, stressors, and neuroendocrine integration of the adaptive response, The 1997 Hans Selye Memorial Lecture, in Stress of Life from Molecules to Man, *Annals of the New York Academy of Sciences*, Vol. 851, Csermely, P., Ed., New York Academy of Sciences, New York, 1998, pp. 311–335.

Chrousos, G.P., Reproductive placental corticotropin-releasing hormone and its clinical implications, *Am. J. Obstet. Gynecol.*, 180 (1), S249–S250, 1999.

Chrousos, G.P., The role of stress and the hypothalamic-pituitary-adrenal axis in the pathogenesis of the metabolic syndrome: neuro-endocrine and target-tissue related causes, *Int. J. Obesity Related Metabolic Disorders*, 24 (S2), S50–S55, 2000.

Chrousos, G.P. and Gold, P.W., The concept of stress and stress system disorders, overview of physical and behavioral homeostasis, *J. Am. Medical Assoc.*, 267 (9), 1244–1252, 1992.

Cohen, S. and Miller, G.E., Stress, immunity, and susceptibility to upper respiratory infection, in *Psychoneuroimmunology*, 3rd ed., Ader, R., Felten, D.L., and Cohen, N., Eds., Academic Press, New York, 2001, pp. 499–509.

Cohen, S., Tyrrell, D.A.J., and Smith, A.P., Psychological stress and susceptibility to the common cold, *New England J. Med.*, 325 (9), 606–612, 1991.

Courtney, J.G., Longnecker, M.P., Theorell, T., and Gerhardsson de Verdier, M., Stressful life events and the risk of colorectal cancer, *Epidemiology*, 4 (5), 407–414, 1993.

Cox, W.I., Holbrook, N.J., and Friedman, H., Mechanisms of glucocorticoid action on murine natural killer cell activity, *J. Natl. Cancer Inst.*, 71 (5), 973–981, 1983.

Cunningham, Jr., E.T., Bohn, M.C., and Sawchenko, L.W., Organization of adrenergic inputs to the paraventricular and supraoptic nuclei of the rat hypothalamus, *J. Comp. Neurol.*, 292 (4), 651–667, 1990.

Deckard, G., Meterko, M., and Field, D., Physician burnout: an examination of personal, professional, and organizational relationships, *Medical Care*, 32 (7), 745–754, 1994.

Dhabhar, F.S. and McEwen, B.S., Stress-induced enhancement of antigen-specific cell-mediated immunity, *J. Immunol.*, 156 (7), 2608–2615, 1996.

Dhabhar, F.S. and McEwen, B.S., Acute stress enhances while chronic stress suppresses cell-mediated immunity *in vivo*: a potential role for leukocyte trafficking, *Brain, Behav., Immunol.*, 11 (4), 286–306, 1997.

Dhabhar, F.S. and McEwen, B.S., Enhancing versus suppressive effects of stress hormones on skin immune function, *Proc. Natl. Acad. Sci. U.S.A.*, 96, 1059–1064, 1999.

Dhabhar, F.S., Miller, A.H., McEwen, B.S., and Spencer, R.L., Stress-induced changes in blood leukocyte distribution: role of adrenal steroid hormones, *J. Immunol.*, 157 (4), 1638–1644, 1996.

Dhabhar, F.S., Satoskar, A., Bluethmann, H., David, J.R., and McEwen, B.S., Stress-induced enhancement of skin immune function: a role for γ interferon, *Proc. Natl. Acad. Sci. U.S.A.*, 97 (6), 2846–2851, 2000.

Dunn, A.J. and Berridge, C.W., Is corticotropin-releasing factor a mediator of stress response? in A Decade of Neuropeptides: Past, Present, and Future, *Annals of The New York Academy of Sciences*, Vol. 597, Koob, G.F., Sandman, C.A., and Strand, F.L., Eds., New York Academy of Sciences, New York, 1990, pp. 183–191.

Ehrhart-Bornstein, M., Hinson, J.P., Bornstein, S.R., Scherbaum, W.A., and Vinson, G.P., Intraadrenal interactions in the regulation of adrenocortical steroidogenesis, *Endocrine Rev.*, 19 (2), 101–143, 1998; published erratum, *Endocrine Rev.*, 19 (3), 301, 1998.

Ekman, P., Levenson, R.W., and Friesen, W.V., Autonomic nervous system activity distinguishes among emotions, *Science*, 221 (4616), 1208–2110, 1983.

Eliot, R.S., *From Stress to Strength?* Bantam Books, New York, 1994.

Eliot, R.S. and Breo, D.L., *Is It Worth Dying For?* Bantam Books, New York, 1989.

Elkabir, D.R., Wyatt, M.E., Vellucci, S.V., and Herbert, J., The effects of separate or combined infusions of corticotrophin-releasing hormone and vasopressin either intraventricularly or into the amygdala on aggressive and investigative behavior in the rat, *Regulatory Peptides*, 28 (2), 199–214, 1990.

Everson, S.A., Kaplan, G.A., Goldberg, D.E., and Salonen, J.T., Hypertension incident is predicted by high levels of hopelessness in Finnish men, *Hypertension*, 35 (2), 561–567, 2000.

Ferry, B., Roozendaal, B., and McGaugh, J.L., Role of epinephrine in mediating stress hormone regulation of long-term memory storage: a critical involvement of the amygdala, *Biological Psychiatry*, 46 (9), 1140–1152, 1999.

Fleshner, M., Nguyen, K.T., Cotter, C.S., Watkins, L.R., and Maier, S.F., Acute stressor exposure both suppresses acquired immunity and potentiates innate immunity, *Am. J. Physiol.*, 275, R870–R878, 1998.

Frasure-Smith, N., Lespérance, F., and Talajic, M., Depression following myocardial infarction, *J. Am. Medical Assoc.*, 270 (15), 1819–1825, 1993.

Friedman, H., Klein, T.W., and Friedman, A.L., *Psychoneuroimmunology, Stress, and Infection*, CRC Press, Boca Raton, FL, 1996.

Ghizzoni, L., Vottero, A., Street, M.E., and Berasconi, S., Dose-dependent inhibition of growth hormone (GH)-releasing hormone-induced GH release by corticotropin-releasing hormone in prepubertal children, *J. Clinical Endocrinol. Metab.*, 81 (4), 1397–1400, 1996.

Girard, M.T., Hjaltadottir, S., Fejes-Toth, A.N., and Guyre, P.M., Glucocorticoids enhance the gamma-interferon augmentation of human monocyte immunoglobulin G Fc receptor expression, *J. Immunol.*, 138 (10), 3235–3241, 1987.

Glaser, R., and Kiecolt-Glaser, J.K., *Handbook of Human Stress and Immunity*, Academic Press, San Diego, 1994.

Gold, P.W. et al., Corticotropin-releasing hormone: relevance to normal physiology and to the pathophysiology and differential diagnosis of hypercortisolism and adrenal insufficiency, *Adv. Biochemical Psychopharmacol.*, 43, 183–200, 1987.

Gruber, B.L., Hersh, S.P., Hall, N.R., Waletzky, L.R., Kunz, J.F., Carpenter, J.K., Kverno, K.S., and Weiss, S.M., Immunological responses of breast cancer patients to behavioral interventions, *Biofeedback Self Regulation*, 18 (21), 1–22, 1993.

Guyre, P.M., Girard, M.T., Morganelli, P.M., and Manganiello, P.D., Glucocorticoid effects on the production and actions of immune cytokines, *J. Steroid Biochem.*, 30 (1–6), 89–93, 1988.

Habib, K.E. et al., Oral administration of a corticotropin-releasing hormone receptor antagonist significantly attenuates behavioral, neuroendocrine, and autonomic responses to stress in primates, *Proc. Natl. Acad. Sci. U.S.A.*, 97 (11), 6079–6084, 2000.

Haidan, A., Bornstein, S.R., Glasow, A., Uhlmann, K., Lubke, C., and Ehrhart-Bornstein, M., Basal steroidogenic activity of adrenocortical cells is increased 10-fold by coculture with chromaffin, *Endocrinology*, 139 (2), 772–780, 1998.

Haidan, A., Bornstein, S.R., Liu, Z., Walsh, L.P., Stocco, D.M., and Ehrhart-Bornstein, M., Expression of adrenocortical steroidogenic acute regulatory (StAR) protein is influenced by chromaffin, *Molecular Cellular Endocrinol.*, 165 (1–2), 25–32, 2000.

Hench, P.S., Kendall, E.C., Slocumb, C.H., and Polley, H.F., The effect of a hormone of the adrenal cortex (17-hydroxycorticosterone: compound E) and of pituitary adrenocorticotropic hormone on rheumatoid arthritis, *Mayo Clinic Proc.*, 24, 181, 1949.

Hetts, S.W., To die or not to die: an overview of apoptosis and its role in disease, *J. Am. Medical Assoc.*, 279 (4), 300–307, 1998.

Holbrook, N.J., Cox, W.I., and Horner, H.C., Direct suppression of natural killer cell activity in human peripheral blood leukocyte cultures by glucocorticoids and its modulation by interferon, *Cancer Res.*, 43 (9), 4019–4025, 1983.

Huang, S.T. and Cidlowski, J.A., Glucocorticoids inhibit serum depletion-induced apoptosis in T lymphocytes expressing Bcl-2, *FASEB J.*, 13 (3), 467–476, 1999.

Ilyinsky, O.B., Surkina, I.D., Gotovtseva, E.P., Shchurin, M.R., and Zozulya, A.A., Immune and opioid systems in stress: participation in healing process, in Neuropeptides and Immunopeptides: Messengers in a Neuroimmune Axis, *Annals of the New York Academy of Sciences*, Vol. 594, O'Dorisio, M.S. and Panerai, A.E., Eds., New York Academy of Sciences, New York, 1990, pp. 461–462.

Jackson, D.C., Malmstadt, J.R., Larson, C.L., and Davidson, R.J., Suppression and enhancement of emotional responses to unpleasant pictures, *Psychophysiology*, 37 (4), 515–522, 2000.

Jamieson, C. and Yammoto, K.R., Crosstalk pathway for inhibition of glucocorticoid-induced apoptosis by T cell receptor signaling, *Proc. Natl. Acad. Sci. U.S.A.*, 97 (13), 7319–7324, 2000.

Januzzi, J.L., Stern, T.A., Pasternak, R.C., and DeSanctis, R.W., The influence of anxiety and depression on outcomes of patients with coronary artery disease, *Arch. Intern. Med.*, 160, 1913–1921, 2000.

Jiang, W. et al., Mental stress—induced myocardial ischemia and cardiac events, *J. Am. Medical Assoc.*, 275 (21), 1651–1656, 1996.

Kavelaars, A., Ballieux, R.E., and Heijnen, C.J., Interaction between corticotropin-releasing hormone and interleukin-1 in the immune system, in Neuropeptides and Immunopeptides: Messengers in a Neuroimmune Axis, *Annals of the New York Academy of Sciences*, Vol. 594, O'Dorisio, M.S. and Panerai, A.E., Eds., New York Academy of Sciences, New York, 1990, pp. 368–370.

Keller, S.E., Schleifer, S.J., and Demetrikopoulos, M.K., in *Psychoneuroimmunology*, 2nd ed., Ader, R., Felten, D.L., and Cohen, N., Eds., Academic Press, New York, 1991, pp. 771–787.

Kerr, J.F., Wyllie, A.R., and Currie, A.R., Apoptosis: a basic biological phenomenon with wide-ranging implications in tissue kinetics, *Br. J. Cancer*, 26 (4), 239–257, 1972.

Khansari, D.N., Murgo, A.J., and Faith, R.E., Effects of stress on the immune system, *Immunol. Today*, 11, 170–175, 1990.

Kiecolt-Glaser, J.K. and Glaser, R., Stress and immune function in humans, in *Psychoneuroimmunology*, 2nd ed., Ader, R., Felten, D.L., and Cohen, N., Eds., Academic Press, New York, 1991, pp. 849–867.

Kiecolt-Glaser, J.K. and Glaser, R., Chronic stress and mortality among older adults, *J. Am. Medical Assoc.*, 282 (23), 2259–2260, 1999.

Kiecolt-Glaser, J.K., Gardner, W., Speicher, C., Penn, G.M., Holliday, J., Glaser, R., Psychosocial modifiers of immunocompetence in medical students, *Psychosomatic Med.*, 46 (1), 7–14, 1984.

Kiecolt-Glaser, J.K., Fisher, L.D., Ogrocki, P., Stout, J.C., Speicher, C.E., and Glaser, R., Marital quality, marital disruption, and immune function, *Psychosomatic Medicine*, 49 (1). 13–34, 1987.

Kiecolt-Glaser, J.K., Kennedy, S., Malkoff, S., Fisher, L., Speicher, C.E., and Glaser, R., Marital discord and immunity in males, *Psychosomatic Med.*, 50 (3), 213–229, 1988.

Kiecolt-Glaser, J.K., Marucha, P.T., Malarkey, W.B., Mercado, A.M., and Glaser, R., Slowing of wound healing by psychological stress, *Lancet*, 346 (8984), 1194–1196, 1995.

Kiecolt-Glaser, J.K., Preacher, K.J., MacCallum, R.C., Atkinson, C., Malarkey, W.B., and Glaser, R., Chronic stress and age-related increases in the proinflammatory cytokine IL-6, *Proc. Natl. Acad. Sci. U.S.A.*, 100 (15), 9090–9095, 2003.

Kiss, A. and Aguilera, G., Participation of alpha-1-adrenergic receptors in the secretion of hypothalamic corticotropin-releasing hormone during stress, *Neuroendocrinology*, 56 (2), 153–160, 1992.

Kiss, A. and Aguilera, G., Role of alpha-1-adrenergic receptors in the regulation of corticotropin-releasing hormone mRNA in the paraventricular nucleus of the hypothalamus during stress, *Cell. Molecular Neurobiol.*, 20 (6), 683–694, 2000.

Kobasa, S.C., Stressful life events, personality, and health: an inquiry into hardiness, *J. Personality Social Psychol.*, 37 (1), 1–11, 1979.

Kobasa, S.C., Effectiveness of hardiness, exercise and social support as resources against illness, *J. Psychosomatic Res.*, 45 (4), 839–850, 1983.

Kobasa, S.C., Personality and social resources in stress resistance, *J. Personality Social Psychol.*, 29 (5), 525–533, 1985.

Kogon, M.M., Biswas, A., Pearl, D., Carlson, R.W., and Spiegel, D., Effects of medical and psychotherapeutic treatment on the survival of women with metastatic breast carcinoma, *Cancer*, 80 (2), 225–230, 1997.

Koopman, C., Hermanson, K., Diamond, S., Angell, K., and Spiegel, D., Social support, life stress, pain and emotional adjustment to advanced breast cancer, *Psychooncology*, 7 (2), 101–111, 1998.

Kop, W.J. et al., Effects of mental stress on coronary epicardial vasomotion and flow velocity in coronary artery disease: relationship with hemodynamic stress responses, *J. Am. Coll. Cardiol.*, 37 (5), 1359–1366, 2001.

Krantz, D.S., Santiago, H.T., Kop, W.J., Bairey Merz, C.N., Rozanski, A., and Gottdiener, J.S., Prognostic value of mental stress testing in coronary artery disease, *Am. J. Cardiol.*, 84 (11), 1292–1297, 1999.

Krantz, D.S., Sheps, D.S., Carney, R.M., and Natelson, B.H., Effects of mental stress in patients with coronary artery disease, *J. Am. Medical Assoc.*, 283 (14), 1800–1802, 2000.

Kumlin, L. et al., Marital status and cardiovascular risk in French and Swedish automotive industry workers—cross sectional results from the Renault–Volvo Coeur study, *J. Intern. Med.*, 249 (4), 315–323, 2001.

Lacey, K., Zaharia, M.D., Griffiths, J., Ravindran, A.V., Merali, Z., and Anisman, H., A prospective study of neuroendocrine and immune alterations associated with the stress of an oral academic examination among graduate students, *Psychoneuroendocrinology*, 25 (4), 339–356, 2000.

Ladwig, K.H., Röll, G., Breithardt, G., Budde, T., and Borggrefe, M., Post-infarction depression and incomplete recovery 6 months after acute myocardial infarction, *Lancet*, 343, 20–23, 1994.

LeDoux, J.E., Emotion, memory and the brain, *Sci. Am.*, (June), 50–57, 1994.

LeDoux, J.E., *The Emotional Brain*, Simon & Schuster, New York, 1996.

Levav, I., Kohn, R., Iscovich, J., Abramson, J.H., Tsai, W.Y., and Vigdorovich, D., Cancer incidence and survival following bereavement, *Am. J. Public Health*, 90 (10), 1601–1607, 2000.

Levin, J., *God, Faith, and Heal: Exploring the Spirituality–Health Connection*, John Wiley & Sons, New York, 2001.

Lupien, S.J. et al., Cortisol levels during human aging predict hippocampal atrophy and memory deficits, *Nat. Neurosci.*, 1 (1), 69–73, 1998.

Markovitz, J.H. and Matthews, K.A., Platelets and coronary heart disease: potential psychophysiologic mechanisms, *Psychosomatic Med.*, 53, 643–668, 1991.

Marucha, P.T., Sheridan, J.F., and Padgett, D., Stress and wound healing, in *Psychoneuroimmunology*, 3rd ed., Ader, R., Felten, D.L., and Cohen, N., Eds., Academic Press, New York, 2001, pp. 613–626.

McClelland, D.C., Ross, G., and Patel, V., The effect of an academic examination on salivary norepinephrine and immunoglobulin levels, *J. Hum. Stress*, 11 (2), 52–59, 1985.

McDonald, T.J. and Nathanielsz, P.W., The involvement of innervation in the regulation of fetal adrenal steroidogenesis, *Horm. Metabolic Res.*, 30 (6–7), 297–302, 1998.

McEwen, B.S., Protective and damaging effects of stress mediators, *New England J. Med.*, 338 (3), 171–179, 1998.

McEwen, B.S., Effects of adverse experiences for brain structure and function, *Biological Psychiatry*, 48 (4), 721–731, 2000a.

McEwen, B.S., The neurobiology of stress: from serendipity to clinical relevance, *Brain Res.*, 886 (1–2), 172–189, 2000b.

McEwen, B.S., Allostasis, allostatic load, and the aging nervous system: role of excitatory amino acids and excitotoxicity, *Neurochemical Res.*, 25 (9–10), 1219–1231, 2000c.

McEwen, B.S., Allostasis and allostatic load: implications for neuropsychopharmacology, *Neuropsychopharmacology*, 22 (2),108–124, 2000d.

McEwen, B.S. and Stellar, E., Stress and the individual: mechanisms leading to disease, *Arch. Intern. Med.*, 153 (18), 2093–2101, 1993.

McMurray, J.E., Linzer, M., Konrad, T.R., Douglas, J., Shugerman, R., and Nelson, K., The work lives of women physicians results from the physician work life study: the SGIM Career Satisfaction Study Group, *J. Gen. Intern. Med.*, 15 (6), 372–380, 2000.

Meier, D.E., Back, A.L., and Morrison, R.S., The inner life of physicians and care of the seriously ill, *J. Am. Medical Assoc.*, 286 (23), 3007–3014, 2001.

Moller, J., Hallqvist, J., Diderichsen, F., Theorell, T., Reuterwall, C., and Ahlbom, A., Do episodes of anger trigger myocardial infarction? A case-crossover analysis in the Stockholm Heart Epidemiology Program (SHEEP), *Psychosomatic Med.*, 61 (6), 842–849, 1999.

Morganelli, P.M. and Guyre, P.M., IFN-gamma plus glucocorticoids stimulate the expression of a newly identified human phagocyte antigen, *J. Immunol.*, 140 (7), 2296–2304, 1988.

Moynihan, J.A. and Stevens, S.Y., Mechanisms of stress-induced modulation of immunity in animals, in *Psychoneuroimmunology*, 3rd ed., Ader, R., Felten, D.L., and Cohen, N., Eds., Academic Press, New York, 2001, pp. 227–249.

Munck, A. and Guyre, P.M., Glucocorticoids and immune function, in *Psychoneuroimmunology*, 2nd ed., Ader, R., Felten, D.L., and Cohen, N., Eds., Academic Press, New York, 1991, pp. 447–474.

Munck, A., Guyre, P.M., and Holbrook, N.J., Physiological functions of glucocorticoids in stress and their relation to pharmacological actions, *Endocrine Rev.*, 5 (1), 25–44, 1984.

Neunan, J.C. and Hubbard, J.R., Stress in the workplace: an overview, in *Stress Medicine, an Organ System Approach*, Neunan, J.C. and Workman, E.A., Eds., CRC Press, Boca Raton, FL, 1998, pp. 232–236.

O'Connor, C.M., Gurbel, P.A., and Serebruany, V.L., Depression and ischemic heart disease, *Am. Heart J.*, 140 (4 suppl.), 63–69, 2000.

Ohl, F., Michaelis, T., Vollmann-Honsdorf, G.K., Kirschbaum, C., and Fuchs, E., Effect of chronic psychosocial stress and long-term cortisol treatment on hippocampus-mediated memory and hippocampal volume: a pilot study in tree shrews, *Psychoneuroendocrinology*, 25 (4), 357–363, 2000.

Orth-Gomer, K., Wamala, S.P., Horsten, M., Schenck-Gustafsson, K., Schneiderman, N., and Mittleman, M.A., *J. Am. Medical Assoc.*, 284 (23), 3008–3014, 2000.

Oya, H. et al., The differential effect of stress on natural killer T (NKT) and NK cell function, *Clinical Experimental Immunol.*, 121 (2),384–390, 2000.

Pacak, K., Stressor-specific activation of the hypothalamic–pituitary–adrenocortical axis, *Physiological Res.*, 49 (S10), S11–S17, 2000.

Pacak, K., Palkovits, M., Kopin, I.J., and Goldstein, D.S., Stress-induced norepinephrine release in the hypothalamic paraventricular nucleus and pituitary–adrenocortical axis and sympathoadrenal activity: *in vivo* microdialysis studies, *Frontiers Neuroendocrinol.*, 16 (2), 89–150, 1995.

Panerai, A.E., Sacerdote, P., Bianchi, M., and Manfredi, B., Intermittent but not continuous footshock stress and intracerebroventricular interleukin-1 similarly affect immune responses and immunocyte beta-endorphin concentrations in the rat, *Int. J. Clinical Pharmacological Res.*, 17 (2–3), 115–116, 1997.

Papanicolaou, D.A., Wilder, R.L., Manolagas, S.C., and Chrousos, G.P., The pathophysiologic roles of interleukin-6 in human disease, *Ann. Intern. Med.*, 128 (2), 127–137, 1998.

Päth, G., Bornstein, S.R., Ehrhart-Bornstein, M., and Scherbaum, W.A., Interleukin-6 and interleukin-6 receptor in the human adrenal gland: expression and effects on steroidogenesis, *J. Clinical Endocrinol. Metab.*, 82 (7), 2343–2349, 1997.

Pignatelli, D., Magalhaes, M.M., and Magalhaes, M.C., Direct effects of stress on adrenocortical function, *Horm. Metabolic Res.*, 30 (6–7), 464–474, 1998.

Planey, S.L. and Litwack, G., Glucocorticoid-induced apoptosis in lymphocytes, *Biochemical Biophysical Res. Commun.*, 279 (2), 307–312, 2000.

Quirarte, G.L., Roozendaal, B., and McGaugh, J.L., Glucocorticoid enhancement of memory storage involves noradrenergic activation in the basolateral amygdala, *Proc. Natl. Acad. Sci. U.S.A.*, 94 (25), 14048–14053, 1997.

Ramirez, A.J., Craig, T.K., Watson, J.P., Fentiman, I.S., North, W.R., and Rubens, R.D., Stress and relapse of cancer, *Br. Medical J.*, 298 (6669), 291–293, 1989.

Rinehart, J.J., Sagone, A.L., Balcerzak, S.P., Ackerman, G.A., and LoBuglio, A.F., Effects of corticosteroid therapy on human monocyte function, *New England J. Med.*, 292 (5), 236–241, 1975.

Rittmaster, R.S., Cutler, Jr., G.B., Brandon, D.D., Gold, P.W., Loriaux, D.L., and Chrousos, G.P., The effects of endogenous vasopressin on ACTH and cortisol secretion in man, *J. Clinical Endocrinol. Metab.*, 64 (2), 371–376, 1987.

Rosch, P.J., Stress and cancer: disorders of communication, control, and civilization, in *Handbook of Stress, Medicine, and Health*, Cooper, C.L., Ed., CRC Press, Boca Raton, FL, 1996, pp. 27–60.

Rozanski, A. et al., Mental stress and the induction of silent myocardial ischemia in patients with coronary artery disease, *New England J. Med.*, 318 (16), 1005–1012, 1988.

Saffran, M. and Schaly, A.V., The release of corticotropin by the anterior pituitary tissue *in vivo*, *Can. J. Biochemistry Physiol.*, 33, 408–415, 1955.

Sapolsky, R.M., Stress in the wild, *Sci. Am.*, (Jan.), 116–123, 1990.

Sapolsky, R.M., *Why Zebras Don't Get Ulcers: a Guide to Stress, Stress-Related Diseases, and Coping*, W.H. Freeman and Co., New York, 1994, p. 36.

Sapolsky, R.M., Krey, L., and McEwen, B.S., The neuroendocrinology of aging: the gluco-corticoid cascade hypothesis, *Endocrine Rev.*, 7 (3), 284–301, 1986.

Schaefer, C., Quesenberry, C.P., and Wi, S., Mortality following conjugal bereavement and the effects of a shared environment, *Am. J. Epidemiol.*, 141 (12), 1177–1178, 1995.

Schaffer, J.W., Duszynski, K.R., and Thomas, C.B., Youthful habits of work and recreation and later cancer among physicians, *J. Clinical Psychol.*, 38 (4), 893–900, 1982a.

Schaffer, J.W., Duszynski, K.R., and Thomas, C.B., Family attitudes in youth as possible precursor of cancer among physicians: a search for explanatory mechanisms, *J. Behav. Med.*, 5 (2), 143–163, 1982b.

Schleifer, S.J., Keller, S.E., Camerino, M., Thornton, J.C., and Stein, M., Suppression of lymphocyte stimulation following bereavement, *J. Am. Medical Assoc.*, 250 (3), 374–377, 1983.

Schrock, D., Palmer, R.F., and Taylor, B., Effects of psychosocial intervention on survival among patients with stage I breast and prostate cancer: a matched case-control study, *Alternative Therapies*, 5 (3), 49–55, 1999.

Selye, H., Effect of ACTH and cortisone on an "anaphylactoid reaction," *Can. Medical Assoc. J.*, 61, 553–556, 1949.

Selye, H., Stress and disease, *Science*, 122, 625–631, 1955.

Shavit, Y., Stress, opioid peptides, and immunity, in *Psychoneuroimmunology*, 2nd ed., Ader, R., Felten, D.L., and Cohen, N., Eds., Academic Press, New York, 1991, pp. 789–806.

Shavit, Y., Terman, G.W., Martin, F.C., Lewis, J.W., Liebeskind, J.C., and Gale, R.P., Stress, opioid peptides, the immunity system, and cancer, *J. Immunol.*, 135 (2), 834S–837S, 1985.

Sheline, Y.I., Wang, P.W., Gado, M.H., and Csernansky, J.G., Hippocampal atrophy in recur-rent major depression, *Proc. Natl. Acad. Sci. U.S.A.*, 93, 3908–3913, 1996.

Smith, E.M., Harbour-McMenamin, D., and Blalock, J.E., Lymphocyte production of endor-phins and endorphin-mediated immunoregulatory activity, *J. Immunol.*, 135 (2), 779S–782S, 1985.

Soloman, G.F. and Benton, D., Psychoneuroimmunologic aspects of aging, in *Handbook of Human Stress and Immunity*, Glaser, R. and Kiecolt-Glaser, J.K., Eds., Academic Press, San Diego, 1994, pp. 341–363.

Soloman, G.F. and Morley, J.E., Psychoneuroimmunology and aging, in *Psychoneuroimmu-nology*, 3rd ed., Ader, R., Felten, D.L., and Cohen, N., Eds., Academic Press, New York, 2001, pp. 710–711.

Spiegel, D., Bloom, J.R., Kraemer, H.C., and Gottheil, E., Effect of psychosocial treatment on survival of patients with metastatic breast cancer, *Lancet*, 2 (8668), 888–89, 1989.

Spiegel, D., Psychosocial aspects of breast cancer treatment, *Semin. Oncol.*, 24 (suppl. 1), S1/36–S1/47, 1997.

Spiegel, D., Healing words: emotional expression and disease outcome, *J. Am. Medical Assoc.*, 281 (14), 1328–1329, 1999.

Spiegel, D., Cancer, in *Encyclopedia of Stress*, Vol. 1, Fink, G., Ed., Academic Press, San Diego, CA, 2000, pp. 368–376.

Spiegel, D. et al., Group psychotherapy for recently diagnosed breast cancer patients: a multicenter feasibility study, *Psychooncology*, 8 (6), 482–493, 1999.

Taylor, A.L. and Fishman, L.M., Corticotropin-releasing hormone, *New England J. Med.*, 319 (4), 213–222, 1988.

Taylor, S.E., Klein, L.C., Lewis, B.P., Gruenewald, T.L., Gurung, R.A., and Updegraff, J.A.,
    Biobehavioral responses to stress in females: tend-and-befriend, not fight-or-flight,
    Psychological Rev., 107 (3), 411–429, 2000.
Thomas, C.B. and McCabe, O.L., Precursors of premature disease and death: habits of nervous
    tension, *Johns Hopkins Medical J.*, 147 (4), 137–145, 1980.
Thomas, C.B., Duszynski, K.R., and Schaffer, J.W., Family attitudes reported in youth as
    potential predictors of cancer, *Psychosomatic Med.*, 41 (4), 287–302, 1979.
Tolosa, E. and Ashwell, J.D., Thymus-derived glucocorticoids and the regulation of antigen-
    specific T-cell development, *Neuroimmunomodulation*, 6 (1–2),90–96, 1999.
Turner-Cobb, J.M., Sephton, S.E., Koopman, C., Blake-Mortimer, J., and Spiegel, D., Social
    support and salivary cortisol in women with metastatic breast cancer, *Psychosomatic
    Med.*, 62 (3), 337–345, 2000.
Turner-Cobb, J.M., Sephton, S.E., and Spiegel, D., Psychosocial effects on immune function
    and disease progression in cancer: human studies, in *Psychoneuroimmunology*, 3rd
    ed., Ader, R., Felten, D.L., and Cohen, N., Eds., Academic Press, New York, 2001,
    pp. 565–582.
Vacchio, M.S., Ashwell, J.D., and King, L.B., A positive role for thymus-derived steroids in
    formation of the T-cell repertoire, in Neuroimmunomodulation Molecular Aspects,
    Integrative Systems, and Clinical Advances, *Annals of the New York Academy of
    Sciences*, Vol. 840, McCann, S.M., Sternberg, E.M., Lipton, J.M., Chrousos, G.P.,
    Gold, P.W., and Smith, C.G., Eds., New York Academy of Sciences, New York, 1998,
    pp. 317–327.
Vale, W., Spiess, J., Rivier, C., and Rivier, J., Characterization of a 41-residue ovine hypo-
    thalamic peptide that stimulates secretion of corticotropin and beta-endorphin, *Sci-
    ence*, 213 (4514), 1394–1397, 1981.
Watson, M., Haviland, J.S., Greer, S., Davidson, J., and Bliss, J.M., Influence of psychological
    response on survival in breast cancer: a population-based cohort study, *Lancet*, 354
    (9187), 1331–1336, 1999.
Webster, E.L., Torpy, D.J., Elenkov, I.J., and Chrousos, G.P., Corticotropin-releasing hormone
    and inflammation, in Neuroimmunomodulation Molecular Aspects, Integrative Sys-
    tems, and Clinical Advances, *Annals of the New York Academy of Sciences*, Vol. 840,
    McCann, S.M., Sternberg, E.M., Lipton, J.M., Chrousos, G.P., Gold, P.W., and Smith,
    C.G., Eds., New York Academy of Sciences, New York, 1998, pp. 21–32.
Weiss, J.M., Psychological factors in stress and disease, *Sci. Am.*, 226 (6), 104–113, 1972.
Weiss, J.M. and Simson, P.E., Neurochemical and electrophysical events underlying stress-
    induced depression in an animal model, *Adv. Experimental Med. Biol.*, 245, 425–440,
    1988.
Wolf, S., Predictors of myocardial infarction over a span of 30 years in Roseto, Pennsylvania,
    Integrative Physiological Behavioral Sci., 27 (3), 246–257, 1992.
Wong, M.L. et al., Pronounced and sustained central hypernoradrenergic function in major
    depression with melancholic features: relation to hypercortisolism and corticotropin-
    releasing hormone, *Proc. Natl. Acad. Sci. U.S.A.*, 97 (1), 325–330, 2000.
Yehuda, R., Biology of posttraumatic stress disorder, *J. Clinical Psychiatry*, 61 (Suppl. 7),
    14–21, 2000.
Yeung, A.C. et al., The effect of atherosclerosis on the vasomotor response of coronary arteries
    to mental stress, *New England J. Med.*, 325 (21), 1551–1556, 1991.

ADDITIONAL RESOURCES

Anda, R.F., Williamson, D.F., Escobedo, L.G., Remington, P.L., Mast, E.E., and Madans, J.H., Self-perceived stress and the risk of peptic ulcer disease, *Arch. Intern. Med.*, 152, 829–833, 1992.

Arnsten, A.F., Mathew, R., Ubriani, R., Taylor, J.R., and Li, B.M., Alpha-1 noradrenergic receptor stimulation impairs prefrontal cortical cognitive function, *Biological Psychiatry*, 45 (1), 26–31, 1999.

Bassett, J. R. and West, S.H., Vascularization of the adrenal cortex: its possible involvement in the regulation of steroid hormone release, *Microsc. Res. Tech.*, 36 (6), 546–557, 1997.

Besedovsky, H.O., del Rey, A., Sorkin, E., Da Prada, M., and Keller, H.H., Immunoregulation mediated by the sympathetic nervous system, *Cell. Immunol.*, 48 (2), 346–355, 1979.

Bonneau, R.H., Experimental approaches to identify mechanisms of stress-induced modulation of immunity to herpes simplex infection, in *Handbook of Human Stress and Immunity*, Glaser, R. and Kiecolt-Glaser, J.K., Academic Press, San Diego, 1994, pp. 125–160.

Chikanza, I.C., Petrou, P., Kingsley, G., Chrousos, G., and Panayi, G.S., Defective hypothalamic response to immune and inflammatory stimuli in patients with rheumatoid arthritis, *Arthritis Rheumatism*, 35 (11), 1281–1288, 1992.

Chikanza, I.C., Petrou, P., Chrousos, G., Kingsley, G., and Panayi, G.S., Excessive and dysregulated secretion of prolactin in rheumatoid arthritis: immunopathogenetic and therapeutic implications, *Br. J. Rheumatol.*, 32 (6), 445–448, 1993.

Chrousos, G.P., The hypothalamic-pituitary-adrenal axis and immune-mediated inflammation, *New England J. Med.*, 332 (20), 1351–1362, 1995.

Chrousos, G.P. and Gold, P.W., Editorial: a healthy body in a healthy mind—and vice versa— the damaging power of "uncontrollable" stress, *J. Clinical Endocrinol. Metab.*, 83 (6), 1842–1845, 1998.

Classen, C., Koopman, C., Angell, K., and Spiegel, D., Coping styles associated with psychological adjustment to advanced breast cancer, *Health Psychol.: Off. J. Div. Health Psychol., Am. Psychological Assoc.*, 15 (6), 434–437, 1996.

Cooper, C.L., Ed., *Handbook of Stress, Medicine, and Health*, CRC Press, Boca Raton, FL, 1996.

DeBellis, M.D. et al., Hypothalamic-pituitary-adrenal axis dysregulation in sexually abused girls, *J. Clinical Endocrinol. Metab.*, 78 (2), 249–255, 1994.

Ehrhart-Bornstein, M. and Hilbers, U., Neuroendocrine properties of adrenocortical cells, *Horm. Metabolic Res.*, 30 (6–7), 436–439, 1998.

Feldman, S. and Weidenfeld, J., Involvement of amygdalar alpha adrenoceptors in hypothalamo-pituitary-adrenocortical responses, *Neuroreport*, 7 (18), 3055–3057, 1996.

Feldman, S. and Weidenfeld, J., The excitatory effects of the amygdala on hypothalamo-pituitary-adrenocortical responses are mediated by hypothalamic norepinephrine, serotonin, and CRF-41, *Brain Res. Bull.*, 45 (4), 389–393, 1998.

Feldman, S., Newman, M.E., Gur, E., and Weidenfeld, J., Role of serotonin in the amygdala in hypothalamo-pituitary-adrenocortical responses, *Neuroreport*, 9 (9), 2007–2009, 1998.

Feldman, S., Newman, M.E., and Weidenfeld, J., Effects of adrenergic and serotonergic agonists in the amygdala on the hypothalamic-pituitary-adrenocortical axis, *Brain Res. Bull.*, 52 (6), 531–536, 2000.

Ferry, B. and Di Scala, G., Basolateral amygdala NMDA receptors are selectively involved in the acquisition of taste-potentiated odor aversion in the rat, *Behavioral Neurosci.*, 114 (5), 1005–1010, 2000.

Ferry, B., Roozendaal, B., and McGaugh, J.L., Basolateral amygdala noradrenergic influences on memory storage are mediated by an interaction between beta- and alpha1-adreno-ceptors, *J. Neurosci.*, 19 (12), 5119–5123, 1999.

Ferry, B., Roozendaal, B., and McGaugh, J.L., Involvement of alpha1-adrenoceptors in the basolateral amygdala in modulation of memory storage, *Eur. J. Pharmacol.*, 372 (1), 9–16, 1999.

Fink, G., Ed., *Encyclopedia of Stress*, Vols. 1–3, Academic Press, San Diego, 2000.

Friedman, E.M. and Irwin, M.R., A role for CRH and the sympathetic nervous system in stress-induced immunosuppression, in Neuroimmunomodulation Molecular Aspects, Integrative Systems, and Clinical Advances, *Annals of the New York Academy of Sciences*, Vol. 840, McCann, S.M., Sternberg, E.M., Lipton, J.M., Chrousos, G.P., Gold, P.W., and Smith, C.G., Eds., New York Academy of Sciences, New York, 1998, pp. 396–418.

Fuggetta, M.P., Graziani, G., Aguino, A., D'Atri, S., and Bonmassar, E., The effect of hydrocortisone on human natural killer activity and its modulation by beta interferon, *Int. J. Immunopharmacol.*, 10 (6), 687–694, 1988.

Fuller, R.W., Serotonin receptors involved in regulation of pituitary-adrenocortical function in rats, *Behavioral Brain Res.*, 73 (1–2), 215–219, 1996.

Geratcioti, Jr., T.D., Orth, D.N., Ekhator, N.N., Blumenkopf, B., and Loosen, P.T., Serial cerebrospinal fluid corticotropin-releasing hormone concentrations in healthy and depressed humans, *J. Clinical Endocrinol. Metab.*, 74 (6), 1325–1330, 1992.

Glaser, R., Kiecolt-Glaser, J.K., Malarkey, W.B., and Sheridan, J.F., The influence of psycho-logical stress on the immune response to vaccines, in Neuroimmunomodulation Molecular Aspects, Integrative Systems, and Clinical Advances, *Annals of the New York Academy of Sciences*, Vol. 840, McCann, S.M., Sternberg, E.M., Lipton, J.M., Chrousos, G.P., Gold, P.W., and Smith, C.G., Eds., New York Academy of Sciences, New York, 1998, pp. 649–655.

Gold, P.W., Goodwin, F.K., and Chrousos, G.P., Clinical and biochemical manifestations of depression, relation to the neurobiology of stress (1), *New England J. Med.*, 319 (6), 384–353, 1988.

Gold, P.W., Goodwin, F.K., and Chrousos, G.P., Clinical and biochemical manifestations of depression, relation to the neurobiology of stress (2), *New England J. Med.*, 319 (7), 413–420, 1988.

Griep, E.N., Boersma, J.W., Lentjes, E.G., Prins, A.P., van der Korst, J.K., and Kloet, E.R., Function of the hypothalamic-pituitary-adrenal axis in patients with fibromyalgia and low back pain, *J. Rheumatol.*, 25 (7), 1374–1381, 1998.

Irwin, M., Hauger, R.L., Brown, M., and Britton, K.T., CRF activates autonomic nervous system and reduces natural killer cell cytotoxicity, *Am. J. Physiol.*, 255 (5), R744–R747, 1998.

Jessop, D.S., Stimulatory and inhibitory regulators of the hypothalamic-pituitary-adrenocor-tical axis, *Baillieres Clinical Endocrinol. Metab.*, 13 (4), 491–501, 1999.

Johnson, E.O., Kamilaris, T.C., Chrousos, G.P., and Gold, P.W., Mechanisms of stress: a dynamic overview of hormonal and behavioral homeostasis, *Neurosci. Biobehavioral Rev.*, 16 (2), 115–130.

Kiecolt-Glaser, J.K., Glaser, R., Gravenstein, S., Malarkey, W.B., and Sheridan, J.F., Chronic stress alters the immune response to influenza virus vaccine in older adults, *Proc. Natl. Acad. Sci. U.S.A.*, 93 (7), 3043–3047, 1996.

Kling, M.A. et al., Cerebrospinal fluid immunoreactive corticotropin-releasing hormone and adenocorticotropin secretion in Cushing's disease and major depression: potential clinical implications, *J. Clinical Endocrinol. Metab.*, 72 (2), 260–271, 1991.

Lentjes, E.G., Griep, E.N., Boersma, J.W., Romijn, F.P., and Kloet, E.R., Glucocorticoid receptors, fibromyalgia and low back pain, *Psychoneuroendocrinology*, 22 (8), 603–614, 1997.

Levenstein, S., Ackerman, S., Kiecolt-Glaser, J.K., and Dubois, A., Stress and peptic ulcer, *J. Am. Med. Assoc.*, 281 (1), 10–11, 1999.

Mastorakos, G., Chrousos, G.P., and Weber, J.S., Recombinant interleukin-6 activates the hypothalamic–pituitary–adrenal axis in humans, *J. Clinical Endocrinol. Metab.*, 77 (6), 1690–1694, 1993.

Michelson, D. et al., Bone mineral density in women with depression, *New England J. Med.*, 335 (16), 1176–1181, 1996.

Moynihan, J.A. et al., Stress-induced modulation of immune function in mice, in *Handbook of Human Stress and Immunity*, Glaser, R. and Kiecolt-Glaser, J.K., Eds., Academic Press, San Diego, 1994, pp. 125–160.

Overton, J.M. and Fisher, L.A., Modulation of central nervous system actions of corticotropin-releasing factor by dynorphin-related peptides, *Brain Res.*, 488 (1–2), 233–240, 1989.

Pacak, K., Palkovits, M., Kvetnansky, R., Yadid, G., Kopin, I.J., and Goldstein, D.S., Effects of various stressors on *in vivo* norepinephrine release in the hypothalamic paraventricular nucleus and on the pituitary–adrenocortical axis, in Stress: Basic Mechanisms and Clinical Implications, *Annals of the New York Academy of Sciences*, Vol. 771, Chrousos, G.P. et al., Eds., New York Academy of Sciences, New York, 1995, pp. 396–418.

Raadsheer, F.C., Hoogendijk, W.J., Stam, F.C., Tilders, F.J., and Swaab, D.F., Increased numbers of corticotropin-releasing hormone expressing neurons in the hypothalamic paraventricular nucleus of depressed patients, *Neuroendocrinology*, 60 (4), 436–444, 1994.

Roy, A., Pickar, D., Paul, S., Doran, A., Chrousos, G.P., and Gold, P.W., CSF corticotropin-releasing hormone in depressed patients and normal control subjects, *Am. J. Psychiatry*, 144 (5), 641–645, 1987.

Seligman, M.E., Weiss, J., Weinraub, M., and Schulman, A., Coping behavior: learned helplessness, physiological change and learned inactivity, *Behav. Res. Ther.*, 18 (5), 459–512, 1980.

Sheridan, J.F. et al., Stress-induced neuroendocrine modulation of viral pathogenesis and immunity, in Neuroimmunomodulation Molecular Aspects, Integrative Systems, and Clinical Advances, *Annals of the New York Academy of Sciences*, Vol. 840, McCann, S.M., Sternberg, E.M., Lipton, J.M., Chrousos, G.P., Gold, P.W., and Smith, C.G., Eds., New York Academy of Sciences, New York, 1998, pp. 803–808.

Simson, P.G., Weiss, J.M., Hoffman, L.J., and Ambrose, M.J., Reversal of behavioral depression by infusion of an alpha-2 adrenergic agonist into the locus coeruleus, *Neuropharmacology*, 25 (4), 385–389, 1986.

Spiegel, D., Sephton, S.E., Terr, A.I., and Stites, D.P., Effects of psychosocial treatment in prolonging cancer survival may be mediated by neuroimmune pathways, in Neuroimmunomodulation Molecular Aspects, Integrative Systems, and Clinical Advances, *Annals of the New York Academy of Sciences*, Vol. 840, McCann, S.M., Sternberg, E.M., Lipton, J.M., Chrousos, G.P., Gold, P.W., and Smith, C.G., Eds., New York Academy of Sciences, New York, 1998, pp. 674–683.

Sternberg, E.M., Chrousos, G.P., Wilder, R.L., and Gold, P.W., The stress response and the regulation of inflammatory disease, *Ann. Intern. Med.*, 117 (10), 854–866, 1992.

Sternberg, E.M. et al., Corticotropin-releasing hormone related behavioral and neuroendocrine responses to stress in Lewis and Fischer rats, *Brain Res.*, 570 (1–2), 54–60, 1992.

Terman, G.W., Shavit, Y., Lewis, J.W., Cannon, J.T., and Liebeskind, J.C., Intrinsic mechanisms of pain inhibition: activation by stress, *Science*, 226, 1270–1278, 1984.

Tsigos, C., and Chrousos, G.P., Stress, endocrine manifestations, and diseases, in *Handbook of Stress, Medicine, and Health*, Cooper, C.L., Ed., CRC Press, Boca Raton, FL, 1996, pp. 61–85.

Weidenfeld, J., Itzik, A., and Feldman, S., Effects of glucocorticoids on the adrenocortical axis response to electrical stimulation and the ventral noradrenergic bundle, *Brain Res.*, 754 (1–2), 187–194, 1997.

Weiss, J.M., Effects of coping responses on stress, *J. Comp. Physiological Psychol.*, 65 (2), 251–260, 1968.

Weiss, J.M. and Glazer, H.I., Effects of acute exposure to stressors on subsequent avoidance-escape behavior, *Psychosomatic Med.*, 37 (6), 499–521, 1975.

Weiss, J.M., Glazer, H.I., Pohorecky, L.A., Brick, J., and Miller, N.E., Effects of chronic exposure to stressors on avoidance-escape behavior and on brain norepinephrine, *Psychosomatic Med.*, 37 (6), 522–534, 1975.

4 The Relaxation System: Theoretical Construct

The concept of total wellness recognizes that every thought, word, and behavior affects our greater health and well-being. And we, in turn, are affected not only emotionally but also physically and spiritually.

Greg Anderson (1964–#)
U.S. basketball player,
NBA forward/center
for San Antonio Spurs and
Atlantic Hawks

CONTENTS

INTRODUCTION

We understand that there is darkness because we know light; we understand that there is light because we know darkness. Likewise, we know stress because we have experienced relaxation and vice versa. Hans Selye introduced us to the stress response and Herb Benson to the relaxation response, both of which, essentially, are epidemiological findings of various physiological responses to stressed or relaxed patient populations, respectively. The autonomic nervous system (ANS), our neural or electrical control center for stress and relaxation, has a sympathetic portion that responds to stress and a parasympathetic portion that is concerned with homeostasis or relaxation. The key is *balance*.

It is universally recognized that there is a stress system, including a set pattern of electrical and hormonal responses, varying in sequence and quality between acute and chronic reactions. We propose that the body not only possesses a stress system but an endogenous relaxation system as well. Would the body only harbor a hormonal cascade for stress and not for relaxation? Logically, there ought to be a hormonal component to both systems. Herein we present, for the first time, evidence of an endogenous relaxation system that both hormonally counterbalances the stress response and, furthermore, integrates the physical response with mental and emotional input. We call the combination of the endogenous relaxation system and the nonphysical input, the *theta healing system*. The term was coined because the effect naturally occurs when the body is relaxed enough to allow the mind to enter a tranquil state. While we have not been able to determine the *sequence* of hormonal release, we have been able to substantiate our theory with reports of both hormones that induce tranquility as well as neuropeptides that are associated with deep relaxation.

> Imagine with me for a moment that you are outside on a clear evening far from city lights. The sky is a rich, dark indigo blue and the stars are brilliantly luminous. You begin to realize that certain areas of the sky hold pictures with discernable images: a bear, a hunter, a crown. You see the dots of light that make up these images, light in the midst of darkness, but there are no lines to connect them. We have located many of these dots of light that belong to the *theta healing system*, and an undeniable picture is beginning to emerge, but not all of the lines have been connected as of yet.

William Devane, who holds a doctorate in pharmacology from the St. Louis University Medical School, made a prodigious discovery while in the midst of completing his doctoral degree. Under the tutelage of cannabinoid researcher Allyn Howlett, Devane found and characterized a cannabinoid, or tetrahydrocannabinol (THC, that is the main active ingredient in marijuana), receptor in the rat brain (Devane et al., 1988). The finding compelled Devane (and numerous others around the world) to search for the endogenous ligand for the THC receptor. An intriguing unsubstantiated story surrounds the discovery. Devane traveled to the Sri Aurobindo ashram (an ashram is a place of Hindu meditation and teaching) in India. While meditating there, he had a vision in which he foresaw that he would be the one to discover the hormone that acted on the cannabinoid receptor. The Sanskrit word for bliss is *ananda*, and Devane thought it a fitting name for the putative ligand. He surmised that the new neuropeptide would be an amide; so long before finding it, he called the molecule *anandamide*, which means the amide of bliss. Devane subsequently traveled to Hebrew University in Jerusalem because he wanted to work on finding the elusive molecule with Raphael Mechoulam, the researcher who had unraveled the molecular structure of THC in the early 1970s (Mechoulam et al., 1972a, 1972b). Four years later, Devane's vision proved prophetic, and he indeed discovered anandamide. As published in *Science* magazine in 1992, these researchers, along with several other colleagues at Hebrew University, succeeded in extracting anandamide from pig brain tissue (Devane et al., 1992).

The story of Devane's discovery of anandamide, although not verified, is reminiscent of the story of the elucidation of the structure of the benzene ring by Friedrich Kekulé in 1866. The well-known story is that Kekulé was in an extremely relaxed state, gazing into his fireplace, when he had a vision of a snake that curled into itself and bit its own tail. He then realized that the benzene structure was actually a ring, a fact that subsequently was shown to be correct. Kekulé's method of discovery, to many people, would seem unusual or creative; nonetheless, it was an insight that would revolutionize the field of chemistry. How fitting that the discovery of the relaxation neuropeptide anandamide would also occur through a vision in a state of deep relaxation.

So, can we deduce from Devane's finding that our body naturally produces a substance that instills calm? It is a far more coherent and logical theory to presume that we have an equally authoritative, but opposing, physiological system to the stress system than to assume that any relaxation response is a haphazard reaction to our mind and emotions. Evidence for the presence of a relaxation system resides, in part, in the endogenous relaxation hormones, such as anandamide, as they are the biochemical basis for a complex, interactive relaxation network. I believe ongoing scientific research in this field is a new frontier of medical science. An understanding of these transmitters of relaxation is the starting point in the elaboration of a human relaxation system. We present the rudimentary, sometimes speculative, but strongly compelling facts that point to the existence of the *theta healing system*. The *theta healing system* involves the integration of the physiological, mental/emotional, and even the spiritual aspects of our being. Furthermore, we define relaxation medicine as any therapy that triggers the theta healing response and then elaborate some of the key components of the *theta healing system*. The next chapter provides an extensive review of relaxation medicine modalities. By the end of this book, you will understand how the *theta healing system* also is a passageway or conduit for experiences of subtle energy, referred to in Eastern systems of medicine as *Qi*.

THE HISTORY

Let us begin with a brief review of the major events in the history of relaxation medicine. Herbert Benson, who is currently an associate professor of medicine at the Mind/Body Medical Institute at Harvard Medical School, has been a pioneer in relaxation research. In the early 1970s, when Benson began studying the physiology of practitioners of transcendental meditation (TM), there were already various relaxation modalities—such as hypnosis, progressive muscle relaxation, autogenic training, and biofeedback (for an extensive review of these techniques, see the respective listing in Chapter 5 on relaxation modalities)—that were quite well known to medical science. The term *relaxation response* was coined in the late 1960s to refer to the general stress-reducing phenomenon resulting from meditation and similar practices.

Benson constructively exploited the term to get physicians and the general population thinking about the benefits of relaxing. He developed a four-step procedure, which he felt elicited the relaxation response (Benson, 1974, 1975). Benson learned that meditation and other modalities induced beneficial physiological responses. For example, subjects consumed 17% less oxygen, had lower heart and respiratory rates, and had lower blood pressure than did control subjects. Other researchers soon began confirming the physical and mental benefits of integrating relaxation techniques and conventional medicine. The salient aspects of meditation techniques were lifted and taught to patients in a manner that involved no philosophical conviction or religious belief. One notable example of this trend took place in the late 1970s with the Lifestyle Heart Trials of Dr. Dean Ornish (Ornish et al., 1983). Ornish's programs include diet, exercise, as well as a TM-type meditation. Results of a 5-year Lifestyle Heart Trial (1986–1992), published in the *Journal of the American Medical Association*, indicate that the experimental group evidenced regression of coronary atherosclerosis at 1 year and had half the cardiac events of the control group (Ornish et al., 1998).

Researcher Jon Kabat-Zinn did for mindfulness meditation what Herbert Benson had done for TM. He took this, essentially Buddhist, practice and secularized it, providing meditation training for medical patients. Unlike TM, which is based on the repetitive use of a mantra, mindfulness-based meditation involves developing a keen sense of moment-to-moment awareness by observing thoughts and sensations. Kabat-Zinn taught chronic pain patients mindfulness meditation, and a 4-year follow-up study indicated good compliance and significant improvement in coping with the pain (Kabat-Zinn et al., 1986). He also worked with patients with anxiety disorders and witnessed significant reduction in anxiety at a 3-year follow-up (Kabat-Zinn et al., 1992). Patients learned to identify anxious thoughts as just thoughts rather than "reality." The intent of mindfulness therapy is not simply to obtain coping skills but to acquire a practice intended to be a way of life. Both studies indicate that there was an ongoing value to patients in having acquired the meditation skills.

While these therapeutic practices undoubtedly have benefited thousands of people, they have taught us little about the actual physiological events that occur inside the body. For instance, *why* is it that heart rate or blood pressure are lowered while meditating? Benson, Ornish, and Kabat-Zinn provide us with epidemiological data, that is, they give us broad pieces of information about disease and health for those who meditate as opposed to those who do not. In the previous chapter, we analyzed the major factors involved in the classic stress system. Similarly, we will now propose a system of hormones and neurotransmitters that make up the *theta healing system*—the first system to be introduced as a coherent system of relaxation.

ENDOGENOUS LIGANDS OF THE RELAXATION RESPONSE

The brain has its own resident neurotransmitters or endogenous ligands. Many endogenous ligands and the precise receptors for them are known; we can assume that there are many yet to be discovered. Neurotransmitters are both the messengers of our nervous system and the chemistry of our emotions. But, what happens when a drug (i.e., an exogenous substance) also fits into a receptor? In some instances, the drug mimics the endogenous ligand; in other instances, it can produce a much stronger or significantly different reaction than the natural chemical.

Drugs can work by blocking actions of neurotransmitters or by interfering with or enhancing the mechanisms associated with the receptor, such as blocking their reuptake and preventing them from doing their job. As discussed in Chapter 1, when a drug or endogenous ligand promotes a known effect, such as relaxation at a benzodiazepine receptor site, it is called an *agonist*. When a drug or endogenous ligand exhibits the ability to block a receptor, it is called an *antagonist*. Antagonists stop the known effects, which, in the case of benzodiazepine receptors, means not permitting a reduction in anxiety. A third type of effect that may occur is sometimes referred to as a *reverse* or *inverse agonist*. This occurs when a drug or endogenous ligand actually produces an outcome that evokes symptoms opposite of those known to occur. What is quite amazing to ponder is that one receptor can interact with all three types of ligands. The communication can become more complex when multiple receptors are activated in response to an agonist. It is not only possible that different agonists for the same receptor elicit diverse magnitudes of response, but that they also select several signaling pathways (Pauwels, 2000).

When it is known that a drug produces a particular effect in humans, researchers go searching to find a receptor into which the drug fits. As soon as the receptor is located, scientists want to know what endogenous ligand fits into the receptor. For many of the hormones, such as anandamide, which are discussed in this chapter, the receptors and endogenous ligands have been located relatively recently. Bear in mind, however, that simply finding a molecule that binds to a known receptor does not establish that there is also a function for that ligand within the human body. As we discussed in the chapter on stress (Chapter 3), oxytocin is a hormone with properties that evoke a response that can be categorized as a relaxation response. In this chapter, we will cover properties of several other hormones that are putatively relaxation ligands, including benzodiazepines and associated ligands, melatonin, the cannabinoids, and *N,N*-dimethyltryptamine.

THE BENZODIAZEPINES

OVERVIEW

We begin our discussion with a review of the benzodiazepines because so many of the relaxation hormones are purported to fit into benzodiazepine receptors or to have actions that mimic the functions of the benzodiazepines. The benzodiazepines are a class of drugs that have had enormous therapeutic impact, particularly for those individuals who have suffered from anxiety or depression. Benzodiazepines also are used for their anticonvulsant, hypnotic, and muscle-relaxing properties, and some of them are used to reduce withdrawal symptoms. They are well-known by their commercial names, such as Valium (diazepam), Xanax (alprazolam), Versed (midazolam), and Librium (chlordiazepoxide). Librium was the prototype for the benzodiazepine compounds.

The location of the benzodiazepine receptor was unknown for many years, yet it had to exist somewhere in our bodies because pharmaceutical companies had found drugs, which they called *benzodiazepines*, with distinctive anxiety-reducing therapeutic properties. Sure enough, in 1977, two teams of researchers simultaneously located specific benzodiazepine receptors (Braestrup and Squires, 1977; Mohler and Okada, 1977). The location of the receptor was vital to the development of the drugs. Researchers found that different types of benzodiazepines bind to the receptors with more or less potency, but the fun part was that this indeed correlated to the observed therapeutic strength of the drug—both in animals and in humans.

Each of the scientists who had located the receptor continued their research, postulating that the benzodiazepine receptors existed primarily in the central nervous system (CNS) (Braestrup and Squires, 1978a, 1978b; Mohler and Okada, 1978; Mohler et al., 1978). Since that time, it has been established that benzodiazepine receptors exist in just about every tissue of the body. They are even present on platelets and monocytes (Moingeon et al., 1984; Ruff et al., 1985). Eventually, it was determined that there are actually two types of benzodiazepine receptors. The original receptors found in the CNS currently are referred to as central receptors and the other type as peripheral receptors—a distinction that no longer is applicable in regard to physiological location.

The major difference between the two receptors types is that one potentiates the inhibitory effects of γ-aminobutyric acid (GABA) and the other does not. Recall that GABA is the primary inhibitory neurotransmitter in the CNS. Even before the central receptors were located, scientists knew that the benzodiazepines bind to the GABA receptor complex, specifically the $GABA_A$ receptors located on the postsynaptic neuron (Haefely et al., 1975). The benzodiazepines increase GABA's ability to inhibit neurotransmission at the postsynaptic binding site by causing the chloride channel to open and allowing chloride to enter the second neuron. This action prevents excessive discharge by reducing the potential excitability of the postsynaptic neuron (Tallman et al., 1980). So, we journey inward and observe the flow of hormonal reactions that contribute to a calming effect.

As mentioned, when scientists know that there is a receptor, they are curious to discover which endogenous ligand also fits into the receptor. In 1983, ligands for both peripheral as well as central benzodiazepine receptors were located. The major ligand for the peripheral receptor is called *diazepam-binding inhibitor* (DBI) because it displaces drugs that have a high affinity for the receptor (see Guidotti et al., 1983; Papadopoulos, 1993, for a review of DBI). There are numerous ligands that have been shown to bind to the central benzodiazepine receptor. Some of the candidates that we will review include β-carboline, nicotinamide, inosine, hypoxanthine, melatonin, and cannabinoids—all potential relaxation hormones. Curiously, in addition to finding agonists and antagonists, researchers also found ligands that acted like inverse agonists, producing anxiety and convulsions, effects opposite to the benzo-diazepines (Braestrup et al., 1983; Prado de Carvalho et al., 1983). Researchers continue to unravel the multifaceted relationship of various ligands to the benzodi-azepine receptor and GABA complex, including receptor subunits, and seem to be endlessly discovering new ligands (Haefely et al., 1993; Rothstein et al., 1992; Teuber et al., 1999).

BENZODIAZEPINES AND THE IMMUNE SYSTEM

Before surveying the putative endogenous ligands for the benzodiazepine receptor, we want to divert for a moment to share with you a little about the role of benzo-diazepines in the immune system. For years, it has been known that benzodiazepine receptors are present on platelets, monocytes, and circulating lymphocytes (Moin-geon et al., 1983, 1984; Ruff et al., 1985). Furthermore, a correlation between an imbalance of benzodiazepine receptor binding (both increased and decreased) and various diseases, including liver disease, brain tumor, epilepsy, heart disease, and leukemia, often has been cited (Basile et al., 1991; Ferrarese et al., 1989; Ishiguro et al., 1987; Mazzone et al., 2000; Mullen et al., 1990; Savic et al., 1988; Venturini et al., 1998).

Recall that when we experience stress, the hypothalamic–pituitary–adrenal axis (HPA) is activated. Remember that during an acute stress response, the HPA has mechanisms by which it stimulates the immune response and arouses the immuno-logical memory. This process becomes skewed, if not destructive, when stress is attenuated. There is now evidence that the anxiety-reducing benzodiazepines play a protective role in stress-induced immune suppression, which is at least partly due to suppression of the HPA (Korneyev, 1997; Rocca et al., 1993; Zavala, 1997). Some of this effect may occur as a result of the ability of benzodiazepines to limit the production and release of corticotropin-releasing hormone (CRH) or adrenocortico-tropic hormone (ACTH) (Rohrer et al., 1994; Skelton et al., 2000). Epidemiological studies support this theory. For example, research shows that diazepam modifies the immune response of rats during acute and chronic swim stress (Salman et al., 2000). This is a striking role that the benzodiazepines play in modulating the immune system—a role that we will see (later in this chapter) is also played by melatonin, the primary hormone of the pineal gland.

We now proceed with a review of some of the significant ligands, detailing their relationship to the benzodiazepines and their role in the *theta healing system*.

β-CARBOLINE, HYPOXANTHINE, INOSINE, AND NICOTINAMIDE

In 1977, when Dr. Claus Braestrup from Denmark located the benzodiazepine receptor, he did so by locating a compound, called *β-carboline-3-carboxylic acid*, in the urine of mentally ill patients. It was soon learned that β-carboline inhibits brain benzodiazepine receptors, and there was much speculation that some derivative of it might be an endogenous ligand for the benzodiazepine receptor (Braestrup et al., 1980). β-carboline actually has a higher affinity for the benzodiazepine receptor than do most benzodiazepines. The only problem is that the molecule that Braestrup found was not really an endogenous ligand but an artifact of the extraction process he used to isolate it. No matter, because it turned out to be profoundly useful anyway, and soon endogenous β-carboline alkaloids were located and found to be benzodiazepine Ligands (Rommelspacher et al., 1981). These alkaloids (primarily harmane and norharmane) were also shown to possess antioxidant properties (Tse et al., 1991). At first, β-carboline was recognized as an antagonist (Beer et al., 1978). However, further testing uncovered its reverse agonist properties, that is, β-carboline can in fact produce anxiety and convulsions in animals and humans (Dorow et al., 1983; Duka et al., 1987; File et al., 1985; Rommelspacher et al., 1981). Because β-carboline does not share a recognition site with diazepam, researchers very early on began to speculate that the benzodiazepine receptor must be a multicomponent complex (Hirsch, 1982). In other words, it was clear that the benzodiazepine receptor site permitted numerous, diverse types of actions at its portal.

Three other endogenous ligands for the benzodiazepine receptor were identified in the late 1970s; they are inosine, hypoxanthine, and nicotinamide (Asano and Spector, 1979; Mohler et al., 1979; Skolnick et al., 1978). Like β-carboline, they competitively bind to benzodiazepine sites but not to other sites with similar actions, such as β-adrenergic or opiate sites. Unlike β-carboline, they bind to the benzodiazepine receptor with a low affinity. Inosine and hypoxanthine increase the inhibiting ability of diazepam, and nicotinamide was shown to potentiate the anticonvulsant properties of barbiturates typically used for epilepsy (Bourgeois et al., 1983; Marangos et al., 1981).

In addition, various other factors have been proposed as endogenous ligands of the benzodiazepine receptor, such as prostaglandins and glutamate (Asano and Ogasawara, 1982; Garthwaite et al., 1988). However, the literature is not consistent on how these various factors function or even whether they actually use the benzodiazepine/GABA receptor complex. And as mentioned, having binding properties does not mean that there is a physiological or therapeutic component. The endogenous benzodiazepine ligands appear to play a role in modulating neuronal actions, and it is my speculation that this may be the clue to their most important function (Skolnick et al., 1978).

MELATONIN

Melatonin (N-acetyl-5-methoxytryptamine) is the principal hormone of the pineal gland, and the pineal is our major transducer of neuroendocrine information. It transforms neural input into endocrine output. The pineal converts light, temperature, and magnetic environmental information into neuroendocrine signals that influence the body's functioning, often via melatonin.

There is an intriguing piece of research on the benzodiazepines that I happened upon over 20 years ago. The researchers discovered that melatonin not only fits into its own receptor, but also into the benzodiazepine receptor (Marangos et al., 1981). We also know that both receptors are modulated by the GABA receptor (Haefely et al., 1975; Li et al., 2001; Monteleone et al., 1989). There are noteworthy similarities between the physiological characteristics of benzodiazepines and melatonin. For example, melatonin, like the benzodiazepines, reduces anxiety, is an antidepressant, and can aid insomnia. However, melatonin often ameliorates the same symptoms with far fewer side effects (Garfinkel et al., 1999; Raghavendra et al., 2000).

Diazepam can suppress melatonin-binding sites in the brain, an action that can be reversed by exogenous melatonin administration, and peripheral benzodiazepine ligands can reverse the antidepressant action of melatonin (Atsmon et al., 1996; Raghavendra et al., 2000). Furthermore, when test animals are administered melatonin or a benzodiazepine (temazepam), similar types and levels of effects (e.g., sleep induction) are elicited (Gilbert et al., 1999; Stone et al., 2000). Consequently, melatonin has been used therapeutically to facilitate benzodiazepine discontinuation with insomnia patients and to enhance the reduction of anxiety in the preoperative period (Garfinkel et al., 1999; Naguib and Samarkandi, 1999, 2000). Clearly, there appears to be a reciprocal and interactive nature between these two molecules.

MELATONIN AND THE IMMUNE AND STRESS SYSTEMS

Over 30 years ago, researchers showed that pinealectomized rodents demonstrate a depressed immune response and that melatonin is, in fact, a fundamental modulator of immune responses in normal mammals (Jankovic et al., 1970; Maestroni et al., 1989). We now know that melatonin has prophylactic functions, immune-enhancing properties, and ameliorates the immune-deteriorating effects of stress. It also plays a fundamental role in immune reactions to viral and bacterial infections.

The prophylactic functions of melatonin are particularly effective during times of stress. Immune system suppression in mice (including reduced antibody production, resistance to virus, gastric ulceration, and lower thymus weight) caused by the exogenous administration of the stress hormone corticosterone can actually be reversed by melatonin (Khan et al., 1990; Maestroni et al., 1986, 1987). The benzodiazepine receptors present on monocytes may be the avenue through which melatonin modulates the immune system (Moingeon et al., 1984; Ruff et al., 1985). Research on rodents and restraint stress reveals that the beneficial effect of melatonin is actually not dependent upon a reduction of corticosteroids, but rather occurs via melatonin's immune-enhancing capability (Maestroni and Conti, 1991). This finding is quite stunning, as it implies that melatonin functions as an ongoing immune-system support. Reinforcing this theory are several experiments showing that the antistress effects of melatonin are only seen in mice that have been primed with antigen (Maestroni et al., 1986; Pierpaoli and Maestroni, 1987). Immune-enhancing functions of melatonin also have been observed in patients with various conditions that depress the immune system, including pharmacological therapies that are typically administered for cancer treatment (Maestroni, 1993, 2001).

Just as melatonin boasts discrete immune-enhancing characteristics, certain immune products, such as γ-interferon, colony-stimulating factors, and interleukin-2 (IL-2), are in turn capable of modulating the synthesis of melatonin in the pineal (Maestroni, 1993). Here again we have one of those remarkable instances of systems interacting in a bidirectional manner reminiscent of the systems integration paradigms reviewed in Chapter 2 (Maestroni, 1999).

So, melatonin ends up being a powerful mediator of stress that works in a subtle manner, via the immune system, perhaps synergistically with the benzodiazepines.

I think that this fact alone gives us pause to suspect that it plays a part in an endogenous system of relaxation hormones. Research is just beginning to show that the stress-reducing and immune-enhancing effects of melatonin are associated with a reduction in both breast and prostate cancer (see Coker, 1999, for a review). In the chapter on the pineal gland (Chapter 6), you will read more about associations between melatonin and disease.

MELATONIN AND MEDITATION

Research performed by the Maharishi University (named after the founder of TM) in Fairfield, IA, identifies numerous physiological associations between a regular practice of meditation and health benefits (e.g., Alexander et al., 1989). When we meditate, electroencephalogram (EEG) measurements are in the alpha–theta frequency range. The Maharishi University researchers have shown that in long-term practitioners of TM, this pattern persists during sleep (Mason et al., 1997). It is as if meditation has become part of the fabric of the lives of these individuals. In other words, there is a correlation between our physical health and the time we spend in a relaxed state of mind. Such research comes under the category of epidemiological types of studies, such as that promoted by Herb Benson and others (Benson, 1974, 1975). However, intriguingly, some newer research has shown that there is a direct correlation between meditation and our endogenous levels of melatonin.

Melatonin levels have been shown to rise during meditation and are higher in those who regularly meditate (see Figure 4.1). Researchers working with Jon Kabat-Zinn at the Stress Reduction and Relaxation Program in Worcester, Massachusetts, found that eight women who regularly practiced mindfulness meditation (graduates of or teachers at the program) had higher melatonin levels (as measured by urinary 6-sulphatoxymelatonin) than did eight female controls who did not meditate (Massion et al., 1995). Another group of researchers in Australia found that melatonin levels measured at midnight are higher immediately following a period of meditation (Tooley et al., 2000). They used experienced meditators from two different traditions, one that practiced for a half hour and the other for an hour. Both groups had significantly higher melatonin levels following their period of meditation than did the controls.

The Australian researchers reasoned that, from a physiological standpoint, it is unlikely and undesirable that meditation during the day could cause melatonin levels to rise. I think their reasoning is spurious. Although it is speculative because the research has not been performed, I think that it is reasonable to assume that daytime melatonin levels could also rise during meditation. Eyes are closed, the room is usually darkened, the body begins to relax—it seems feasible that levels could rise. For most meditators, it may only be a modest elevation. However, it is my contention that the slight increase in melatonin begins a hormonal cascade that we have chosen to call the *theta healing system*. In support of this premise is research that shows that the physiological parameters that occur during meditation are very different from those of subjects during eyes-closed rest (Jevning et al., 1992). So, we have fairly solid evidence that melatonin, one of our putative hormones of healing, is in fact correlated to a primary experience of relaxation.

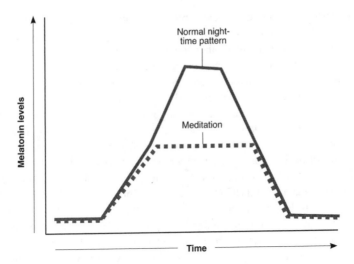

FIGURE 4.1 Meditation and levels of melatonin.

THE CANNABINOIDS

CANNABINOID RECEPTORS

As reviewed in the beginning of this chapter, William Devane found and characterized a cannabinoid or THC receptor in the rat brain (Devane et al., 1988). A couple of years later, researchers at the National Institute of Mental Health (NIMH) located the rat gene that encodes the THC receptor and soon learned that the receptor influences several major functional areas of the brain, including sensory, motor, cognitive, limbic, and autonomic (Matsuda et al., 1990, 1993). It was also in 1990 that cannabinoid receptors were localized in human brains. The work again occurred at the NIMH and was led by Miles Herkenham and included Ross Johnson and Lawrence Melvin, who had worked with Howlett and Devane on the original receptor study (Herkenham et al., 1999).

Studies have shown (as with the benzodiazepines) that other categories of psychoactive drugs (e.g., opiates) have no effect at these receptor sites. The NIMH researchers determined that cannabinoid receptors are most dense in the hippocampus, the cerebellum, and the outflow areas of the basal ganglia. Conversely, they are extremely sparse in the lower brainstem areas that control the heart and respiratory function, which may likely be why high doses of THC are not lethal. We will not cover the issue here, but suffice it to say that the relationship is a complex one regarding THC and the respiratory system, with chronic use of marijuana being associated with increased symptoms for asthmatics and injury to the lungs (e.g., Calignano et al., 2000; Sarafian et al., 2001).

There are actually three receptor subtypes, designated CB1, CB1A, and CB2, for the cannabinoid receptor (see Axelrod and Felder, 1998; Felder and Glass, 1998; Matsuda, 1997, for reviews). CB1 receptors are largely expressed in the nervous system, and CB2 receptors are expressed in the lymphoid organs (Hajos et al., 2001).

Sometimes different endogenous cannabinoid ligands respond in discrete ways to the CB1 and CB2 receptors. For example, anandamide suppresses norepinephrine release at the CB1 receptor, but another endogenous ligand, sn-2 arachidonylglycerol (2-AG), increases the release of norepinephrine (Kurihara et al., 2001). The CB1 receptor can exhibit the same action or function with more than one ligand, such as modulation of food intake (Di Marzo et al., 2001).

There is almost no information available regarding cannabinoid interaction with other receptor types. In 1986, a brief article was published revealing that eight of nine test subjects had elevated melatonin blood levels after smoking a 1% THC cigarette but not after smoking a tobacco cigarette (Lissoni et al., 1986). Because the ninth subject had a very different profile with inhibition of melatonin, the researchers speculated that THC may regulate the pineal in some way. They called for more research, but it was not forthcoming. Over 10 years later, another study found that in bovine tissue, anandamide decreases 5-HT (a melatonin precursor) receptor binding, but had no effect on benzodiazepine receptor binding (Kimura et al., 1998). These scientists speculated that anandamide might be mediated via the 5-HT receptor. We have been unable to confirm any of this work, but at the very least, it does point to some interaction between the cannabinoids and melatonin.

CANNABINOID LIGANDS

As of this writing, there are five known endogenous ligands for the cannabinoid receptor. They are referred to as endocannabinoids, as they are endogenous cannabinoids. First, anandamide, as stated, was discovered in 1992. Next, in 1995, 2-AG was identified simultaneously by Mechoulam's group in Israel and by a group in Japan led by Takayuki Sugiura. Then, the endogenous ligand, 2-arachidonoyl-glycerol ether, which the researchers call noladin ether, was located through the efforts of Mechoulam and colleagues in Israel (Devane et al., 1992; Hanus et al., 2001; Mechoulam et al., 1995; Sugiura et al., 1995). Finally and most recently, virodhamine and N-arachidonoyldopamine have been located, but very little has been published on either of them (Chu et al., 2003; Porter et al., 2002; Walker et al., 2002). Parenthetically, there are also numerous synthetic agonists and novel analogs that have been developed for research purposes (e.g., Hanus et al., 1999; Priller et al., 1995; Suhara et al., 2001). We will not cover these agonists, as our work is directed toward understanding the hormones involved in the *theta healing system*.

Anandamide

Devane and colleagues in Israel worked for over 2 years to obtain the first drop of the purified compound of anandamide (Devane et al., 1992). Devane then returned to the United States and began work at the NIMH with Julius Axelrod who, with Richard Wurtman, had been instrumental in determining the synthesis and catabolism of melatonin in the 1970s (see Chapter 6 on the pineal gland). By 1996, anandamide had been isolated from the human brain, heart, and spleen. Its minor presence in the blood and cerebrospinal fluid (CSF) led researchers to conclude that the majority of its action most likely occurs right where it is synthesized, and this insight opened the door to speculation that anandamide might participate in systems regulation (Felder et al., 1996; Piomelli, 2000). Furthermore, anandamide is part of a novel class of lipid neurotransmitters and, like melatonin, is highly lipophilic, which means that it easily passes in and out of cell membranes (Axelrod and Felder, 1998). The lipophilic quality makes it likely that anandamide is a neuromodulator, as it can travel in a retrograde direction as well (Devane and Axelrod, 1994; Di Marzo, 1999; Felder et al., 1996; Piomelli et al., 2000).

Along with other NIMH researchers, Devane and Axelrod continued to learn more about the anandamide ligand, confirming its role as an endogenous THC receptor ligand and establishing its similarities to exogenous THC, its predominantly inhibitory actions, and its therapeutic actions (Crawley et al., 1993; Felder et al., 1993). The therapeutic actions of anandamide include amelioration of pain, nausea produced by chemotherapeutic agents, wasting syndrome (particularly in cancer and AIDS patients), and brain damage (Di Marzo, 1999; Mechoulam, 1999; Walker et al., 1999a, 1999b). Both its ability to modulate neurotransmission and its distinct therapeutic functions are key to our theory of a *theta healing system* and anandamide's role in modulating the effects of stress.

2-AG

As mentioned previously, 2-AG was identified in 1995 by two research groups who isolated it from rat brain and canine intestine (Mechoulam et al., 1995; Sugiura et al., 1995). The endogenous ligand 2-AG is a unique lipid molecule that has the capability to calm neuronal function via a negative feedback system, inhibiting neurotransmission at cannabinoid receptors (Sugiura and Waku, 2000). This function is crucially important to the relaxation system because sustained activation of neurons, as we discussed in the chapter on stress (Chapter 3), is correlated to cellular exhaustion and apoptosis. The 2-AG ligand is present at 170 to 800 times the concentration of anandamide in the brain, giving rise to claims that it, and not anandamide, is the primary endogenous ligand for the cannabinoid receptor (Stella et al., 1997; Sugiura et al., 1999; Sugiura and and Waku, 2000). Some researchers speculate that 2-AG and anandamide perform complementary functions. However, one of its most distinctive functions, speeding recovery from head injury, may be exclusive to this ligand (Panikashvili et al., 2001).

Noladin Ether

Raphael Mechoulam has been involved in the identification of the three initial endogenous ligands for the cannabinoid receptor. Noladin ether, the most recently identified cannabinoid ligand, was isolated from porcine brain and binds far more strongly to the CB1 than to the CB2 receptor (Hanus et al., 2001). Little is currently known about it, but the researchers speculate that it will have a more narrow profile of activity because of its very weak binding to the CB2 receptor. In a personal communication, Dr. Mechoulam said that a few of his colleagues were rather skeptical about the compound, in part because it is an ether derivative, which is a new, unprecedented type of cannabinoid ligand. Mechoulam said that his collaborator, Dr. Lumir Hanus, successfully repeated its identification in the labs at the National Institutes of Health (NIH). "So, it's for real!" he exclaimed. So far, Mechoulam has found that noladin ether in rabbits is an excellent agent for the reduction of intraocular pressure, which is obviously a model for glaucoma, and that research on its effects on the immune system have had very encouraging preliminary results.

FUNCTIONS OF CANNABINOIDS IN THE STRESS AND IMMUNE SYSTEMS

The available research on stress and the cannabinoids is seemingly contradictory. On the one hand, there are several reports that exogenous and endogenous cannabinoids activate the HPA axis (Hao et al., 2000; Murphy et al., 1998; Weidenfeld et al., 1994). This sets the stress response in motion, which, as we have emphasized in previous chapters, can be beneficial on a short- but not long-term basis. On the other hand, there are studies indicating that there are various antistress properties of the cannabinoids, such as ameliorating ulcers, possessing antioxidant mechanisms that modulate B-lymphocyte growth and survival, and reducing anxiety and stress-induced pain (Chen and Buck, 2000; Germano et al., 2001; Giuliani et al., 2000; Valverde et al., 2000). One interesting study looked at structural changes in the hippocampus resulting from extended cannabinoid administration. The researchers found that patterns of change looked similar to those seen with toxic damage, but opposite to that observed with chronic stress (Lawston et al., 2000).

When the CB2 receptor was identified, it was located in macrophages of the spleen (which, among other immune functions, stores lymphocytes). Subsequently, researchers learned that the CB2 receptors are expressed in far higher quantities in the peripheral blood mononuclear cells than are the CB1 receptors (Munro et al., 1993; Nong, 2001). The CB2 receptor appears to be a predominantly immune-related receptor. However, CB1 receptors were also identified as being involved in the immune system via functions of the brain (Sinha et al., 1998). While anandamide has been shown to have some immune-modulating factors, such as potentiating the release of IL-6, it is 2-AG that seems to play the larger role in the immune system (Berdyshev et al., 2001; Molina-Holgado et al., 1998). The 2-AG ligand has been shown to inhibit lymphocyte response, the formation of antioxidants, the production of *in vitro* tumor necrosis factor, and the T- and B-cell response—all depressing the immune system (Gallily et al., 2000; Lee et al., 1995).

One of the main issues limiting the use of exogenous cannabinoids for therapeutic purposes is that they induce psychotropic side effects. Another is that exogenous THC, particularly marijuana, is associated with modulation of the immune system (including T and B lymphocytes, natural killer cells, and macrophages) in such a manner as to depress its ability to fight disease (Klein et al., 2001; Schwarz et al., 1994). While we know that cannabinoids play a role in modulating the immune response, the exact role they play remains unclear, which is evidenced by the contradictory research results that can be found (Klein et al., 2001; Lynn and Herkenham, 1994; Salzet et al., 2000; Zimmer et al., 1999). Endocannabinoids may depress the immune system via their ability to inhibit cytokine secretion or modulate inflammation, although, again, the results are conflicting (Klein et al., 2000, 2001; Salzet et al., 2000). The most promising area for therapeutic use of cannabinoids may well be as analgesics. Endocannabinoids appear to be natural modulators of pain, suppressing pain receptors at the level of the spinal cord and thalamus (Iversen and Chapman, 2002; Walker et al., 2001, 2002). Work needs to be done to cull out the factors of how and when the cannabinoids do and do not support the immune system. There is obviously a missing factor or, more likely, factors. It is possible that one kind of cannabinoid-induced reaction occurs during stress and another when the mind is calm.

THE CANNABINOID AND THE *THETA HEALING SYSTEM*

We now present further compelling medical evidence for the *theta healing system*. Recall from the prior benzodiazepine discussion that the benzodiazepines increase GABA's ability to inhibit neurotransmission at the postsynaptic binding site by causing the chloride channel to open, thus allowing chloride to enter the second neuron. This effect is typical of the way in which neurons pass on or inhibit a message. However, unlike the benzodiazepines, the cannabinoids work at the site of the presynaptic neurons and their actions involve calcium channels. For over a decade, it has been known that calcium can induce a retrograde inhibition at presynaptic terminals (Llano et al., 1991). The less-conventional retrograde signaling involves a message being returned to the neuron that sent it (i.e., the presynaptic neuron), and the message is: "Stop producing neurotransmitter." Consequently, the presynaptic cell causes an inhibition of the neurotransmitter at the postsynaptic neuron (Vincent and Marty, 1993). It eventually became clear that a receptor on the presynaptic cell, most likely a cannabinoid receptor, is central to the calcium-channel–induced inhibition of the neurotransmitter (Sullivan, 1999; Twitchell et al., 1997). Most interestingly, these experiments were performed on the hippocampus, which is not only central to learning and memory, but is also a critical link to the limbic system, our central processing station for emotion.

Researchers named this process of retrograde inhibition of neuron activity *depolarization-induced suppression of inhibition* (DSI), and they determined that it not only occurs in the hippocampus, but also in the cerebellum (a part of the brain that is central to cooridinated movement). They knew the mechanism and the putative receptor, but not the messenger itself. In 2001, two seminal but little-known studies were published that identified the messenger. First, Rachel Wilson, a graduate student of Rodger Nicoll's at the University of California, San Francisco, determined that endocannabinoids are in fact the elusive messenger.

Activated, depolarized hippocampal neurons release the cannabinoids as postsynaptic calcium levels rise. Both the synthesis and the release of the cannabinoids are calcium dependent, which actually had been known for some time (Di Marzo et al., 1994). The cannabinoid receptor CB1 is expressed largely by GABA-mediated neurons. Wilson figured out that when the endocannabinoids, anandamide and 2-AG, are released, they send a message backward, across the synapse, to the presynaptic neuron and tell GABA to slow down (Wilson et al., 2001). It means that the cannabinoids are telling inhibitory neurons to stop inhibiting quite so much, thus, paradoxically, increasing excitation. This finding was simultaneously made by a group in Japan and published in the same month (Ohno-Shosaku et al., 2001). Wilson showed that the process occurred in a very rapid fashion in hippocampal cells, providing discrete evidence of a neuromodulatory role for the cannabinoids.

As she states, "Our study represents the first identification of a physiological process mediated by endogenous brain cannabinoids."

The identification of a second physiological function mediated by cannabinoids came right on the heels of Wilson's report. Some researchers in the neurobiology department at Harvard's medical school heard that Wilson had identified the cannabinoids as the messenger in DSI. They concluded that the cannabinoids might well be the elusive retrograde messenger in a process of neuromodulation that is similar to DSI, which they named *depolarization-induced suppression of excitatory inputs* (DSE). Working with cerebellar Purkinje cells, researchers Antol Kreitzer and Wade Regehr determined that the DSI process of postsynaptic depolarization and the increase of calcium that causes a release of endocannabinoids, via the retrograde mechanism, can also inhibit excitatory neurons, not just the inhibitory ones that Wilson had identified (Kreitzer and Regehr, 2001a). The researchers make the point that the retrograde mechanism is important to both synaptic strength and rapid time scales. Later that year, Kreitzer and Regehr published another study that confirmed Wilson's DSI work but went on to show that the DSI signaling mechanism functions in the cerebellum in addition to the hippocampus (Kreitzer and Regehr, 2001b). The diffusible and short-lived endocannabinoids, therefore, have a notable role in modulation of both inhibitory and excitatory neuronal communication. In fact, it ends up looking a bit like a mechanism of homeostatic regulation.

The obvious issue, given that DSI and DSE occur in hippocampal tissue, is the role of the cannabinoids in memory and learning, and by extension, of the limbic system in our emotional well-being. It is known that the exogenous cannabinoid marijuana reduces memory and learning functions. Mechoulam and colleagues emphasize that there are significant pharmacological differences between the exogenous and the endogenous cannabinoid ligands (Martin et al., 1999). It is likely that marijuana overwhelms the receptors and results in a physiological picture very different from endocannabinoids, including deficient memory processes. Is it possible that the endocannabinoids, via the subtle DSI and DSE modulations, could actually enhance memory? There is research that points in this direction. By observing a spectrum of behavior in CB1 knock-out mice (i.e., mice without the CB1 receptor), researchers in Spain determined that activation of the CB1 receptor by endocannabinoids controls memory and learning as well as emotional behavior (Martin et al., 2002). This study is epidemiological evidence for DSI/DSE-facilitated cannabinoid modulation.

There is one other study that we want to share with you because it is related to the hippocampus. A group of scientists at the Institute of Experimental Medicine, which is part of the Hungarian Academy of Sciences, have done work on the cannabinoids (Hajos et al., 2000, 2001). They found that the gamma oscillations of the hippocampus, which are synchronous, could be reduced in amplitude by a particular CB1 receptor agonist (with the lively name of CP 55,940). The reduced amplitude occurs in a DSI/DSE manner, with activation of presynaptic CB1 receptors decreasing calcium-dependent GABA release. So, picture your hippocampus, like the pendulum of a grandfather's clock, perpetually oscillating. A little anandamide comes along and modulates the synchronicity of the hippocampus.

Another thing happens with DSI that we have not spoken about yet. When GABA inhibition is slowed, it causes long-term potentiation of glutamatergic synapses—a condition that facilitates learning. The same Hungarian group performed a similar study on the amygdala and found that the agonists (CP 55,940 plus one called WIN55,212-2) modulate specific elements of the amygdala nuclei via the same retrograde synaptic signaling action (Katona et al., 2001). These results leave wide open the possibility that the endocannabinoids play a part in expression of emotion and, in particular, might participate in the regulation of fear (perhaps correlated to the reported symptoms of paranoia with some marijuana users). DSI can only occur when there is robust depolarization; therefore, cannabinoids probably are released only when there is a strong external stimulus. What sort of stimuli could cause an increase in the endocannabinoids? It appears that the factors could range from experiences of intense peace to significant fear.

SPECULATING ABOUT THE ROLE OF CANNABINOIDS IN THE RELAXATION RESPONSE

So, let us translate all of this theory into the potential practical applications in human functioning. When the synchronous gamma oscillations of the hippocampus are reduced in amplitude by a CB1 receptor agonist we surmise that the individual is in a state of deep relaxation and that cannabinoids are being secreted. Most people are in alpha and theta when they meditate or engage in any number of other of the modalities you will read about in the next chapter. Therefore, it makes logical sense that the cannabinoid ligands are potentially neuropeptides of deep relaxation. When one goes into a deeply meditative state at the alpha–theta interface, it is possible that anandamide and 2-AG are facilitating that sense of inner calm of which meditators speak. It is a balancing act, not a surging hormonal expression. However, the physiological effect may leave the individual in a state of deep and profound tranquility. The body seems to dissolve, and the mind is balanced. In Chapter 8, we will describe the neurological complement to this hormonal phenomenon. This whole area of research on DSI/DSE receptors, in my opinion, is nothing short of landmark. We now have the first biochemical verification for the physiological underpinnings, not only of relaxation medicine, but also for energy medicine, which will be discussed in Chapter 7.

N,N-DIMETHYLTRYPTAMINE (DMT)

Another possible relaxation hormone is DMT, an endogenous molecule with hallucinogenic properties that is found in the brain, urine, blood, and CSF. It can be actively transported across the blood–brain barrier. The psychedelic effects of DMT were first discovered by Dr. Stephen Szára in the mid-1950s when he injected the substance into himself. Dr. Szára started his work in Budapest and then worked at the U.S. National Institute on Drug Abuse in Washington, D.C. In 1972, Julius Axelrod, who was working at the National Institutes of Health, found DMT in human blood. In response to an antipsychedelic sentiment sweeping the country in the late 1960s, Congress passed a law in 1970 that put many of the psychedelic drugs into a legal category that highly restricted their use for research. Concerns of inducing short-term psychosis in normal volunteers, as well as the recreational use and abuse of lysergic acid diethylamide (LSD), conspired to virtually end research on psychedelic substances. This moratorium continued until 1990 when a physician, Rick Strassman, was given the go-ahead to research DMT (Strassman, 2001).

Strassman wanted to understand more about the hallucinogenic nature of DMT. He used intravenous (IV) injections on his volunteers because enzymes called *monoamine oxidases* (MAOs), which are plentiful in the stomach, quickly break down DMT and prevent its hallucinogenic effects from occurring. The IV route bypasses the MAOs' ability to degrade DMT. DMT is probably diffused via the CSF because MAOs could just as easily break it down in the blood. In general, the volunteers had classic stress responses to DMT (e.g., elevated blood pressure and heartbeat); a few had lasting personal or spiritual insights; while most had little obvious benefit from the DMT. Several subjects described seeing clowns, lights, colors, and encounters with other "beings." While Strassman concluded that DMT is "the spiritual molecule," he unequivocally felt that it had no therapeutic value.

Strassman reasoned that the pineal gland is the endogenous source of DMT because serotonin, a crucial precursor to DMT, has its highest concentrations in the pineal. However, serotonin is also the precursor to melatonin, and I would speculate that DMT is very closely related to melatonin because the functional manifestations have significant similarities. Strassman himself had spent years of his life researching melatonin in his quest for "a biological basis of spiritual experience." He stopped his research on melatonin, feeling it was not the "spiritual molecule," and shifted his focus to carry out the studies on DMT.

β-carboline, as previously discussed, is another possible hormone of relaxation, which also may be synthesized in the pineal and bind to L-tryptophan, a precursor similar to that of melatonin (Fekkes et al., 2001). β-carboline increases melatonin production and inhibits the MAOs from breaking down DMT (Rommelspacher, 1994). β-carboline is the reason why the DMT-active South American drink, called *ayahuasca*, can be ingested and still be psychoactive. The ayahuasca concoction includes plants that contain β-carboline. Drinking ayahuasca results in psychoactive effects that are of longer duration and milder intensity than those of IV-administered DMT (Riba et al., 2001). The presence of β-carboline in our bodies is important because having a hallucinogenic-type experience while we are engaged in daily functions would be extremely disruptive. In fact, there has been a whole line of research investigating the relationship between DMT and schizophrenia. One study reported that after, but not before, ingesting ayahuasca, hallucinogenic compounds were detected in the healthy subjects' urine samples. These compounds were the same substances found in urine samples from acutely psychotic patients who were not taking any type of medication (Pomilio et al., 1999).

Most of the hard science is yet to be performed, but it makes medical and intuitive sense to me that there could be a synergistic relationship between DMT, melatonin, and possibly β-carboline, just as there is among other hormones of relaxation. Perhaps, the association is akin to the reciprocal relationship between norepinephrine and epinephrine, which organically resemble one another yet have distinct operational components. Similarly, there is a likeness between the chemical makeup of melatonin and DMT (e.g., they both appear to derive from the tryptamine molecule), and an analysis of their behavioral expression reveals some fascinating associations. However, available published medical studies on Strassman's research indicate that melatonin levels are unaffected by the IV administration of DMT (Strassman and Qualls, 1994). So, if there is a synergistic relationship, it has to be that melatonin reaches a threshold that triggers the synthesis of DMT and not the opposite, and we can be certain that the actions of endogenous DMT are far more moderate than those of any exogenous administration.

It has already been established that melatonin is secreted during meditation, even of the alpha-wave frequency. Could it be that endogenous DMT is released during deep states of meditation? Yes, I think so. The energetic similarities between melatonin and DMT beg the question of why they are found together in the pineal gland. It is my feeling that while melatonin is secreted first, DMT is released in deeper states of meditation, culminating in visions and other experiences that could be interpreted as hallucinogenic.

PLACEBO

We spoke about nocebo and what we call voodoo medicine in Chapter 3. Physicians, family, and friends all have the power to support or seriously hinder the patient in his or her efforts to heal. But, is there really a placebo response? Researchers Hróbjartsson and Gøtzsche from Denmark compared 114 randomized clinical trials that used both a placebo group and an untreated group and found that placebos had no more effect than not providing treatment (Hróbjartsson and Gotzsche, 2001). The researchers made sweeping conclusions about there being no justification for placebos outside of their use for clinical trials. In doing so, they swept under the carpet the fact that they had found a correlation between placebo and pain and that the reviewed studies may have been too few to provide the statistical power to elucidate other such small subgroups. It did make for a dramatic, media-catching publication, however. Paradoxically, I agree, the placebo no longer exists because we now can call it *psychoneuroimmunology*. PNI research has demonstrated that our minds can alter the actions of hormones and neurotransmitters, potentially evoking physiological responses that result in either immune suppression (nocebo) or healing (placebo).

What are the implications? Physicians hold tremendous power for healing their patients. Helping patients to believe that some type of "healing" can happen in their lives directs the course of both the mental and physical aspects of the disease. Caregivers, families, and friends all hold similar power to support the patient and foster wholeness. Faith represents the ultimate placebo response. A placebo only works if you believe in it. As you will recall from the introduction to this book, it kept Steve alive for 10 years.

THE *THETA HEALING SYSTEM* AND LIMBIC THERAPY

The research still needs to be performed, but it is my strong belief that eventually a pattern of hormonal action and interaction (much like the stress system, in which

ACTH actually decreases with chronic stress, while cortisol remains elevated) will be established for a relaxation response. The known hormones already point us toward an endogenous relaxation system. I do not know whether you have taken note of it, but there is a distinct interweaving of the hormones of relaxation. The research is not yet all there, as it is for the stress response, but what is known so far is intriguing.

Let us look at how the various hormones of relaxation overlap. First, like lipophilic melatonin and the endogenous cannabinoids, DMT is able to cross the blood–brain barrier. Second, GABA, our body's most powerful inhibitory neurotransmitter, influences and/or is influenced by benzodiazepines, melatonin, and the endogenous cannabinoids. It would make sense that DMT, which potentially guides us to more profound relaxation or spiritual experiences, would not be in this group. Third, the MAOs increase melatonin levels but quickly break down DMT levels (Murphy et al., 1986; Strassman, 2001). Meanwhile, β-carboline increases melatonin production and inhibits the MAOs from breaking down DMT. Then consider that β-carboline, nicotinamide, inosine, hypoxanthine, melatonin, and the cannabinoids all share actions, if not receptors, with the benzodiazepines. Furthermore, anandamide and THC appear to be modulated via a melatonin precursor (5-HT receptor) in some unknown manner. And finally, melatonin and the benzodiazepines seem to have at least somewhat similar mechanisms of action, as they each reduce stress in a manner that is dependent upon bolstering the immune system. We do not yet have the exact hormonal sequence or the corresponding physiological repercussions that have been established for the stress system. We also do not know exactly how the various hormones contribute to the relaxation system, but it seems very likely that each are contributing members of a complex network of relaxation hormones.

Undoubtedly, the most dramatic finding is that the endogenous cannabinoid ligands have the ability to influence the relaxation system in a retrograde manner and modulate both inhibition and excitation. Not only is it the first time that we have had concrete physiological evidence of a putative relaxation hormone, but we also have evidence that the retrograde action drives the body toward an alpha–theta state, which is the frequency of meditation. We have our first confirmed picture of how the neuroendocrine system operates during relaxation. It is my contention that deep relaxation places humans within a "target zone" for the endogenous release of any of the family of neuropeptides of relaxation. The target zone is a state of alpha brain resonance, while the interface, sometimes referred to as a state of hypnagogic reverie, is the bull's eye of the deep healing process. I like to refer to the interface as limbic therapy because the theta resonance is the "healing zone" in which traumatic and repressed memories can be neutralized.

It is noteworthy, both for DMT and the cannabinoids, that the exogenous versions, for the most part, appear to overwhelm our receptors. In Western society, we want a quick fix. If it doesn't happen immediately and powerfully, it must not be good. If a little is good, a lot must be better. While the neurons that facilitate an endogenous relaxation response can individually fire rapidly, the hormones work in retrograde and localized fashions. Slow and steady is their modus operandi, often taking years to reset our patterns of neuronal firing. Their mode of action reflects what happens to us as we try to live more peaceful lives. Sometimes it can take years to change just one aspect of your personality with which you are not pleased. A whole new of hormonal reactions must be secreted in situations that previously caused stress, anxiety, fear, or whatever the emotion. Giving the mind and the body more time to practice relaxation, such as periods of meditation, promotes the endogenous learning of how to instigate a cascade of relaxation rather than stress hormones.

We know what chronic stress can do to the body. Have you ever wondered what prolonged relaxation—true, deep relaxation—could do for your physical health? In the chapter on stress (Chapter 3), we discussed the concept of encoded engrams, which stem from repressed or imbalanced emotions that create an energetic imbalance and may result in functional pathology. Encoded trauma and memories that promote fear or reduce our self-worth are engrams, which are very hard to change. They crystallize, but we now have a schematic of the endogenous hormonal pattern that can change them.

Experiences of deep peace, as encountered in the theta range, allow us to release the pain associated with memories (i.e., engrams) in a detached manner and permit us to make life choices with freedom rather than as slaves to our emotions. We see, from a physiological perspective, how it is possible to change one's response to the memories. I call it limbic therapy because the emotion associated with the memory, which has been encoded in the hippocampus, can actually be released. As we train our minds to observe our reactions, we can learn to mitigate our responses to stress. In the next chapter, we will review numerous techniques that can engender this state of relaxation. The braver you are in facing the night, the more stars you will be able to discern, until someday you will note a distinct, discernible pattern in the sky and will experience a peace of which mystics speak, a peace that passes understanding.

REFERENCES

Alexander, C.N., Langer, E.J., Newman, R.I., Chandler, H.M., and Davies, J.L., Transcendental meditation, mindfulness, and longevity: an experimental study with the elderly, *J. Personality Soc. Psychol.*, 57 (6), 950–964, 1989.

Asano, T. and Ogasawara, N., Prostaglandins A as possible endogenous ligands of benzodiazepine receptor, *Eur. J. Pharmacol.*, 80 (2–3), 271–274, 1982.

Asano, T. and Spector, S., Identification of inosine and hypoxanthine as endogenous ligands for the brain benzodiazepine-binding sites, *Proc. Natl. Acad. Sci. U.S.A.*, 76 (2), 977–981, 1979.

Atsmon, J. et al., Reciprocal effects of chronic diazepam and melatonin on brain melatonin and benzodiazepine binding sites, *J. Pineal Res.*, 20 (2), 65–71, 1996.

Axelrod, J. and Felder, C.C., Cannabinoid receptors and their endogenous agonist, anandamide. *Neurochemical Res.*, 23 (5), 575–581, 1998.

Basile, A.S. et al., Elevated brain concentrations of 1,4-benzodiazepines in fulminant hepatic failure, *New England J. Med.*, 325 (7), 473–478, 1991.

Beer, B., Klepner, C.A., Lippa, A.S., and Squires, R.F., Enhancement of 3H-diazepam binding by SQ 65,396: a novel anti-anxiety agent, *Pharmacol., Biochem., Behav.*, 9 (6), 849–851, 1978.

Benson, H., The relaxation response, *Psychiatry*, 37 (1), 37–46, 1974.

Benson, H., *The Relaxation Response*, William Morrow and Co., New York, 1975.

Berdyshev, E.V., Schmid, P.C., Krebsbach, R.J., and Schmid, H.H., Activation of PAF receptors results in enhanced synthesis of 2-arachidonoylglycerol (2-AG) in immune cells, *FASEB J.: Off. Publ. Fed. Am. Soc. Experimental Biol.*, 15 (12), 2171–2178, 2001.

Bourgeois, B.F., Dodson, W.E., and Ferrendelli, J.A., Potentiation of the antiepileptic activity of phenobarbital by nicotinamide, *Epilepsia*, 24 (2), 238–244, 1983.

Braestrup, C. and Squires, R.F., Specific benzodiazepine receptors in rat brain characterized by high-affinity (3H)diazepam binding, *Proc. Natl. Acad. Sci. U.S.A.*, 74 (9), 3805–3809, 1977.

Braestrup, C. and Squires, R.F., Brain specific benzodiazepine receptors, *Br. J. Psychiatry; J. Mental Sci.*, 133, 249–260, 1978a.

Braestrup, C. and Squires, R.F., Pharmacological characterization of benzodiazepine receptors in the brain, *Eur. J. Pharmacol.*, 48 (3), 263–270, 1978b.

Braestrup, C., Nielsen, M., and Olsen, C.E., Urinary and brain beta-carboline-3-carboxylates as potent inhibitors of brain benzodiazepine receptors, *Proc. Natl. Acad. Sci. U.S.A.*, 77 (4), 2288–2292, 1980.

Braestrup, C., Nielsen, M., Honore, T., Jensen, L.H., and Petersen, E.N., Benzodiazepine receptor ligands with positive and negative efficacy, *Neuropharmacology*, 22 (12B), 1451–1457, 1983.

Calignano, A. et al., Bidirectional control of airway responsiveness by endogenous cannabinoids, *Nature*, 408 (6808), 96–101, 2000.

Chen, Y. and Buck, J., Cannabinoids protects cells from oxidative cell death: a receptor-independent mechanism, *J. Pharmacol. Experimental Ther.*, 293 (3), 807–812, 2000.

Chu, C.J., Huang, S.M., De Petrocellis, L., Bisogno, T., Ewing, S.A., Miller, J.D., Zipkin, R.E., Daddario, N., Appendino, G., Di Marzo, V., and Walker, J.M., N-oleoyldopamine, a novel endogenous capsaicin-like lipid that produces hyperalgesia, *J. Biol. Chem.*, 278(16), 13633–13639, 2003.

Coker, K.H., Meditation and prostate cancer: integration a mind/body intervention with traditional therapies, *Semin. Urologic Oncol.*, 17 (2), 111–118, 1999.

Crawley, J.N., Corwin, R.L., Robinson, J.K., Felder, C.C., Devane, W.A., and Axelrod, J., Anandamide, an endogenous ligand of the cannabinoid receptor, induces hypomotility and hypothermia *in vivo* in rodents, *Pharmacol., Biochem., Behav.*, 46 (4), 967–972, 1993.

Devane, W.A. and Axelrod, J., Enzymatic synthesis of anandamide, an endogenous ligand for the cannabinoid receptor, by brain membranes, *Proc. Natl. Acad. Sci. U.S.A.*, 91 (14), 6698–6701, 1994.

Devane, W.A., Dysarz, III, F.A., Johnson, M.R., Melvin, L.S., and Howlett, A.C., Determination and characterization of a cannabinoid receptor in rat brain, *Molecular Pharmacol.*, 34 (5), 605–613, 1988.

Devane, W.A. et al., Isolation and structure of a brain constituent that binds to the cannabinoid receptor, *Science*, 258 (5090), 1946–1949, 1992.

Di Marzo, V., Biosynthesis and inactivation of endocannabinoids: relevance to their proposed role as neuromodulators, *Life Sci.*, 65 (6–7), 645–655, 1999.

Di Marzo, V. et al., Formation and inactivation of endogenous cannabinoid anandamide in central neurons, *Nature*, 372 (6507), 686–691, 1994.

Di Marzo, V. et al., Leptin-regulated endocannabinoids are involved in maintaining food intake, *Nature*, 410 (6830), 822–825, 2001.

Dorow, R., Horowski, R., Paschelke, G., and Amin, M., Severe anxiety induced by FG 7142, a beta-carboline ligand for benzodiazepine receptors, *Lancet*, 2 (8341), 98–99, 1983.

Duka, T., Stephens, D.N., Krause, W., and Dorow, R., Human studies on the benzodiazepine receptor antagonist β-carboline ZK 93 426: preliminary observations on psychotropic activity, *Psychopharmacology*, 93 (4), 421–427, 1987.

Fekkes, D., Tuiten, A., Bom, I., and Pepplinkhuizen, L., Trytophan: a precursor for the endogenous synthesis of norharman in man, *Neurosci. Lett.*, 303 (3), 145–148, 2001.

Felder, C.C. and Glass, M., Cannabinoid receptors and their endogenous agonists, *Ann. Rev. Pharmacol. Toxicol.*, 38, 179–200, 1998.

Felder, C.C., Briley, E.M., Axelrod, J., Simpson, J.T., Mackie, K., and Devane, W.A., Anandamide, an endogenous cannabimimetic eicosanoid, binds to the cloned human cannabinoid receptor and stimulates receptor-mediated signal transduction, *Proc. Natl. Acad. Sci. U.S.A.*, 90 (16), 7656–7660, 1993.

Felder, C.C. et al., Isolation and measurement of the endogenous cannabinoid receptor agonist, anandamide, in brain and peripheral tissues of human and rat, *FEBS Lett.*, 16 (2–3), 231–235, 1996.

Ferrarese, C., Appollonio, I., Frigio, M., Gaini, S.M., Piolti, R., and Frattola, L., Benzodiazepine receptors and diazepam-binding inhibitor in human cerebral tumors, *Ann. Neurol.*, 26 (4), 564–568, 1989.

File, S.E., Pellow, S., and Braestrup, C., Effects of the beta-carboline, FG 7142, in the social interaction test of anxiety and the holeboard: correlations between behaviour and plasma concentrations, *Pharmacol., Biochem., and Behav.*, 22 (6), 941–944, 1985.

Gallily, R., Breuer, A., and Mechoulam, R., 2-Arachidonyglycerol, an endogenous cannabinoid, inhibits tumor necrosis factor-alpha production in murine macrophages, and in mice, *Eur. J. Pharmacol.*, 406 (1), R5–R7, 2000.

Garfinkel, D., Zisapel, N., Wainstein, J., and Laudon, M., Facilitation of benzodiazepine discontinuation by melatonin: a new clinical approach, *Arch. Intern. Med.*, 159 (20), 2456–2460, 1999.

Garthwaite, J., Charles, S.L., and Chess-Williams, R., Endothelium-derived relaxing factor release on activation of NMDA receptors suggests role as intercellular messenger in the brain, *Nature*, 336 (6197), 385–388, 1988.

Germano, M.P. et al., Cannabinoid CB1-mediated inhibition of stress-induced gastric ulcers in rats, *Naunyn-Schmiedeberg's Arch. Pharmacol.*, 363 (2), 241–244, 2001.

Gilbert, S.S., van den Heuvel, C.J., and Dawson, D., Daytime melatonin and temazepam in young adult humans: equivalent effects on sleep latency and body temperatures, *J. Physiol.*, 514 (Pt 3), 905–914, 1999.

Giuliani, D., Ferrari, F., and Ottani, A., The cannabinoid agonist HU 210 modifies rat behavioural responses to novelty and stress, *Pharmacological Res.: Off. J. Ital. Pharmacological Soc.*, 41 (1), 45–51, 2000.

Guidotti, A., Forchetti, C.M., Corda, M.G., Konkel, D., Bennett, C.D., and Costa, E., Isolation, characterization, and purification to homogeneity of an endogenous polypeptide with agonistic action on benzodiazepine receptors, *Proc. Natl. Acad. Sci. U.S.A.*, 80 (11), 3531–3535, 1983.

Haefely, W., Kulcsar, A., Mohler, H., Pieri, L., Polc, P., and Schaffner, R., Possible involvement of GABA in the central actions of benzodiazepines, *Adv. Biochemical Psychopharmacol.*, 14, 131–151, 1975.

Haefely, W.E., Martin, J.R., Richards, J.G., and Schoch, P., The multiplicity of actions of benzodiazepine receptor ligands, *Can. J. Psychiatry*, 38 (suppl. 4), S102–S108, 1993.

Hajos, N., Ledent, C., and Freund, T.F., Novel cannabinoid-sensitive receptor mediates inhibition of glutamatergic synaptic transmission in the hippocampus, *Neuroscience*, 106 (1), 1–4, 2001.

Hajos, N. et al., Cannabinoids inhibit hippocampal GABAergic transmission and network oscillations, *Eur. J. Neurosci.*, 12 (9), 3239–3249, 2000.

Hanus, L. et al., HU-308: a specific agonist for CB(2), a peripheral cannabinoid receptor, *Proc. Natl. Acad. Sci. U.S.A.*, 96 (25), 14228–14233, 1999.

Hanus, L. et al., 2-Arachidonyl glyceryl ether, an endogenous agonist of the cannabinoid CB(1) receptor, *Proc. Natl. Acad. Sci. U.S.A.*, 98 (7), 3662–3665, 2001.

Hao, S., Avraham, Y., Mechoulam, R., and Berry, E.M., Low dose anandamide affects food intake, cognitive function, neurotransmitter and corticosterone levels in diet-restricted mice, *Eur. J. Pharmacol.*, 392 (3), 147–156, 2000.

Herkenham, M. et al., Cannabinoid receptor localization in brain, *Proc. Natl. Acad. Sci. U.S.A.*, 87 (5), 1932–1936, 1990.

Hirsch, J.D., Photolabeling of benzodiazepine receptors spares [3H]propyl beta-carboline binding, *Pharmacol., Biochem., Behav.*, 16 (2), 245–248, 1982.

Hróbjartsson, A. and Gotzsche, P.C., Is the placebo powerless? An analysis of clinical trials comparing placebo with no treatment, *New England J. Med.*, 344 (21), 1594–1602, 2001.

Ishiguro, K., Taft, W.C., DeLorenzo, R.J., and Sartorelli, A.C., The role of benzodiazepine receptors in the induction of differentiation of HL-60 leukemia cells by benzodiazepines and purines, *J. Cellular Physiol.*, 131 (2), 226–234, 1987.

Iversen, L. and Chapman, V., Cannabinoids: a real prospect for pain relief, *Curr. Opinion Pharmacol.*, 2 (1), 50–55, 2002.

Jankovic, B.D., Isakovic, K., and Petrovic, S., Effect of pinealectomy on immune reactions in the rat, *Immunology*, 18 (1), 1–6, 1970.

Jevning, R., Wallace, R.K., and Beidebach, M., The physiology of meditation: a review; a wakeful hypometabolic integrated response, *Neurosci. Biobehavioral Rev.*, 16 (3), 415–424, 1992.

Kabat-Zinn, J., Lipworth, L., and Burney, R., Four-year follow-up of a meditation-based program for the self-regulation of chronic pain: treatment outcomes and compliance, *Clinical J. Pain*, 2 (3), 159–173, 1986.

Kabat-Zinn, J., Massion, A.O., and Kristeller, J., Effectiveness of a mindfulness-based stress reduction program in the treatment of anxiety disorders, *Am. J. Psychiatry*, 149 (7), 936–943, 1992.

Katona, I. et al., Distribution of CB1 cannabinoid in the amygdale and their role in the control of GABAergic transmission, *J. Neurosci.: Off. J. Soc. Neurosci.*, 21 (23), 9506–9518, 2001.

Khan, R., Daya, S., and Potgieter, B., Evidence for a modulation of the stress response by the pineal gland, *Experientia*, 46 (8), 860–862, 1990.

Kimura, T., Ohta, T., Watanabe, K., Yoshimura, H., and Yamamoto, I., Anandamide, an endogenous cannabinoid receptor ligand, also interacts with 5-hydroxytryptamine (5-HT) receptor, *Biological Pharm. Bull.*, 21 (3), 224–226, 1998.

Klein, T.W., Lane, B., Newton, C.A., and Friedman, H., The cannabinoid system and cytokine network, *Proc. Soc. Experimental Biol. Med.*, 225 (1), 1–8, 2000.

Klein, T.W., Newton, C.A., and Friedman, H., Cannabinoids and the immune system. *Pain Res. Manage.: J. Can. Pain Soc.*, 6 (2), 95–101, 2001.

Korneyev, A.Y., The role of the hypothalamic-pituitary-adrenocortical axis in memory-related effects of anxiolytics, *Neurobiol. Learning Memory*, 67 (1), 1–13, 1997.

Kreitzer, A.C. and Regehr, W.C., Retrograde inhibition of presynaptic calcium influx by endogenous cannabinoids at excitatory synapses onto Purkinje cells, *Neuron*, 29 (3), 567–570, 2001a.

Kreitzer, A.C. and Regehr, W.G., Cerebellar depolarization-induced suppression of inhibition is mediated by endogenous cannabinoids, *J. Neurosci.: Off. J. Soc. Neurosci.* 21 (20), RC174, 2001b.

Kurihara, J. et al., 2-Arachidonoylglycerol and anandamide oppositely modulate norepinephrine release from the rat heart sympathetic nerves, *Jpn. J. Pharmacol.*, 87 (1), 93–96, 2001.

Lawston, J., Borella, A., Robinson, J.K., and Whitaker-Azmitia, P.M., Changes in hippocampal morphology following chronic treatment with synthetic cannabinoid WIN 55,212-2, *Brain Res.*, 877 (2), 407–410, 2000.

Lee, M., Yang, K.H., and Kaminski, N.E., Effects of putative cannabinoid receptor ligands, anandamide and 2-arachidonyl-glycerol, on immune function in B6C3F1 mouse splenocytes, *J. Pharmacol. Experimental Ther.*, 275 (2), 529–536, 1995.

Li, G.L., Li, P., and Yang, X.L., Melatonin modulates gamma-aminobutyric acid(A) receptor-mediated currents on isolated carp retinal neurons, *Neurosci. Lett.*, 301 (1), 49–53, 2001.

Lissoni, P. et al., Effects of tetrahydrocannabinol on melatonin secretion in man, *Horm. Metab. Res.*, 18 (1), 77–78, 1986.

Llano, I., Leresche, N., and Marty, A., Calcium entry increases the sensitivity of cerebellar Purkinje cells to applied GABA and decreases inhibitory synaptic currents, *Neuron*, 6 (4), 565–574, 1991.

Lynn, A.B. and Herkenham, M., Localization of cannabinoid receptors and nonsaturable high-density cannabinoid binding sites in peripheral tissues of the rat: implications for receptor-mediated immune modulation by cannabinoids, *J. Pharmacol. Experimental Ther.* 268 (3),1612–1623, 1994.

Maestroni, G.J., The immunoneuroendocrine role of melatonin, *J. Pineal Res.*, 14 (1), 1–10, 1993.

Maestroni, G.J., MLT and the immune-hematopoietic system, *Adv. Experimental Med. Biol.*, 460, 395–405, 1999.

Maestroni, G.J., The immunotherapeutic potential of melatonin, *Expert Opinion Investigational Drugs*, 10 (3), 467–476, 2001.

Maestroni, G.J.M. and Conti, A., Role of the pineal neurohormone melatonin in the psycho-neuroendocrine-immune network, in *Psychoneuroimmunology*, 2nd ed., Ader, R., Felten, D.L., and Cohen, N., Eds., Academic Press, San Diego, 1991, pp. 495–513.

Maestroni, G.J., Conti, A., and Pierpaoli, W., Role of the pineal gland in immunity: circadian synthesis and release of melatonin modulates the antibody response and antagonizes the immunosuppressive effect of corticosterone, *J. Neuroimmunol.*, 13 (1), 19–30, 1986.

Maestroni, G.J., Conti, A., and Pierpaoli, W., Role of the pineal gland in immunity: II, melatonin enhances the antibody response via an opiatergic mechanism, *Clinical Experimental Immunol.*, 68 (2), 384–391, 1987.

Maestroni, G.J.M., Conti, A., and Pierpaoli, W., Melatonin, stress, and the immune system, in *Pineal Research Reviews*, Vol. 7, Reiter, R.J., Ed., Alan R. Liss, New York, 1989, pp. 203–226.

Marangos, P.J., Trams, E., Clark-Rosenberg, R.L., Paul, S.M., and Skolnick, P., Anticonvulsant doses of inosine result in brain levels sufficient to inhibit [3H] diazepam binding, *Psychopharmacology*, 75 (2), 175–178, 1981.

Martin, B.R., Mechoulam, R., and Razdan, R.K., Discovery and characterization of endogenous cannabinoids, *Life Sci.*, 65 (6–7), 573–595, 1999.

Martin, M., Ledent, C., Parmentier, M., Maldonado, R., and Valverde, O., Involvement of CB1 cannabinoid receptors in emotional behaviour, *Psychopharmacology*, 159 (4), 379–387, 2002.

Mason, L.I. et al., Electrophysiological correlates of higher states of consciousness during sleep in long-term practitioner of the transcendental meditation program, *Sleep*, 20 (2), 102–110, 1997.

Massion, A.O., Teas, J., Herbert, J.R., Wertheimer, M.D., and Kabat-Zinn, J., Meditation, melatonin and breast/prostrate cancer: hypothesis and preliminary data, *Medical Hypotheses*, 44 (1), 39–46, 1995.

Matsuda, L.A., Molecular aspects of cannabinoid receptors, *Crit. Rev. Neurobiol.*, 11 (2–3), 143–166, 1997.

Matsuda, L.A., Lolait, S.J., Brownstein, M.J., Young, A.C., and Bonner, T.I., Structure of a cannabinoid receptor and functional expression of the cloned cDNA, *Nature*, 346 (6248) 561–564, 1990.

Matsuda, L.A., Bonner, T.I., and Lolait, S.J., Localization of cannabinoid receptor mRNA in rat brain, *J. Comp. Neurol.*, 327 (4), 535–550, 1993.

Mazzone, A. et al., Increased expression of peripheral benzodiazepine receptors on leukocytes in silent myocardial ischemia, *J. Am. Coll. Cardiol.*, 36 (3), 746–750, 2000.

Mechoulam, R., Recent advantages in cannabinoid research, *Forschende Komplementarmedizin*, 6 (suppl. 3), 16–20, 1999.

Mechoulam, R., Braun, P., and Gaoni, Y., Synthesis of 1-tetrahydrocannabinol and related cannabinoids, *J. Am. Chemical Soc.*, 94 (17), 6159–6165, 1972a.

Mechoulam, R., Varconi, H., Ben-Zvi, Z., Edery, H., and Grunfeld, Y., Synthesis and biological activity of five tetrahydrocannabinol metabolites, *J. Am. Chemical Soc.*, 94 (22), 7930–7931, 1972b.

Mechoulam, R. et al., Identification of an endogenous 2-monoglyceride, present in canine gut, that binds to cannabinoid receptors, *Biochemical Pharmacol.*, 50 (1), 83–90, 1995.

Mohler, H. and Okada, T., Benzodiazepine receptor: demonstration in the central nervous system, *Science*, 198 (4319), 849–851, 1977.

Mohler, H. and Okada, T., The benzodiazepine receptor in normal and pathological human brain, *Br. J. Psychiatry; J. Mental Sci.*, 133, 261–268, 1978.

Mohler, H., Okada, T., Heitz, P., and Ulrich, J., Biochemical identification of the site of action of benzodiazepines in human brain by 3H-diazepam binding, *Life Sci.*, 22 (11), 985–995, 1978b.

Mohler, H., Polc, P., Cumin, R., Pieri, L., and Kettler, R., Nicotinamide is a brain constituent with benzodiazepine-like actions, *Nature*, 278 (5704), 563–565, 1979.

Moingeon, P., Bidart, J.M., Alberici, G.F., and Bohuon, C., Characterization of a peripheral-type benzodiazepine binding site on human circulating lymphocytes, *Eur. J. Pharmacol.*, 92 (1–2), 147–149, 1983.

Moingeon, P. et al., Benzodiazepine receptors on human blood platelets, *Life Sci.*, 35 (20), 2003–2009, 1984.

Molina-Holgado, F., Molina-Holgado, E., and Guaza, C., The endogenous cannabinoid anandamide potentiates interleukin-6 production by astrocytes infected with Theiler's murine encephalomyelitis virus by a receptor-mediated pathway, *FEBS Lett.*, 433 (1–2), 139–142, 1998.

Monteleone, P., Forziati, D., Orazzo, C., and Maj, M., Preliminary observations on the suppression of nocturnal plasma melatonin levels by short-term administration of diazepam in humans, *J. Pineal Res.*, 6 (3), 253–258, 1989.

Mullen, K.D., Szauter, K.M., and Kaminsky-Russ, K., "Endogenous" benzodiazepine activity in body fluids of patients with hepatic encephalopathy, *Lancet*, 336 (8707), 81–83, 1990.

Munro, S., Thomas, K.L., and Abu-Shaar, M., Molecular characterization of a peripheral receptor for cannabinoids, *Nature*, 365 (6441), 61–65, 1993.

Murphy, D.L., Garrick, N.A., Tamarkin, L., Taylor, P.L., and Markey, S.P., Effects of antidepressants and other psychotropic drugs on melatonin release and pineal gland function, *J. Neural Transmission. Supplementum*, 21, 291–309, 1986.

Murphy, L.L., Munoz, R.M., Adrian, B.A., and Villanua, M.A., Function of cannabinoid receptors in the neuroendocrine regulation of hormone secretion, *Neurobiol. Disease*, 5 (6), 432–446, 1998.

Naguib, M. and Samarkandi, A.H., Premedication with melatonin: a double-blind, placebo-controlled comparison with midazolam, *Br. J. Anaesthesia*, 82 (6), 875–880, 1999.

Naguib, M. and Samarkandi, A.H., The comparative dose-response effects of melatonin and midazolam for premedication of adult patients: a double-blinded, placebo-controlled study, *Anesthesia Analgesia*, 91 (2), 473–479, 2000.

Nong, L., Newton, C., Friedman, H., and Klein, T.W., CB1 and CB2 receptor MRNA expression in human peripheral blood mononuclear cells (PBMC) from various donor types, *Adv. Experimental Med. Biol.*, 493, 229–233, 2001.

Ohno-Shosaku, T., Maejima, T., and Kano, M., Endogenous cannabinoids mediate retrograde signals from depolarized postsynaptic neurons to presynaptic terminals, *Neuron*, 29 (3), 729–738, 2001.

Ornish, D. et al., Effects of stress management training and dietary changes in treating ischemic heart disease, *JAMA: J. Am. Medical Assoc.*, 249 (1), 54–59, 1983.

Ornish, D. et al., Intensive lifestyle changes for reversal of coronary heart disease, *JAMA: J. Am. Medical Assoc.*, 280 (23), 2001–2007, 1998.

Panikashvili, D. et al., An endogenous cannabinoid (2-AG) is neuroprotective after brain injury, *Nature*, 413 (6855), 527–531, 2001.

Papadopoulos, V., Peripheral-type benzodiazepine/diazepan binding inhibitor receptor: biological role in seroidogenic cell funcion. *Endocr. Rev.*, 14(2), 222–240, 1993.

Pauwels, P.J., Diverse signaling by 5-hydroxytryptamine (5-HT) receptors, *Biochemical Pharmacol.*, 60 (12), 1743–1750, 2000.

Pierpaoli, W. and Maestroni, G.J., Melatonin: a principal neuroimmunoregulatory and anti-stress hormone: its anti-aging effects, *Immunol. Lett.*, 16 (3–4), 355–361, 1987.

Piomelli, D., Giuffrida, A., Calignano, A., and Rodriguez de Fonseca, F., The endocannabinoid system as a target for therapeutic drugs, *Trends Pharmacological Sci.*, 21 (6), 218–224, 2000.

Pomilio, A.B., Vitale, A.A., Ciprian-Ollivier, J., Cetkovich-Bakmas, M., Gomez, R., and Vazquez, G., Ayahuasca: an experimental psychosis that mirrors the transmethylation hypothesis of schizophrenia, *J. Ethnopharmacol.*, 65 (1), 29–51, 1999.

Porter A.C., Saver, J.M., Knierman, M.D., Becker, G.W., Berner, M.J., Bao, J., Nomikos, G.G., Carter, P., Bymaster, F.P., Leese, A.B., and Felder, C.C., Characterization of a novel endocannabinoid, virodhame, with antagonist activity at the CB1 receptor, *J. Pharmacol. Exp. Ther.*, 301(3), 1020–1024, 2002.

Prado de Carvalho, L.P., Grecksch, G., Chapouthier, G., and Rossier, J., Anxiogenic and non-anxiogenic benzodiazepine antagonists, *Nature*, 301 (5895), 64–66, 1983.

Priller, J., Briley, E.M., Mansouri, J., Devane, W.A., Mackie, K., and Felder, C.C., Mead ethanolamide, a novel eicosanoid, is an agonist for the central (CB1) and peripheral (CB2) cannabinoid receptors, *Molecular Pharmacol.*, 48 (2), 288–292, 1995.

Raghavendra, V., Kaur, G., and Kulkarni, S.K., Anti-depressant action of melatonin in chronic forced swimming-induced behavioral despair in mice, role of peripheral benzodiazepine receptor modulation, *Eur. Neuropsychopharmacol.: J. Eur. Coll. Neuropsychopharmacol.*, 10 (6), 473–481, 2000.

Riba, J. et al., Subjective effects and tolerability of the South American psychoactive beverage Ayahuasca in healthy volunteers, *Psychopharmacology*, 154 (1), 85–95, 2001.

Rocca, P., Bellone, G., Benna, P., Bergamasco, B., Ravizza, L., and Ferrero, P., Peripheral-type benzodiazepine receptors and diazepam binding inhibitor-like immunoreactivity distribution in human peripheral blood mononuclear cells, *Immunopharmacology*, 25 (2), 163–178, 1993.

Rohrer, T., von Richtofen, V., Schulz, C., Beyer, J., and Lehnert, H., The stress-, but not corticotropin-releasing hormone-induced activation of the pituitary-adrenal axis in man is blocked by alprazolam, *Horm. Metab. Res.*, 26 (4), 200–206, 1994.

Rommelspacher, H., Nanz, C., Borbe, H.O., Fehske, K.J., Muller, W.E., and Wollert, U., Benzodiazepine antagonism by harmane and other beta-carbolines *in vitro* and *in vivo*, *Eur. J. Pharmacol.*, 70 (3), 409–416, 1981.

Rommelspacher, H., May, T., and Salewski, B., Harman (1-methyl-beta-carboline) is a natural inhibitor of monoamine oxidase type A in rats, *Eur. J. Pharmacol.*, 252 (1), 51–59, 1994.

Rothstein, J.D., Garland, W., Puia, G., Guidotti, A., Weber, R.J., and Costa, E., Purification and characterization of naturally occurring benzodiazepine receptor ligands in rat and human brain, *J. Neurochem.*, 58 (6), 2102–2115, 1992.

Ruff, M.R., Pert, C.B., Weber, R.J., Wahl, L.M., Wahl, S.M., and Paul, S.M., Benzodiazepine receptor-mediated chemotaxis of human monocytes, *Science*, 229 (4719), 1281–1283, 1985.

Salman, H. et al., Effect of diazepam on the immune response of rats exposed to acute and chronic swim stress, *Biomed. Pharmacother.*, 54 (6), 311–315, 2000.

Salzet, M., Breton, C., Bisogno, T., and Di Marzo, V., Comparative biology of the endocannabinoid system: possible role in the immune response, *Eur. J. Biochem./FEBS*, 267 (16), 4917–4927, 2000.

Sarafian, T.A., Tashkin, D.P., and Roth, M.D., Marijuana smoke and Delta(9)-tetrahydrocannabinol promote necrotic cell death but inhibit Fas-mediated apoptosis, *Toxicol. Appl. Pharmacol.*, 174 (3), 264–272, 2001.

Savic, I., Persson, A., Roland, P., Pauli, S., Sedvall, G., and Widen, L., *In-vivo* demonstration of reduced benzodiazepine receptor binding in human epileptic foci, *Lancet*, 2 (8616), 863–866, 1988.

Schwarz, H., Blanco, F.J., and Lotz, M., Anandamide, an endogenous cannabinoid receptor agonist inhibits lymphocyte proliferation and induces apoptosis, *J. Neuroimmunol.*, 55 (1), 107–115, 1994.

Sinha, D., Bonner, T.I., Bhat, N.R., and Matsuda, L.A., Expression of the CB1 cannabinoid receptor in macrophage-like cells from brain-tissue: immunochemical characterization by fusion protein antibodies, *J. Neuroimmunol.*, 82 (1), 13–21, 1998.

Skelton, K.H., Nemeroff, C.B., Knight, D.L., and Owens, M.J., Chronic administration of the triazolobenzodiazepine alprazolam produces opposite effects on corticotropin-releasing factor and urocortin neuronal systems, *J. Neurosci.*, 20 (3), 1240–1248, 2000.

Skolnick, P., Marangos, P.J., Goodwin, F.K., Edwards, M., and Paul, S., Identification of inosine and hypoxanthine as endogenous inhibitors of [3H] diazepam binding in the central nervous system, *Life Sci.*, 23 (14), 1473–1480, 1978.

Stella, N., Schweitzer, P., and Piomelli, D., A second endogenous cannabinoid that modulates long-term potentiation, *Nature*, 388 (6644), 773–778, 1997.

Stone, B.M., Turner, C., Mills, S.L., and Nicholson, A.N., Hypnotic activity of melatonin, *Sleep*, 23(5), 663–669, 2000.

Strassman, R.J. and Qualls, C.R., Dose-response study of *N,N*-dimethyltryptamine in humans: I, neuroendocrine, autonomic, and cardiovascular effects, *Arch. Gen. Psychiatry*, 51 (2), 85–97, 1994.

Strassman, R., *DMT: The Spirit Molecule*, Park Street Press, Rochester, VT, 2001.

Sugiura, T. and Waku, K., 2-Arachidonoylglycerol and the cannabinoid receptors, *Chem. Phys. Lipids*, 108 (1–2), 89–106, 2000.

Sugiura, T. et al., 2-Arachidonoylglycerol: a possible endogenous cannabinoid receptor ligand in brain, *Biochemical Biophysical Res. Commn.*, 215 (1), 89–97, 1995.

Sugiura, T. et al., Evidence that the cannabinoid CB1 receptor is a 2-arachidonoylglycerol receptor: structure-activity relationship of 2-arachidonoylglycerol, ether-linked analogues, and related compounds, *J. Biological Chem.*, 274 (5), 2794–2801, 1999.

Suhara, Y. et al., Synthesis and biological activities of novel structural analogues of 2-arachidonoylglycerol, an endogenous cannabinoid receptor ligand, *Bioorganic Medicinal Chem. Lett.*, 11 (15), 1985–1988, 2001.

Sullivan, J.M., Mechanisms of cannabinoid-receptor-mediated inhibition of synaptic transmission in cultured hippocampal pyramidal neurons, *J. Neurophysiol.*, 82 (3), 1286–1294, 1999.

Tallman, J.F., Paul, S.M., Skolnick, P., and Gallager, D.W., Receptors for the age of anxiety: pharmacology of the benzodiazepines, *Science*, 207 (4428), 274–281, 1980.

Teuber, L., Watjens, F., and Jensen, L.H., Ligands for the benzodiazepine binding site—a survey, *Curr. Pharm. Design*, 5 (5), 317–343, 1999.

Tooley, G.A., Armstrong, S.M., Norman, T.R., and Sali, A., Acute increases in night-time plasma melatonin levels following a period of meditation, *Biological Psychol.*, 53 (1), 69–78, 2000.

Tse, S.Y., Mak, I.T., and Dickens, B.F., Antioxidative properties of harmane and beta-carboline alkaloids, *Biochemical Pharmacol.*, 42 (3), 459–464, 1991.

Twitchell, W., Brown, S., and Mackie, K., Cannabinoids inhibit N- and P/Q-type calcium channels in cultured rat hippocampal neurons, *J. Neurophysiol.* 78 (1), 43–50, 1997.

Valverde, O., Ledent, C., Beslot, F., Parmentier, M., and Roques, B.P., Reduction of stress-induced analgesia but not of exogenous opioid effects in mice lacking CB1 receptors, *Eur. J. Neurosci.*, 12 (2), 533–539, 2000.

Venturini, I. et al., Up-regulation of peripheral benzodiazepine receptor system in hepatocellular carcinoma, *Life Sci.*, 63 (14), 1269–1280, 1998.

Vincent, P. and Marty, A., Neighboring cerebellar Purkinje cells communicate via retrograde inhibition of common presynaptic interneurons, *Neuron*, 11 (5), 885–893, 1993.

Walker, J.M., Hohmann, A.G., Martin, W.J., Strangman, N.M., Huang, S.M., and Tsou, K., The neurobiology of cannabinoid analgesia, *Life Sci.*, 65 (6–7), 665–673, 1999a.

Walker, J.M., Huang, S.M., Strangman, N.M., Tsou, K., and Sanudo-Pena, M.C., Pain modulation by release of the endogenous cannabinoid anandamide, *Proc. Natl. Acad. Sci. U.S.A.*, 96 (21), 198–203, 1999b.

Walker, J.M., Strangman, N.M., and Huang, S.M., Cannabinoids and pain, *Pain Res. Manage.: J. Can. Pain Soc.*, 6 (2), 74–79, 2001.

Walker, J.M., Krey, J.F., Chu, C.J., and Huang, S.M., Endocannabinoids and related fatty acid derivatives in pain modulation, *Chem. Phys. Lipids*, 121 (1–2), 159–172, 2002.

Weidenfeld, J., Feldman, S., and Mechoulam, R., Effect of the brain constituent anandamide, a cannabinoid receptor agonist, on the hypothalamo-pituitary-adrenal axis in the rat, *Neuroendocrinology*, 59 (2), 110–112, 1994.

Wilson, R.I., Kunos, G., and Nicoll, R.A., Presynaptic specificity of endocannabinoid signaling in the hippocampus, *Neuron*, 31 (3), 453–462, 2001.

Zavala, F., Benzodiazepines, anxiety and immunity, *Pharmacol. Ther.*, 75 (3), 199–216, 1997.

Zimmer, A., Zimmer, A.M., Hohmann, A.G., Herkenham, M., and Bonner, T.I., Increased mortality, hypoactivity, and hypoalgesia in cannabinoid CB1 receptor knockout mice, *Proc. Natl. Acad. Sci. U.S.A.*, 96 (10), 5780–5785, 1999.

ADDITIONAL RESOURCES

Kabat-Zinn, J., *Full Catastrophe Living*, Delacorte, New York, 1990.

Kabat-Zinn, J. et al., Influence of a mindfulness meditation-based stress reduction intervention on rates of skin clearing in patients with moderate to severe psoriasis undergoing phototherapy (UVB) and photochemotherapy (PUVA), *Psychosomatic Med.*, 60 (5), 625–632, 1998.

Stress Reduction Clinic, University of Massachusetts Memorial Medical Center, Worcester, MA; available on-line at http://nccam.nih.gov/fcp/classify.

5 The Relaxation System: Therapeutic Modalities

CONTENTS

INTRODUCTION

This chapter presents a review of various healing modalities. The National Center for Complementary and Alternative Medicine (NCCAM), which is part of the National Institutes of Health (NIH), designates five major domains of complementary and alternative medical practices: (1) alternative medical systems, (2) mind–body interventions, (3) biologically based treatments, (4) manipulative and body-based methods, and (5) energy therapies. Each of these categories is comprised of numerous individual systems and treatments for which the NIH provides research support. We have chosen to organize our review by beginning with the mechanical modalities and then continuing to those that are subtler in nature, or the so-called energy therapies. However, note the correlation between our categories and those of the NIH. Techniques of healing that correspond to each category are described in our review. If after perusing the chapter, you may want to research a particular technique and the bibliography provides a variety of resources.

MECHANICAL ENERGY

The following subsections provide some examples of manual medicine or body manipulation.

OSTEOPATHY

Andrew Taylor Still, a physician and an ordained minister, developed the diagnostic and therapeutic techniques of osteopathy after losing three of his children to cerebrospinal meningitis in 1864. Feeling that conventional medical practice was inadequate for the effective treatment of most illnesses, he introduced his concepts of osteopathy 10 years later and opened the first school of osteopathy in 1892 in Kirksville, Missouri. Still based his new methodology on the principle that the body is structurally and functionally one reciprocally interrelated system. Still felt strongly that the body has an inherent ability to repair itself and believed that the healthy body is a homeostitic unit, no a collection of functioning parts. It appears that medical science today is once again coming to terms with that fact.

Still's diagnostic techniques included an evaluation of posture, joint function, the network of myofascial tissue, as well as the respiratory and lymphatic systems. For many years osteopathy was primarily known for, the osteopathic manipulations he developed to restore the body's homeostasis. The high-velocity, low-frequency technique (a thrust with an audible "pop") is the best known manipulation and has been sanctioned by chiropractors as well as osteopaths. Other techniques involve palpating the skin or muscle to release muscle spasm or myofascial tissue and to permit lymphatic drainage. However, osteopathy also incorporates a spectrum of therapeutic techniques, including nutrition, physical therapy, and conventional allopathic medical modalities such as pharmaceuticals and surgery.

A doctor of osteopathy (DO) has full medical licensing and practicing ability in the United States today. Yet, for the last 50 years or so, most DOs have divorced themselves from the classic osteopathic manipulation techniques and have largely practiced conventional medicine. It is notable that although doctor remuneration by insurance companies for the manipulation techniques are currently inadequate, there is a small group of DOs who are bringing back what is nearly a lost art of osteopathic manipulation (e.g., Magnus and Gamber, 1997). Osteopathic manipulation, coupled with the broader spectrum of osteopathic care, is currently used for numerous musculoskeletal injuries, childhood otitis media, and various respiratory conditions. Published research largely involves reviews, case studies, description of techniques, or warnings of neurological complications. The few efficacy studies that can be found appear to be quite mixed, but they do seem to be strongest for musculoskeletal conditions (Bronfort et al., 2001b; Jarski et al., 2000; Jermyn, 2001; Pratt-Harrington, 2000; Richards et al., 1999; Tettambel, 2001; Van Buskirk, 1996; Vicenzino et al., 1996; Williams, 1997).

CRANIOSACRAL THERAPY

The craniosacral system involves the brain, spinal cord, and cerebrospinal fluid (CSF). In the late 19th century, William Garner Sutherland, who was a DO, discovered that the joints between skull bones have a small but palpable range of motion, as do all other joints throughout the body. He also discovered that the dural membranes that cover the CNS have a palpable range of motion. The dura is connected to the sacral and cranial bones, where a similar range of motion can be detected. Furthermore, Sutherland determined that there is a subtle rhythm, which he termed the cranial rhythmic impulse (CRI), that is part of a physiological and mechanistic structure concerned with the body's inherent motility, called the *primary respiratory mechanism* (PRM). The CRI emanates throughout the body via the fascia (connective tissue) and the CSF (Magoun, 1976). The CRI cannot be detected on cadavers; it is an energetic phenomenon of life. To the skilled professional who can detect the delicate tactile impression, it is the palpable manifestation of the cyclic fluctuation (rather than circulating flow) of the CSF. It is a resonance that spreads throughout the body, meaning that the CRI that can be felt in the head occurs in conjunction with a fluctuation throughout the body. Cranial osteopathy involves gentle manipulation to the cranial area. A book published by the Sutherland Cranial Teaching Foundation explains that the therapeutic manipulations change the rate and amplitude of the fluctuation of the CSF and thus may have profound therapeutic effects (Magoun, 1976). Effects that extend to other parts of the body via the fascia often produce release of suppressed, emotionally laden memories. An energy transfer is said to occur between the practitioner and the patient, restoring balance to physical or emotional dysfunction.

While researchers found that both the subject's and the practitioner's CRI rhythms are not related to their respective respiratory or heart rates, the CRI rate of a patient, determined by two practitioners, is generally not the same. However, one practitioner can quite consistently palpate a CRI in the same patient at a consistent rate (Hanten et al., 1998). This study, in spite of its curious findings, states that "it is possible that the perception of CSR [craniosacral rhythm] is illusory." Most of the few other scientific studies belay the authors' skeptical attitudes, and much of the literature appears to be unable to validate Sutherland's findings (e.g., Green et al., 1999; Rogers et al., 1998). One study supporting the use of craniosacral therapy proposes that the functional origin of CRI is the harmonizing of electrical signals from various body functions, particularly from signals between the sympathetic and parasympathetic systems. This palpable harmonization is an entrainment of multiple biological oscillators. The researchers go on to speculate that skilled practitioners, who are versed with centering techniques, can also entrain their bodies with the patient's, accessing the patient's CRI for therapeutic benefit (McPartland and Mein, 1997).

In the 1970s, John Upledger, DO, created craniosacral therapy based on Sutherland's discoveries. The technique is taught to a variety of healthcare professionals, from medical doctors to those performing various types of bodywork, and requires no medical licensing. Craniosacral therapy is said to be useful for the alleviation of pain from accidents, for stress-related symptoms, for sensory disorders, and to promote overall health.

The Cranial Academy was established by Sutherland's students to teach, research, and advance the techniques of cranial osteopathy. The Academy distinguishes itself by certifying only osteopathic doctors, medical doctors, or doctors of dentistry and by requiring approved courses in cranial osteopathy. Cranial osteopathy is based on the same principles of osteopathic care, which emphasize treating the whole body and not any one symptom.

CHIROPRACTIC

Chiropractic treatment is a complementary modality with a long history of prejudice against its use. Daniel David Palmer, who restored hearing to a man by adjusting his thoracic vertebrae, developed the treatment in the 1880s. The profession was essentially legalized in 1987 when an injunction against the American Medical Association (AMA) ordered the AMA to cease its discriminatory practices against chiropractic care, a decision that the Supreme Court let stand in 1990. Chiropractic treatment involves manipulating the spine in order to correct structural imbalances, thus restoring nerve function. A misalignment in the spine is thought to cause a subluxation, which is a slight dislocation of bones within a joint. Currently, the term is used to refer to any type of vertebral blockage, but most often nerve entrapment. Chiropractors believe that such neurophysiological imbalances not only create pain in the body, but also reduce the effective functioning of the body's immune system, leaving the individual more susceptible to disease. Thus, proper alignment of the spine results in optimal health. Currently, chiropractic treatment is prescribed for a variety of conditions, including injury, asthma, migraine and other forms of headache, and neck or back pain, with results of mixed efficacy (Balon et al., 1998; Bove and Nilsson, 1998; Bronfort et al., 2001a; Conway, 2001; Jordan et al., 1998; Meade et al., 1990; Nelson et al., 1998; Tuchin et al., 2000). While complications may occur (Stevinson et al., 2001), studies generally show distinct improvement for some types of disorders as well as a reduction in overall side effects when compared with the side effects of pharmaceuticals (Freeman and Lawlis, 2001; Nelson et al., 1998).

MASSAGE

Massage, which appears to be as old as recorded history, is a manipulation of the soft tissues (i.e., skin, muscles, and fascia) of the body. The tissues are loosened and proper blood supply restored to these areas, resulting in a state of total body relaxation. Massage is also known to promote venous and lymphatic drainage (Freeman and Lawlis, 2001). In addition massage benefits the muscles, skeleton, and nervous system. It affects the ANS, which may reduce pain, support the immune system, and reduce anxiety (Chen and Chen, 1998; Cherkin et al., 2001; Zeitlin et al., 2000). Currently there are a variety of massage techniques used, but most originate from the work of Pehr Henrik Ling and his "Swedish massage" therapy. While, historically speaking, massage is considered effective for pain relief and relaxation, it is also known to elicit feelings and memories of emotional trauma. Several bodywork techniques have evolved in recent years that directly address the issue of the mind–body interface in bodywork, acknowledging the correlation between manipulation of the body and the releasing of deep emotions. Rolfing and the Trager method are just two examples of such approaches.

ROLFING®

Rolfing was named after Ida Rolf, who developed the technique of manipulating connective tissue, or fascia, to restore the body to a state of equilibrium in relationship to the earth's gravitational forces. Her theory is based on the premise that if the body's weight transmission is in a vertical central axis, it will move more efficiently and gracefully. Treatment requires ten sessions, each scheduled about a week apart. As the body is brought to this vertical position, it is thought that the sensations of pain that occur are the sites at which the body has stored emotional trauma. The practitioner applies sufficient force to stretch and move tissue, liberating old patterns of holding myofascial tissue and releasing emotions. The treatment can release lifelong patterns of tension. The result is often a more balanced manner of moving, which is mirrored by an increase in vitality and emotional well-being (Rolf Institute, 1976).

TRAGER® METHOD

Dr. Milton Trager developed the Trager approach to bodywork in 1927. The technique is intended to help the patient release patterns of tension held in the body. The first part of the therapy involves a treatment called *psychosocial integration*, which entails light rhythmic rocking intended to produce a pleasurable experience and meditative state called the *hookup*. The mind–body interface promotes deep relaxation and the release of old pains and improves the patient's flexibility and range of motion. Unlike Rolfing, the focus of treatment is on the psyche of the individual rather than the physiological changes. The Trager method sees the body as a vehicle to help the psyche achieve a sense of well-being. The second part of treatment, called *mentastics*® or *mental gymnastics*, involves learning exercise movements that can be performed at home. The movements are often free-flowing or dancelike. The exercise has repetitive components that are both physically and mentally relaxing and that reinforce the work of the practitioner (Trager and Hammond, 1987).

CHEMICAL ENERGY

PHARMACEUTICALS

Whether plant-derived or synthetically manufactured, pharmaceuticals today are central to conventional medical treatment, but that was not always so. Two significant events occurred in the latter half of the 19th century that changed the course of medicine. First, the AMA successfully established state licensing laws for physicians, and by 1900 these laws had been enacted in every state. Second, medical education and practice were swept up in scientifically based laboratory research capable of identifying the causes of infectious diseases. Then, in 1910, medicine as we now know it was resolutely established with the publication of a paper, "Medical education in the United States and Canada," by Abraham Flexner (funded by the Carnegie Foundation) espousing that all U.S. medical schools use a scientific-based curriculum or be shut down. Natural substances (e.g., herbs) continued to be used in a cause-and-effect manner until the 1930s, when researchers synthesized the first pharmaceuticals, which resulted in a process of phasing out natural substances. The entire perspective toward medicine changed from a focus on all aspects of the individual's health (i.e., mind, body, and spirit) to reductionism and a mechanistic view of the human body. While the understanding of microbes and the development of drugs that could expunge diseases that had killed thousands of people through the ages were enormous contributions to the welfare of all people, it unfortunately came at the cost of losing sight of the whole person.

HERBS

Pharmacognosy (i.e., the scientific study of the therapeutic uses of plants) is the predecessor of the modern pharmaceutical industry. Sometimes referred to as phytomedicine, the use of plants to effectively relieve ailments is an integral part of the indigenous cultures in every part of the world (e.g., aspirin, which is derived from the white willow bark [*Salix alba*], was used to relieve pain for many years before its chemical properties were understood). Attempts to assess the active ingredient of an herb are often a challenge. The difficulty arises because the plant itself may have more than one active ingredient, or its efficacy may result from the interaction of various ingredients. For over 1500 years, physicians have kept records of plants and their healing properties in books called *Materia Medica*. Today the most accurate and authoritative source of information on medicinal plants, both for efficacy and safety, is *The Complete German Commission E Monographs: Therapeutic Guide to Herbal Medicines*, which was translated and published in English in 1998 (Blumenthal, 1998).

SUPPLEMENTS

Supplements include vitamins, minerals, amino acids, and enzymes. While the efficacy of some supplements has been scientifically tested, most decisions concerning the use of supplements are made by the consumer. Recommended dietary allowances (RDAs) of vitamins and minerals were first established in the United States in 1943. As a result, fortified foods generally ensured that the vast majority of the population would receive levels of these supplements adequate to avoid diseases such as rickets. The RDAs originally were intended only to prevent diseases caused by gross deficiency. Health Canada and the Institute of Medicine of the Academy of Science in the United States are currently revising and replacing RDAs with dietary reference intakes (DRIs). The DRIs are based on myriad scientific studies of cellular and molecular functions of vitamins and micronutrients. These new adequacy criteria are intended to help prevent the development of chronic degenerative diseases such as osteoporosis, which generally take decades to manifest (Institute of Medicine, 1999, 2000; McDermott, 2000; Trumbo et al., 2001). The new levels, however, neither take into account environmental or lifestyle factors that destroy vital nutrients nor consider increasing the levels in the presence of serious disease. Currently, therapeutic use of supplements is not commonly practiced by conventional physicians, which is primarily due to lack of knowledge. Therapeutic prescription of supplements largely remains in the hands of naturopaths, herbalists, or the rare physician who has knowledge of alternative medicine.

LIGHT MODALITIES

The divine light illuminates the soul of man.

Proverbs 20:27

FULL-SPECTRUM AND BRIGHT-LIGHT THERAPY

Full-spectrum light, like sunlight, includes all wavelengths of light, from infrared to ultraviolet (UV). Bright light includes all but the UV end of the full spectrum. In 1984 Dr. Norman E. Rosenthal first defined the condition of seasonal affective disorder (SAD), and in 1985 he described the first application of bright artificial light for its treatment (Rosenthal et al., 1984, 1985). SAD appears to stem from dysfunction in secretion patterns of melatonin from the pineal gland and from abnormally low wintertime secretions of serotonin in the CNS. Research has shown that patients with SAD have abnormally delayed circadian rhythms (Sack et al., 1990). In other words, they do not secrete melatonin at the appropriate nighttime hour. Bright or full-spectrum light, but not ordinary indoor light, can advance (i.e., shift to an earlier time) the onset of nighttime melatonin production in humans. Recent research has shown that morning light treatment (administered in circadian time at 8.5 hours after melatonin is endogenously released) is more effective than late morning or evening treatment (Terman et al., 2001). Light therapy appears to be most effective at 10,000 lux for at least 30 minutes but takes about 3 weeks for therapeutic benefit to occur (Eastman et al., 1998; Terman et al., 1998). Bulbs producing bright white light, lacking the UV end of the spectrum, are sometimes used as they are just as effective for depression, but they avoid side effects of sunburn and eye damage (Lam et al., 1992). However, some technicians selling therapeutic light products claim that sunburn and eye damage is an issue created by researchers and not a side effect that their clients ever encounter. Technicians receive complaints of glare with bright light but not with full spectrum.

Other research has indicated that infrared may be just as effective as bright light in the amelioration of SAD (Meesters, 1999). In addition to relieving depression, light therapy reduces symptoms that often accompany SAD, such as poor vision and skin irritation (Terman and Terman, 1999). Light therapy also reduces suicidal ideation but not symptoms of bulimia nervosa, which is frequently comorbid in women with SAD (Lam et al., 2000, 2001). Michael and Jiuan Su Terman, who have been central to the research on SAD, have shown that in addition to bright light, high-density negative air ionization also appears to be effective for SAD. The National Institute of Mental Health (NIMH) is currently conducting a clinical trial to assess the efficacy of both bright light boxes and negative ion generators. There are various devices that deliver full-spectrum or bright light are available for home use (Breiling, 1996).

ULTRAVIOLET (UV) THERAPY

The UV radiation spectrum is composed of three wavelengths: UVB (the short-wavelength spectrum of 238 to 320 nm, which can cause sunburn), UVA (the long-wavelength spectrum of 320 to 400 nm, which can produce tanning without sunburn), and UVC (a wavelength spectrum of 100 to 280 nm, which is lethal to pathogenic organisms). UV radiation does not penetrate deeply into human tissues, so the risk of injury is confined chiefly to the skin and eyes.

Until the advent of antibiotic drugs, high-mountain sunshine was an accepted and widely used form of therapy for many sufferers of tuberculosis. UV light is the primary mode by which the body receives adequate levels of active vitamin D (unless ingested), which is crucial to calcium absorption. Today UV light therapy is used for patients with atopic dermatitis, psoriasis, scleroderma, psoriasis, and lupus erythematosus (Asawanonda et al., 2000; Krutmann, 2000; Morita et al., 2000; Polderman et al., 2001). Sometimes UV light is used with a drug called psoralen, and the combination of treatments is highly effective for controlling psoriasis.

Psoralen enhances sensitivity to light, stops division of diseased cells, binds to DNA in the skin, and sensitizes it to the effects of UVA. Various studies indicate beneficial effects of exposure to UV for the heart, including reduced blood pressure and cholesterol. While too much long-wave UV light can lead to the development of various types of skin cancer, some exposure is crucial to optimal health and should be considered as necessary as any vitamin or mineral that the body requires (Lieberman, 1991). Unfortunately, there is no definitive research on how much exposure is beneficial and how much is harmful.

COLOR THERAPY

Color therapy uses colors to treat both physical and emotional injury. The theory holds that specific colors correlate to a particular disease or condition and can stimulate the sympathetic or parasympathetic nervous system. Colors are also believed to correlate to particular body parts, which are associated with discrete emotions (Lieberman, 1991). Colored light experienced through the retina is believed to induce states of relaxation and release of emotional trauma. Controlled studies have not been performed to the best of our knowledge. Research in the 1970s found correlation between discrete colors and mood (Jacobs and Seuss, 1975; Reeves et al., 1978). Color produces an effect on physiology and thus on mood.

LASER ACUPUNCTURE

Laser is an acronym for "light amplification by stimulated emission of radiation." For therapeutic use, the laser acupuncture instrument is made up of only one wavelength and consists of helium and neon emissions. Laser acupuncture, also called *cold laser therapy*, is effective for wound healing, ulcers, burns, pain, including pain related to temporomandibular joints (TMJ). In a trial that compared the use of drug therapy (desmopressin) and laser acupuncture for children ($n = 10$) 5 years or older with nocturnal enuresis, 75% of the children taking the pharmaceutical were dry at 6 months, while 65% of those receiving laser acupuncture were dry—offering an effective, noninvasive, alternative therapy (Radmayr et al., 2001). Interestingly, one study showed that laser acupuncture of the left foot at the point called "Bladder 67" activated the cuneus corresponding to Brodmann Area 18, as detected by functional magnetic resonance imaging, while placebo stimulation had no effect (Siedentopf et al., 2002). Further research in this area is warranted and is likely to be promising. Low-energy laser beams are used to stimulate traditional acupuncture points without the use of needles. The laser is applied for 15 to 90 seconds in a continuous or a pulsed manner (Kahn, 1994; Lieberman, 1991).

AURICULOTHERAPY

Auriculotherapy, or auricular therapy, has been used by the Chinese since antiquity and was given new life by a French physician, Paul Nogier, in the late 1940s. The theory holds that points on the ear correlate to various locations throughout the body (Chen, 1993). In its original form, traditional acupuncture needles are applied to the ears to treat pain, dyslexia, and addictions. Many practitioners in Russia apply lasers to acupuncture points on the ear to reduce pain at distal sites. While in some instances needle auricular acupuncture may be more effective than laser, laser has the benefit of being pain free and nontraumatic, particularly for children (Brockhaus and Elger, 1990; Schlager et al., 1998; Wong and Fung, 1991). Most of the research that has been conducted on the technique is related to pain reduction, including pain from cancer (Alimi et al., 2000; King et al., 1990; Lewis et al., 1990). Auriculotherapy may be effective for SAD as well as stress syndrome.

SOUND MODALITIES

Oh the sisters of mercy they are not departed or gone.
They were waiting for me when I thought that I just can't go on.
They brought me their comfort and later they brought me their song.
I hope you run into them, you who've been traveling so long.

Leonard Cohen, 1975

MUSIC THERAPY

Music therapy uses music in a controlled manner to influence the well-being of an individual with physiological or emotional symptoms. Music therapy facilitates the release of repressed emotions, reduces stress, relieves depression, and promotes relaxation. The music is selected to match the patient's state of mind and is then slowly altered to encourage a pleasurable or harmonious state of mind. Music preferred by the patient is considered the least therapeutic because it matches their depressed mood. This finding correlates with studies showing that musical entrainment is the most effective type of music therapy (see next section). Studies, which sometimes involve both imagery and music therapy, have shown a decrease in blood pressure, cortisol, mood disturbance, and anxiety and pain in critical care patients and in patients before and after surgery (McKinney et al., 1997; Salmore and Nelson, 2000; White, 2000). Similarly, sound therapy, which reproduces sounds from nature and simply singing release emotion and reduce anxiety (Dewhurst-Maddock, 1993).

MUSICAL ENTRAINMENT

Musical entrainment occurs when two rhythms become perfectly coupled and attain the same frequency. Therapeutic musical entrainment uses music to bring the patient from one state to another healthier state. As with music therapy, the patients begin by listening to music that somewhat matches their current state of mind. The music is then altered to bring the individual to a more positive state. Some studies have shown increased β-endorphin levels resulting from musical entrainment (McKinney et al., 1997). Entrainment tapes have been used for developmental delays, stroke, anxiety, pain, and neurological problems after trauma.

MEDICAL RESONANCE THERAPY MUSIC®

Medical Resonance Therapy Music was developed from the music of classical composer Peter Hübner (spelled Huebner in some English translations). Hübner has studied the natural laws of musical harmony as a means to promote healing by employing the inherent structures of music. He uses subliminal sounds to create electroencephalogram (EEG) patterns to evoke healing of a particular disease. The concept is based on the work of Pythagoras, the 16th century philosopher, astronomer, physician, mathematician, and musicologist. Pythagoras postulated that the laws of the harmony of music are the same as those governing humans. Hübner writes, "Pythagoras believed very strongly that all natural systems could be shown to be interrelated in some concordant fashion, and coined the term *Cosmos* to describe this orderly and harmonious universe." Pythagoras wrote about the ability of music to foster health by activating an internal, natural law of harmony. Hübner's intention is to tap the healing potential inherent in the naturally structured laws of music. Based on this theory, Hübner has composed various pieces of music to treat specific types of mental or physical conditions. He explains, "It is not the music that achieves the medical result—it is the inaudible harmonic information within what we can call music which by its resonance helps the listener's biological system." The effects of Medical Resonance Therapy Music are believed to result from a precise harmony that resonates inside the human, traveling from the ears to the brain, and then to the various organs. The harmony residing in the music is thought to stimulate a resetting of the body's biological order, gradually bringing the entire body toward rejuvenation as well as preventing potential illness. In Germany there are approximately 22,000 pharmacies, each called a Digital Pharmacy®, that distribute listening plans structured for various medical conditions. Hübner's Medical Resonance Therapy Music is currently widely used in Germany. There is no research that has been performed on the modality, except for that produced by the company.

BIOACOUSTICS

Bioacoustics, or life sounds, is a technique that employs both music therapy and biofeedback. It is akin to music therapy in that specific combinations of low-frequency sounds are used, and it is similar to biofeedback in that these sounds are used to elicit specific biological and emotional responses. Sharry Edwards, M.Ed., developed the technique in 1982. Voice spectral analysis is used diagnostically to interpret the complicated frequency interactions within the body and then to determine the physical and emotional health of the individual. Computerized analysis of the voice displays a graphic representation of the individual's strengths and weaknesses.

Bioacoustics claims that vocal analysis can identify the frequency equivalents of structural components, muscles, as well as biochemical and nutrient compounds within the body. Ideally, there is coherence to one's voice patterns; however, disease is said to result when the patterns become discordant.

Edwards explains that every portion of the body has a Frequency Equivalent™ that can be mathematically calculated. She asserts, "This provides the foundation for the concept that the body's ability to heal itself can originate as frequency interactions between the molecular signals of the entire body" (Bioacoustics: www.soundhealthinc.com). Sound formula sets or sound presentation, which are constructed specifically for each individual (often with the aid of objective data, such as blood pressure or temperature readings), help the patient overcome problem areas and promote structural and emotional integrity. The patient listens to the sounds in a planned sequence of sessions, which continues at home. The goal of treatment is to entrain brain waves to healthier patterns. Edwards writes: "The principles of BioAcoustics originate with the idea that the brain perceives and generates impulse patterns that can be measured as brain wave frequencies; which in turn are delivered to the body by way of nerve pathways. The theory incorporates the assumption that these frequency impulses serve as directives that sustain structural integrity and emotional equilibrium. When these patterns are disrupted the body seeks to reveal the imbalance by manifesting symptoms that are interpreted as disease and stress" (Edwards, 1997).

Bioacoustics is used for nutritional diagnosis, sports injury, pain management, structural problems, and tissue regeneration. Sharry Edwards and her company, Sound Health, Inc., have carried out the only studies performed to date.

TOMATIS

A French physician, Albert Tomatis, developed sound therapy to correct learning dysfunction and improve self-esteem. The Tomatis method is based on Tomatis's finding that the larynx can emit only the harmonics that the ear can hear or, as Tomatis was fond of saying, "The voice reproduces only what the ear hears." This fact was proven at the Sorbonne in 1957 and is now known as the Tomatis effect. Tomatis determined that when we sing or speak, we condition our own ears to our own sound. He developed devices that allowed the subject to become unconsciously conditioned to new sound. Tomatis also felt that the ears affected the entire body. He claimed that when one speaks, sound "inundates and spreads over your whole body ... syllable waves break and wash over you. Your entire body surface marks their progress through the skin's sensitivity, as if controlled by a keyboard that is receptive to acoustic touch." Billie Thompson, Ph.D., a certified consultant in the Tomatis method and translator of two of his books, describes the technique as "a sound stimulation and educational intervention that improves listening, language, motivation, attention, learning, self image, awareness, musical ability and appreciation, audio–vocal control, and posture" (Tomatis, 1996). The Tomatis method claims to correct poor functioning, but not organic or neural damage. Correcting the ear to function properly allows it to hear wanted sounds and to shut out unwanted sounds and to produce a more pleasant quality of voice. Tomatis felt that an impaired ability to listen can result in low self-esteem as well as slowed learning and intellectual development.

The Tomatis method is carried out in three phases. The first phase teaches a patient to hear the entire harmonic range of sound information being presented, which teaches him or her to listen better in general. The second phase allows a period of time to integrate the fuller spectrum of sound that the individual can now hear. The final phase teaches the patient to articulate the new sounds that he or she can now hear, producing a voice (speaking or singing) that is more pleasant to hear (Tomatis, 1996).

BIOELECTROMAGNETIC MODALITIES

If humans are indeed wired for God, and benefit from spirituality in the same important ways that every generation past and every generation to come will, how are we to incorporate this new fact of physiology?

Dr. Herbert Benson, 1996

We will first offer a brief review of the mechanics of electromagnetic properties to aid the understanding of the various modalities that follow. Inside the nucleus of an atom there are protons, which are positively charged, and neutrons, which are neutral and have no charge. Electrons, which are negatively charged, rotate in defined orbits around the nucleus. For a current of electricity to occur, there must be an imbalance in the ratio of electrons to protons, usually as a result of a surplus of electrons. An electrical pathway, or current, is created by a flow of electrons to a source that is positively charged (i.e., something that has a predominance of protons). This pathway is called an *electrical circuit*. Electrical interactions and circuits are important to our health at both the cellular and the systems levels. This is where scientific Western and Eastern theories of human physiology unmistakably intersect.

Magnetism is largely known by its properties. Its main property is a polarity that can be arranged to either attract or repel two objects. Furthermore, where there is electricity, there is magnetism, and where there is magnetism, there is electricity. Typically, when a magnetic field comes in contact with an electrical pathway, it produces an electrical current. Conversely, when there is an electrical current flowing, it will have a magnetic field that is at a 90° angle to the current. The interaction of the electrical and magnetic energy results in a 360° electromagnetic field that continues traveling (theoretically infinitely) outward, in concentric circles, at the speed of light. The track of the outward expansion is typically lost as it integrates with other more powerful electromagnetic fields. The electromagnetic field is called a *force field*. The earth's electromagnetic field is an example of a force field. Various human-made objects from medical devices to power lines also generate electromagnetic fields. These localized, human-made fields are generally stronger than the Earth's electromagnetic field.

Electromagnetic fields oscillate at various frequencies. Light, as we know it, is the only frequency at which electromagnetic fields are visible to most humans. Examples of low-frequency fields (i.e., oscillating at slower speeds) are radio frequency and microwave (see below), and examples of high-frequencies fields (i.e., oscillating at faster speeds) are x-rays and gamma rays. Low-frequency fields are associated with levels of radiation that generally are considered safer for humans than high-frequency fields. However, recent research has brought into question the safety of long-term exposure to low-frequency fields, such as those produced by power lines. What makes electromagnetic fields harmful to humans is ionization, a process that occurs when frequencies of electromagnetic energy are high enough to dislodge electrons from the atom. Persistent exposure of the body to ionization, especially in the higher frequency range, might cause cancer or other serious disease because of the generation of free radicals, which are harmful to tissues. So-called nonionizing forms of electromagnetic energy are used for medical purposes. As indicated below, some of them involve heat (see the section on thermal therapies) and some do not (see the section on nonthermal therapies).

Many biomedical researchers now agree that electromagnetic fields surround the body. Electricity flows through the body, with the heart registering the highest electrical activity (emitting 2.5 watts, it produces 40 to 60 times more electricity than the brain). The electrical activity of the heart and nervous system interacts and affects one another. The heart is correlated with the highest magnetic activity as well. According to what we have just reviewed, the heart must then also be a force field that extends out in a theoretically infinite manner. In fact, this is not only true for the heart, but also for the electromagnetic field of the entire body. There are other endogenous electromagnetic fields. The brain is the next strongest, but it is hundreds of times weaker than the heart. Research performed at the Lawrence Berkeley laboratory reveals that pulsed, nonthermal electromagnetic fields influence calcium-channel regulation and signaling in lymphocytes. The impact varies depending on lymphocyte cell status and electromagnetic field intensity (Walleczek, 1992; Walleczek and Budinger, 1992). Researchers are investigating the interaction between exogenous and endogenous electromagnetic fields and the use of various frequencies of electromagnetic energy as a conduit for healing. It is likely that some energy fields are so subtle that they cannot be detected by existing instrumentation, yet they may have significant long-term effects on our health.

Two individuals who have produced landmark work in the field of electromagnetic energy warrant mentioning. The first is Dr. Robert O. Becker, an orthopedic surgeon whose renowned work on the regeneration of salamander limbs forms the basis for the use of electromagnetic energy in medicine today (Becker and Selden, 1985). Becker determined that when a limb is amputated from a salamander, there is continuous electric current that flows from the CNS to the injured limb. He made the fascinating discovery that the electric potential at the site of injury was briefly positive, reversed to a negative potential, and then gradually drifted back to a neutral potential by the time the limb was healed. Becker demonstrated that the human body has a positive polarity that travels along a central axis and a negative polarity along the periphery. He showed that humans likewise exhibit a positive polarity at the site of injury, until healing occurs. Curiously, he also determined that there is a reversal of polarity during altered states, such as anesthesia and hypnosis. Becker, along with Charles Andrew Loockerman Bassett, established the efficacy of using electromagnetic energy for bone healing, and today they are credited with the widespread application of electromagnetic devices for bone healing, particularly for refractory non-union fractures. Becker also developed theories of the analgesic effects of acupuncture, cellular capacitors for the body's electrical system, and the deleterious effects of electrical forces on the environment.

Another individual who has produced landmark work in the field of electromagnetic energy is Dr. Björn Nordenström, formerly director of diagnostic radiology at the Karolinska Institute in Stockholm, Sweden (unquestionably, the most prestigious position attainable in Sweden in this field). Nordenström is a brilliant man who developed balloon catheterization and needle biopsy techniques and who chaired the Nobel Prize committee that selects laureates for medicine. Since the mid-1960s, Nordenström has developed a revolutionary theory of the human body's electrical system and has illustrated the existence of biologically closed electrical circuits (BCEC) within the body (see Figure 5.1). While I find that there is much validity to his theory and believe that it will be an integral part of medicine of the future, his work has neither been widely accepted by the medical establishment nor replicated by colleagues. Nordenström, unfortunately, is one of those unique pioneers who is well ahead of his time and whose work is far too cutting edge for most researchers to put their time into exploring its validity. He is now in his 80s, and I am concerned that this milestone in electromagnetic research might be lost or obscured.

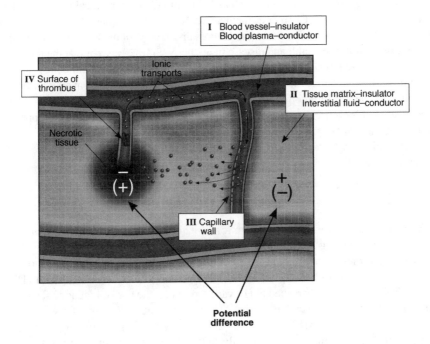

FIGURE 5.1 Biologically closed electrical circuits. (From Nordenström, B.W., *Exploring BCEC Systems*, Nordic Medical Publications, Stockholm, Sweden, 1998. With permission.)

Out of sheer curiosity as to why some malignant tumors had coronas around them, Nordenström discovered that when the body is injured, there is a fluctuation between positive and negative electrical currents until healing occurs. He learned that our veins and arteries act like insulated cables (whose electrical resistance is

200 times that of blood), which effectively shuttle products between injured and healthy cells. Blood and interstitial fluid serve as conductors, and enzymes serve as electrodes, which provides you all the necessary components of an electrical circuit. White blood cells (WBCs), the body's premier immune fighter, carry a negative electrical charge, so Nordenström places a positive electrode within the tumor mass to draw WBCs to the tumor. He simultaneously places a negative electrode just outside the tumor and allows the current to flow in both electrodes for about an hour. The change in the electrical fields causes an acidic-like buildup of particles to occur around the tumor. The buildup of particles prevents red blood cells and oxygen from reaching the tumor, which starves the tumor. Furthermore, Nordenström postulates that the positive electrical field forces water out of the tumor, causing swelling in the surrounding tissue and shrinkage of the tumor, further blocking blood flow to the tumor.

Nordenström's technique has been effective in treating isolated malignant tumors that are 4 cm or smaller. Much work needs to be done to design systematic studies to confirm his findings (Nordenström, 1998). It is possible that Nordenström's electrical circuits are the elusive meridians or channels of the Chinese medical system of acupuncture. As we saw in Chapter 2, medical science now has a basic understanding of the mechanisms of action of neurotransmitters and how various drugs fit into discrete receptors to influence health and disease in the body. Similarly, we are at the threshold of understanding how internal and external electromagnetic energy influences health. It is my firm belief that the next frontier in medical research will involve an understanding of the profound effects that electromagnetic energy has on health. Someday scientists will look back upon Becker's and Nordenström's work with deep appreciation for their notable professional and personal contributions to the field.

The following two sections review the major thermal and nonthermal electromagnetic therapies.

THERMAL THERAPIES

Thermal therapies are used in conventional medicine, although some of them may be considered cutting-edge therapies. However, clinical results of various types of thermal therapies for malignant unresectable hepatic tumors now exceed those for chemotherapy and radiation and are slowly becoming a standard treatment (Dodd et al., 2000). A study performed at Harvard reports on the use of magnetic resonance imaging (MRI) with thermal therapies: "The temperature sensitivity of several intrinsic parameters enables MRI to visualize and quantify the progress of ongoing thermal treatment. MRI is sensitive to thermally induced changes resulting from the therapies, giving the physician a method to determine the success or failure of the treatment" (McDannold and Jolesz, 2000). Thermal therapies also include infrared devices that provide deep-heating treatments, which are commonly used by physical therapists for relief from muscle spasms, strains, and sprains.

LASER SURGERY

Laser surgery is a minimally invasive thermal therapy presently used to treat many different conditions. For example, it is used to heat small solid tumors through implanted optical fibers and eradicate the lesions with little tissue charring. One of the most promising indications for laser surgery is its use for small unresectable hepatomas, metastatic tumors, and other conventionally inoperative tumors. Laser surgery also improves the rate of being able to perform a resection on colorectal liver metastases (Shankar et al., 2001). Studies show good tumor eradication rates, low complication rates, and appear to improve survival time.

The excimer laser was approved by the Food and Drug Administration (FDA) in 1995 for corneal surgery. The more popularly known laser-assisted in situ keratomileusis (LASIK) involves cutting and lifting a superficial corneal flap, after which the excimer laser removes a small amount of tissue to reshape the cornea and correct refractive errors. Healing is rapid because re-epithelialization of the cornea is not needed. Laser surgery is also employed for transmyocardial revascularization, a relatively new procedure to control refractory angina. The laser creates several small channels in areas of the heart that are still viable but where proper blood flow is impeded. Studies show that the procedure can effectively reduce angina and increase the quality of life for patients for whom angioplasty and bypass surgery have failed to relieve symptoms. The procedure is palliative rather than curative (Jones, 2001). In addition, lasers have been used for both diabetic retinopathy and macular degeneration (Akduman and Olk, 1999; Bandello et al., 1999; Miller et al., 1999; Petrovic and Bhisitkul, 1999 [for diabetic retinopathy]; Roider et al., 1999 [for macular degeneration]).

RADIO-FREQUENCY SURGERY

A phase 2 study has been completed on the efficacy of radio-frequency surgery for interstitial tissue ablation prior to surgical resection for patients with hereditary small renal tumors. A positive treatment effect was noted in 10 of the 11 lesions, and no toxicity was detected. Further evaluation is needed (Walther et al., 2000). While the technique was previously thought to be primarily palliative, a recent study showed that nearly 80% of medium (3.1 to 5.0 cm) and large (5.1 to 9.5 cm) malignant hepatocellular tumors of patients with cirrhosis or chronic hepatitis attained either complete necrosis or partial necrosis. Noninfiltrating tumors had a higher rate of necrosis than infiltrating tumors (Livraghi et al., 2000). Other studies on hepatocellular tumors have yielded similar results (e.g., Yamasaki et al., 2001). Occlusion of blood-supply and radio-frequency ablation are also effective treatments for medium to large hepatic tumors (Rossi et al., 2000). At the Mayo Clinic, physicians have performed atrioventricular node ablation using radio-frequency surgery for patients with atrial fibrillation. When there is no underlying heart disease, expected survival is equal to that of the general population, and the need for lifetime drug use is obviated (Ozcan et al., 2001). A recent study also showed radio-frequency surgery to be very effective in knee reconstruction, significantly reducing intra-articular bleeding (Camillieri et al., 2001).

RADIO-FREQUENCY DIATHERMY

Continuous short-wave diathermy permits the uniform elevation of temperature in deep tissue. It is used to reduce inflammation, relieve joint and muscle pain, and promote vasodilation (Goats, 1989). Pulsed short-wave diathermy is used to encourage tissue repair and reduce pain. Although some consider it a nonthermal therapy, recent research shows that as pulse repetition rates are increased, so is the temperature of the skin (Murray and Kitchen, 2000). It is also useful in the treatment of acute lesions.

RADIO-FREQUENCY HYPERTHERMIA

Radio-frequency hyperthermia is typically used for the ablation of malignant tumors of the liver, prostate, and areas where tumors are unresectable (Falk and Issels, 2001; Hurwitz et al., 2001; Livraghi et al., 2000; Yamamoto and Tanaka, 1997). For the past 10 years, Stanford University has used the Stanford 3D hyperthermia treatment planing system, which makes use of patient-specific computer simulations to determine the best amplitude and frequency at which a tumor deep within the body should be heated (Sullivan et al., 1993). Similar procedures are in place at Massachusetts Institute of Technology (MIT) to ensure treatment that avoids regions of the body at which high temperature treatment would be detrimental (Fenn and King, 1994). Research on rats shows that the addition of neutrophils enhances the efficacy of radio-frequency hyperthermia. Rats that were given recombinant human granulocyte colony-stimulating factor increased the antitumor response, and conversely, an injection that decreased the rat neutrophil antibody also decreased the antitumor response (Kokura et al., 1996).

NONTHERMAL THERAPIES

In 1965, researchers Melzack and Wall introduced the "gate control theory" of pain (Melzack and Wall, 1965). This theory postulates that electrical stimulation administered at a level above the area where neurons carrying the pain information enter the spinal cord can effectively close a spinal "gate." The peripheral pain messages attempting to ascend the spinal-thalamic tract to the brain then cannot reach the brain. This theory fostered the development of surgically implanted stimulators to reduce pain. Various electrical stimulators, such as cardiac pacemakers, are implanted in the body to manage arrhythmia and other conditions. Some electrical stimulation devices, such as those described below, are designed to alter or eliminate the pain message by inducing healing at the pain site through stimulation of cutaneous nerves located at a level above the entry of the pain stimulation.

TRANSCUTANEOUS ELECTRICAL NERVE STIMULATION (TENS)

TENS is a modality used by many physical therapists since the early 1970s to relieve both acute and chronic pain. Dr. C. Norman Shealy developed TENS for pain management. The procedure involves attaching two electrodes to the skin. The electrodes are connected to an electricity-generating device that delivers a low-voltage current to the nerves in the vicinity of the pain. TENS works by stimulating endorphin production and by interrupting or blocking the neurological communication pathway of the pain (Kahn, 1994). It is commonly used in physical therapy but also can be used at home. There are over 100 FDA-approved types of units available. Several studies have shown TENS to be less effective than acupuncture for pain control (e.g., Freeman and Lawlis, 2001; Lehmann et al., 1986).

CRANIAL ELECTRICAL STIMULATION (CES)

CES uses an even lower voltage electrical current than TENS (less than 1.5 mA compared with 60 mA for TENS), and the electrodes are attached to the scalp. This very low voltage gently nudges the neuroendocrine system back into a homeostatic state, releasing the individual from a state of chronic stress and its associated diseases. CES was first called *electrosleep*, which is a term derived from researchers in Russia and other Eastern Bloc countries. In 1978, the FDA renamed it cranial electrical stimulation (CES) because the electricity is pulsed across the head. In the late 1970s, the FDA approved its use for treatment of drug addiction, as there was strong evidence for its effectiveness in abolishing withdrawal symptoms. CES proponents have since been embroiled in controversy with the FDA for its approval for use for other conditions (Kirsch, 1999). Nonetheless, CES is used to treat depression, pain, insomnia, headache, anxiety, and depression (George et al., 1999; Kirsch, 1999). Research performed by one manufacturer showed increased levels of β-endorphins, serotonin, and melatonin as well as diminished levels of cortisol and tryptophan (Liss and Liss, 1996). Dr. Shealy (see TENS above) worked with Dr. Saul Liss, developer of the Liss Cranial Electrical Stimulator™ apparatus, and determined that TENS worked more effectively with patients with comorbid depression if they were first treated with CES (Rosch, 1997).

TRANSCRANIAL MAGNETIC STIMULATION (TMS)

TMS is a noninvasive technique that uses powerful magnetic fields to alter brain activity. In one study, lateral stimulation exciting the left frontal cortex using higher frequencies (≥ 10 Hz) and slow (1 Hz) stimulation inhibiting the right prefrontal cortex were both shown to have antidepressant effects (George et al., 1999; Klein et al., 1999). Side effects include tension headache and seizure (never reported with low frequency, ≤ 1 Hz). TMS is unpleasant and painful at higher frequencies. However, it is a favorable alternative for those patients refractory to other treatment. In another study, low-frequency (1 Hz) TMS significantly reduced auditory hallucinations in schizophrenic patients. All patients remained on antipsychotic medication, but those also needing to take anticonvulsant drugs did not respond as well to the treatment (Hoffman et al., 2000).

MAGNETIC BIOSTIMULATION

Magnets have been used as adjuncts to acupuncture for hundreds of years, especially in China (Lawrence et al., 1998). The American public, as evidenced by millions of dollars in sales each year, has embraced the use of magnets to treat sensory and motor dysfunction. Yet, there is a striking paucity of scientific research on its effectiveness. Two small but well-designed pilot studies evidence impressive results and call for the validation of the therapy with larger, more comprehensive studies. One study involving the use of magnetic insoles (a novel approach in the history of the use of magnets) showed a 75% improvement for patients with diabetic neuropathy and a 50% improvement for those with neuropathy without diabetes (Weintraub, 1999). Other research showed strong improvement in sway and lateral stance with the use of magnetic insoles with older adults. While promising, the number of subjects in the study was too small to be definitive (Suomi and Koceja, 2001). Another study on the use of magnets for chronic pelvic pain showed that long-term use improved symptoms, but once again, the sample size was too small to reach statistical significance (Brown et al., 2000).

QI MACHINE™

The Qi Machine was developed by Dr. Shizuo Inoue of Japan to provide a way to oxygenate the body without exercise-related stress or injury. Dr. Inoue researched the correlation between levels of oxygen and health in the human body and deduced that insufficient oxygen is the main factor in most human disease. He looked to nature, particularly the undulating motions of goldfish, to develop the Qi Machine, which is placed under the ankles to rhythmically rock the legs, the spinal cord, and the muscles surrounding it, as well as the entire body, which improves efficient blood circulation. The patient is asked to relax and breathe deeply while the machine rocks the body. Up to 60% of the Qi Machine's benefits occur after the machine stops, during an approximately 3-minute period in which the individual is asked to remain still. It is felt that the Qi Machine massages the internal organs, loosens fascial restrictions, moves lymph fluids, opens bronchioles, aligns the spine, and improves the immune and nervous systems. The Qi Machine is said to have psychological health benefits, including increased vitality and a sense of well-being, as the state of deep relaxation reduces chronic physical tension and mental stress. The machine is not recognized in the United States as a therapeutic appliance, but it has been certified by Japan's Medical Affairs Bureau. Its use is not recommended during pregnancy, after surgery or bone fracture, with serious bleeding or infection, or for those individuals suffering from epilepsy or heart disease. In our review, we failed to find any peer-reviewed medical studies on the Qi Machine.

MICROWAVE THERAPY

Microwave therapy has been used for 20 years, primarily in Russia and the Ukraine (see Jovanović-Ignjatić and Raković, 1999, for a review). The therapy is a non-ionizing level of electromagnetic energy that is used at a nonthermal intensity, either pulsed or continuous. Microwave therapy is used for the treatment of various conditions, including asthma, bronchitis, ulcers, hepatocellular tumors, and atherosclerosis as well as for reparation of immune cells for postoperative lung cancer patients (Babak and Honcharova, 1995; Drobyshev et al., 2000; Dziublik et al., 1989; Ishikawa et al., 2000; Kuz'menko, 1998; Shevchenko, 2000; Shibata et al., 2000;

Shimada et al., 1998). Studies have shown that the treatment is safe and nontoxic, and researchers have produced clear, positive results.

PULSED ELECTROMAGNETIC FIELD THERAPY (PEMF) AND PULSED SIGNAL THERAPY (PST)

PEMF, an extremely low, nonionizing frequency of electromagnetic energy, employs pulsed electromagnetic fields, utilizing a direct current with a constantly repeating signal at a predetermined intensity and frequency. Adenosine triphosphate (ATP), the enzyme that is key to producing high amounts of chemical energy and is stored as energy for many physiological functions, is needed to heal injured cells. PEMF most likely works by amassing ATP in the region of injury by facilitating the influx of potassium into the cells (Rosch, 1997). The Food and Drug Administration has approved the use of PEMF for treating nonunion fractures that do not heal, muscle re-education, and relaxation of muscle spasm (e.g., Trock, 2000). However, PEMF also is used to treat Parkinson's disease, multiple sclerosis, Tourette's syndrome, migraines, and SAD (Sandyk et al., 1991; Sandyk, 1992, 1997a, 1997b, 1998, 1999).

Like PEMF, PST is performed at a low, nonionizing frequency, but it operates by changing pulses (i.e., instead of a constantly repeating signal), which are transmitted in a programmed alternating fashion that mimics the body's natural electrical potentials. Treatment typically is for 1 hour. Proponents of PST feel that the damaged cells, after a relatively short period of time, do not perceive a constantly repeating stimulus, such as is used in PEMF. Beneficial effects of PST are most often reported for osteoarthritis. With osteoarthritis, the chondrocyte (a mature cartilage cell embedded in a lacuna within the cartilage matrix) can no longer receive physiological signals because of pathological changes in the matrix. PST allows the chondrocyte to receive signals in the cartilage matrix, which allows regeneration and growth of the cartilage. Similar results have been achieved with arthritic joints and tendons. Extensive studies by Richard Markoll, M.D., Ph.D., of BioMagnetic Therapy Systems in Boca Raton, Florida, and one of the leading researchers on the effects of PST, indicate that PST is also effective for tinnitus that is not responsive to other therapies. A study published in Russia followed pulse low-frequency electromagnetic field treatment for 25 patients with tinnitus that was refractory to other treatment, and the results support Markoll's findings. The study showed that noise was eliminated in 2 patients and reduced noticeably (by 60%) in 19 patients. The effect persisted at 6- and 12-month follow-up evaluations (Patiakina et al., 1998).

PSYCHOLOGICAL MODALITIES

COUNSELING

We will not review the myriad psychological therapies (e.g., Freudian, Jungian, behavioral, cognitive, etc.), as this information is well covered in numerous other sources. However, it is my contention that work on both the mind and the body is essential for full health.

HYPNOTHERAPY

Hypnosis, a technique of deep concentration that suspends certain states of active awareness. It has been used for hundreds of years and dons a colorful history (Dossey, 2000). It is used for treatment of both psychological maladies and physical problems. Physiological parameters change in a manner consistent with other types of stress-reduction exercises (e.g., reduced respiratory rate, heart rate, and oxygen consumption). Typically hypnosis is used with some form of psychotherapy to reduce psychological or physical symptoms, including pain. Hypnosis can access memory and alter perception or mood, or increases the subject's ability to experience imagery and creativity. A willingness to participate is crucial to its success, but suggestibility does not imply compliance against one's will. However, hypnotic susceptibility has been shown to increase effectiveness of treatment, such as reducing pain (Spinhoven and ter Kuile, 2000). Dr. Milton Erickson's experiments with hypnosis in the first half of the 20th century brought hypnosis into the realm of clinical practice. Erickson recognized the integration of the mind and body many years before psychoneuroimmunology experiments were being carried out. He saw that the unconscious mind was a rich source of information for providing physical and emotional healing. There is evidence that hypnosis is most effective when the mind is in the theta state (see Chapter 1 for information on the theta state). Today various studies attest that hypnosis benefits relaxation and anesthesia (Ashton et al., 1995; Ashton et al., 1997; Defechereux et al., 1999).

AUTOGENIC TRAINING

In autogenic training, a type of self-hypnosis, the patient is taught six "formulas" to repeat in a specific pattern and then use at home. The concept that each of the formulas is tied to major bodily systems, such as the cardiovascular system and the musculature, is key to evoking a physiological relaxation response. Table 5.1 is a typical list of formulas with the corresponding area of the body that each is intended to affect:

TABLE 5.1

Six Formulas for Evoking Relaxation Response in Major Body Systems

Formula No.	State of Mind	Perception of Body Area	Intended Effect
1	I am completely calm	My right arm is heavy	Muscular relaxation
2	I am completely calm	My right arm is warm	Vascular dilation
3	I am completely calm	My heart beats calmly and regularly	Heart function regulation
4	I am completely calm	My breathing is calm and regular...it breathes me	Breathing regulation
5	I am completely calm	My abdomen is flowingly warm	Visceral organ regulation
6	I am completely calm	My forehead is pleasantly cool	Regulation of blood flow to the head

Autogenic training is most efficacious when the patient is in the theta state (Spinhoven and ter Kuile, 2000). It has been shown to be a more effective treatment for motion sickness than intramuscular injections of promethazine. Testing at NASA showed that motion-sickness tolerance was significantly increased with autogenic training. Subjects reported fewer or no symptoms at higher rotational velocities, and there was significantly less heart-rate and skin-conductance variability during motion sickness tests in the group receiving autogenic training (Cowings and Toscano, 2000). While there are plausible claims that autogenic training is effective for reducing anxiety and stress, studies to date generally are methodologically flawed and do not always use the classical autogenic training formulas (Ernst and Kanji, 2000).

HYPNAGOGIA

Hypnagogia is an experience of psychological and physical withdrawal or relaxation at the threshold of sleep; the technique incorporates intense visual and sometimes auditory experiences. Hypnagogia, a hypnoticlike state of consciousness that hovers between being awake and being asleep, involves a loosening of ego boundaries and a conscious participation in the experience. The technique incorporates intense visual and sometimes auditory experiences. It is the conscious experience of being in the theta state and can be intentionally prolonged to promote mental clarity and insight. Hypnagogia induces experiences that are physiologically similar to the spiritual experiences of advanced meditators, with subjects showing decreases in heart rate and oxygen consumption as well as a shift from alpha to theta on the EEG. The technique also induces experiences that are psychologically similar to those reported by advanced meditators, having the two key features of intense concentration and the dissolution of a sense of self as distinct from a sense of otherness (Mavromatis, 1987).

MEDITATION

Training for many types of meditation techniques is available in the United States. Meditation facilitates entry into both the alpha and theta states. These states are important for deep relaxation and stress reduction, but they also provide opportunities for profound insight. Some people can benefit from and handle the insights without outside intervention; for others, greater gain and personal growth require working with a spiritual or psychological counselor to more fully understand the issues that arise. I offer you one word of caution: think carefully about what technique and what aspects of the technique are best for you. It is my experience that even meditation techniques that claim to have no dogma and allege only to disseminate spiritual truth are actually littered with dogmatic rules and regulations. Even rules that may have some inherent health benefits, such as not drinking alcohol, can be a dogma that binds group members in the belief that they stand on higher moral ground than those who are not part of their group. Ultimately, these individuals have missed the point, which is that all of us are part of a common energy (see Chapter 8). The meditation group becomes a way of life, perhaps even providing a false sense of security or structure in one's life instead of a serious personal inner journey. The practitioner is bound by what the leader says instead of taking the more courageous and deeper journey of an independent discovery of one's inner nature and inherent truth.

There are clear health benefits to the daily practice of meditation. As previously mentioned, meditation raises levels of melatonin and possibly anandamide. Meditation also may, very possibly, cause the rise of N,N-dimethyltryptamine (DMT), which is discussed in Chapter 8. Research has also shown that regular practice of meditation leads to an increased EEG-recorded alpha coherence in the frontal lobe, a significantly lower systolic blood pressure and ambulatory diastolic blood pressure, as well as long-term endocrine changes, for example, decreases in serum thyroid-stimulating hormone (TSH), growth hormone, and prolactin levels (Dillbeck and Bronson, 1981; Travis and Wallace, 1999; Wallace et al., 1983; Wenneberg et al., 1997; Werner et al., 1986). One of the most comprehensive reviews of research on the various physical effects of meditation is published by the Institute of Noetic Sciences, an organization dedicated to "the development of human consciousness through scientific inquiry" (Murphy and Donovan, 1997).

IMAGERY

Imagery is pervasive in our lives, occupying our thoughts and memories, providing visions during our meditation or prayer, and filling our daytime and nighttime dreams. Although imagery can seriously harm us, as occurs with the repetitive and intrusively recurring imagery that accompanies posttraumatic stress disorder, imagery also can be effective for recovery from various medical conditions, for decreasing physical pain, and for sundry emotional issues, such as the reduction of anxiety (Achterberg and Lawlis, 1978; Achterberg, 1985; Achterberg et al., 1989; Simonton and Sherman, 1998). Imagery is frequently used with other modalities, including biofeedback, hypnosis, psychotherapy, and sound or music therapy. It is a vehicle that has the potential of providing us with insights about ourselves and developing our personal and spiritual awareness. In a deeply relaxed state of mind, guided or self-directed imagery can help replace negative or destructive mental patterns with healthy images that can effectively change attitudes and behavior. One of the most prominent researchers of imagery for healing is Jeanne Achterberg, Ph.D., who has published numerous studies on the topic (Achterberg, 1985). Achterberg says, "You may think of imagery…as the way what we call 'mind' and what we call 'body' communicate" (Achterberg, 1999). Achterberg feels that imagery is a bridge between the mind and the body. Emotions and traumas, which are encoded in our bodies, are brought to a conscious state through the use of imagery.

HEARTMATH® THERAPY

HeartMath therapy is a process of reducing stress and unwanted emotion by focusing on the heart to help restore equilibrium to the body. In the ancient literature of many religions, the heart is the site of both intuition and wisdom. HeartMath combines this physiological understanding of the wisdom of love with some very solid medical science to formulate several techniques for reducing stress in both our personal and our work lives. There is solid evidence of health benefits from using this technique, including reduced blood pressure and heart rate as well as benefits to the immune system (Childre, 1994; Childre et al., 1999).

HeartMath is based on medical evidence that the heart has a nervous system sophisticated enough to qualify as an independent "brain." The heart is capable of relaying vital information back and forth to the brain but will not necessarily take its marching orders from the brain. Various types of information (e.g., chemical, electromagnetic) are constantly being relayed between the two organs. According to HeartMath, focusing on the heart and feelings of love or appreciation can actually shift these patterns of information and the heart's rhythms.

How does this occur? The HeartMath research team analyzed heart rate variability (HRV) and found a correlation between the HRV pattern and the emotional state of the subject, with positive emotions evidencing a coherent and ordered pattern and negative emotions displaying a random chaotic pattern. HRV is strikingly responsive to our emotions. In addition, the HeartMath research team discovered that when one person touches another person, there is transference of electromagnetic energy from the person's heart who touches to the other person's brain. The brain-wave pattern, as represented on an EEG, mimics the heart pattern as recorded by an electrocardiogram (EKG). This is called *entrainment* (see Figure 5.2). So what is occurring in our hearts is affecting those around us, whether or not we are aware of it (Childre et al., 1999).

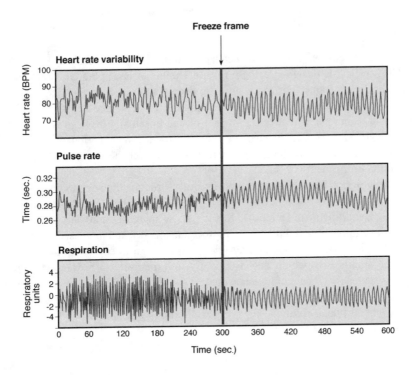

FIGURE 5.2 HeartMath entrainment.

HeartMath researchers found that a similar entrainment occurs *within* our own bodies. The researchers tracked patterns between the HRV and brain-wave patterns while the subjects were engaged in specific HeartMath techniques (see below). Our hearts and minds actually have the ability to entrain one another. Consequently, we experience a subjective sense of balance or harmony when our bodies are entrained because the body is working in harmony. This is the basis for the theory of the heart's intelligence.

There are five basic steps to the HeartMath technique:

1. Recognize that you are stressed and freeze-frame® the moment, which basically means to try to stop the feeling by following the next four steps. It is a technique that allows you to stop your emotions long enough to determine how best to handle the situation.
2. Put your attention on the area around your heart and imagine that your heart is breathing; really try to feel as if your heart is breathing—in and out, in and out.
3. Shift your focus to a positive memory.
4. Using both intuition and common sense, ask your heart to help you determine a response that will minimize stress from resulting in other similar situations.
5. HeartMath says, "Listen to what your heart says in answer to your question." It should provide you with a new perspective on the issues around which you experience stress (Childre, 1994; Childre et al., 1999).

HeartMath also offers two advanced techniques, CUT-THRU and HEART LOCK-IN. CUT-THRU is designed to help release emotional issues that still remain after practicing freeze-frame. For most, undoing deeply engrained negative patterns (e.g., those of anger, insecurity, worthlessness, guilt, etc.) will take years. CUT-THRU provides a technique to reduce the impact of and eventually dissolve some of these feelings. HEART LOCK-IN involves focusing for a longer period of time on the cultivation of feelings of love and appreciation and on the creation of a stronger connection to the heart (Childre et al., 1999).

Instructors of HeartMath have successfully brought their techniques to major corporations and government agencies (e.g., Motorola, Shell, Hewlett Packard, and the U.S. Department of Defense). Results show increases not only in employee health and empowerment, but also in improved teamwork and increased productivity. HeartMath has also provided police officers with a tool to cope with the extremely stressful situations in which they frequently find themselves. A HeartMath police study indicates that the technique has made a significant difference in these people's lives. The research on individuals as well as in social settings reveals that focusing on our inherent heart rhythms may very well entrain our physiology to a healthier, more harmonious life (Childre et al., 1999).

BIOFEEDBACK

Beginning in the 1960s, Barbara Brown, a pioneer in the use of EEGs, was involved in research concerning the voluntary self-regulation of bodily functions that are generally considered to be part of the involuntary nervous system or ANS (Brown, 1966; Brown, 1970). The idea that subjects could *voluntarily* control autonomic functions was novel then. Biofeedback therapy was subsquently derived from these experiments, and as other mechanistic tools were developed that could provide bodily feedback (e.g., the EKG), they, too were applied to the therapy of biofeedback. At a conference in 1969, which Brown sponsored for researchers involved in similar endeavors, the term *biofeedback* was first used, but some argue that it was the research scientist and widely recognized father of biofeedback, Dr. Elmer Green, who coined the word.

Elmer and his late wife, Alyce Green, who did much to promote the concept of biofeedback as a tool for learning bodily self-regulation, defined biofeedback as "the continuous monitoring, amplifying, and displaying to a person ... of an ongoing internal physiological process." Figure 5.3 shows Green's schematic of the mechanism of biofeedback. The Greens also made the point that "becoming aware of normally *involuntary* physiological processes is linked with becoming aware of normally *unconscious* psychological processes" (Green and Green, 1977). The Greens were early advocates for performing research on the mind–body connection. To borrow from stress research, one can say that biofeedback endeavors to teach the patient to bring the body back to homeostasis by learning to perceive internal cues. Biofeedback continues to be used for relaxation or stress control (Edwards et al., 2000; Moser et al., 1997; Nakao et al., 1997; Pages et al., 2001; Weaver and McGrady, 1995; Wiesel et al., 2001). In some instances, biofeedback is used as an adjunct to conventional treatment (e.g., pharmaceuticals and physical therapy).

Various modalities are used for biofeedback, some of which are more effective for one condition than another. In each instance, the goal of therapy is that patients can eventually monitor their condition without the feedback of the modality. Perhaps the most widely used biofeedback modality today is the electromyograph (EMG), which measures muscle activity. Muscles emit an electrical charge when there is any movement, and the EMG can measure this electrical activity. Electrodes are placed at the site of the disorder, such as on the forehead for a tension headache, and the patient learns to be aware when the muscle is engaged. Obviously, the technique is more useful when there is a distinct muscle group involved. Similarly, EEG devices, typically referred to as neurofeedback devices, are used for attention deficit disorder (ADD) in children and for fibromyalgia and other conditions. Another type of bio-feedback therapy is finger-pulse biofeedback, which is accomplished by attaching an electrode to the finger. The electrode measures heart rate and blood pressure and is therefore most effective with cardiovascular ailments (e.g., hypertension and arrhyth-mia) and anxiety. Vascular biofeedback records thermal changes on the skin, as mea-sured by a temperature-sensitive device, which is generally taped to the finger or toe.

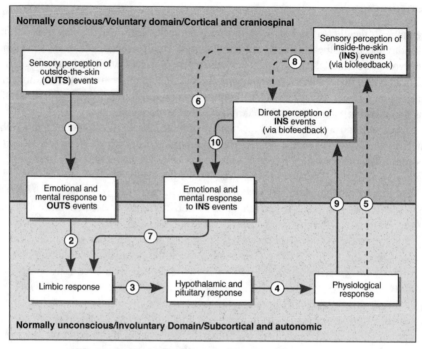

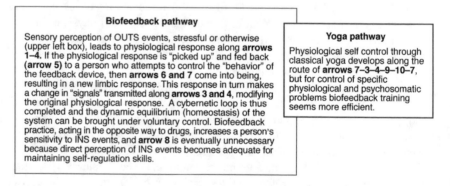

FIGURE 5.3 Elmer Green's schematic of the mechanism of biofeedback.

Low skin temperature, which occurs during stress, corresponds to a decrease in blood flow; as vessels dilate and blood flow increases, which occurs with relaxation, so does skin temperature. Thermal biofeedback is practical for Raynaud's disease, migraine headaches, hypertension, and anxiety. A final example of a biofeedback therapy is the use of sensors to train the patient in better breathing habits that encourage deeper breathing and utilize abdominal muscles. This modality is effective for respiratory conditions such as asthma, and, once again, is used for anxiety.

ART THERAPY

Art therapy is an excellent modality to reveal unconscious emotions, particularly for individuals who are visually oriented and for children who do not yet have the verbal skills to articulate all that they experience. Art therapy uses various media, such as sculpture, painting, drawing, or watercolor. The technique provides an avenue for both children and adults undergoing medical procedures to express their subconscious fears, loss, pain, or other emotions. This application of art therapy is now often referred to as "medical art therapy." Art programs established for inner-city youth, such as Artists for Humanity in Boston, Massachusetts, provide studio art classes for urban teenagers along with staff who are trained and available to discuss personal issues.

DANCE

Dance therapy, much like art therapy, is used to help the individual uncover unexpressed or blocked emotions. The modality is particularly suited to the person who is more sensate oriented, but may be inappropriate for some patients with extreme physical limitations or those who are in a weakened physical state. There is not a great deal of research available on dance and health; however, a few studies indicate that dance is effective for both physical and psychological parameters, including improvements in aerobic ability, depression, anxiety, fatigue, and tension, but not joint status for patients with rheumatoid arthritis (e.g., Noreau et al., 1995). A study of African-American and Hispanic adolescents conducted at the Stanford University Medical School indicates that a dance program coupled with a culturally sensitive health curriculum can be effective in improving health and awareness of the importance of physical exercise for this population (Flores, 1995). The long-range impact of this type of program could be significant, as cardiovascular disease is the major cause of death among adults in both of these ethnic groups. Another intriguing study indicates a significant reduction in anxiety for students participating in a modern-dance class compared with controls participating in physical education, music, or math classes (Leste and Rust, 1984).

Twyla Tharp, framed dancer, director, and choreographer, has brought the world over 30 years of dance that expresses innovative freshness. Ms. Tharp's productions convey the infectious playfulness and vibrant inner spiritual expression from which she creates her dance. In her forthcoming book, Ms. Tharp will share her view that dance is ultimately a spiritual statement, a declaration of the soul conveyed through movement. She advocates using dance in various healthcare settings, including hospitals and hospices. A woman who, in her life and work, has always pushed the boundaries of dance, Ms. Tharp now wants to bring that same attitude to dance as an avenue for health and well-being.

EYE-MOVEMENT DESENSITIZATION AND REPROCESSING (EMDR)

EMDR uses a combination of clinician-directed physical stimuli (primarily a set of specific eye movements but also hand tapping and finger clicking) coupled with mental focus. The mental focus begins first on a trauma, painful memory, or negative belief and then shifts to a positive sentiment. Francine Shapiro, who developed the technique, felt that the physical stimulation (e.g., eye movement) somehow triggers the portion of the brain involved in information processing and thus activates an inherent adaptive response that has gone awry, possibly as a result of the intensity of the trauma (Shapiro, 1995). I would speculate that the mechanism underlying EMDR involves neural pathways that connect the extraocular muscles (i.e., the muscles responsible for eye movement) with the limbic system (i.e., the area most central in processing emotion). The release of traumatic memories may be a positive therapeutic ramification of the programmed movements of EMDR. Ideally, both desensitization to the negative issue and an adaptive resolution can occur.

NEURO-LINGUISTIC PROGRAMMING (NLP)

In the early 1970s, John Grinder, a linguistics professor at UC Santa Cruz, and Richard Bandler, a psychology and mathematics student at the same institution, joined forces to investigate the behavioral patterns of prominent psychotherapists of that time. What they learned is that (1) voice tone, breathing, posture, and eye movements all reveal unconscious thought patterns that correlate to emotional states and (2) once the patterns are identified, they can be altered by reprogramming. *A Pocket Guide to NLP*, written by the NLP Comprehensive, now one of the prominent NLP training centers in the United States, describes NLP in the following words: "NLP is the study of the structure of subjective experience. NLP holds that people think and act based on their internal representations of the world and *not on the world itself*. Once we understand specifically *how* we create and maintain our inner thoughts and feelings, it is a simple matter for us to change them to more useful ones" (NLP Comprehensive, 1991). NLP is a technique that applies language and sensory processing to the thought patterns that are unhelpful to our emotional well-being. Negative patterns of organizing and processing internal and external sensory information can be reprogrammed and replaced with healthier patterns. NLP is used for building self-esteem, eliminating phobias, developing productive relationships, and resolving conflicts in both personal and employment situations.

HUMOR/LAUGHTER

Well before studies were being published on psychoneuroimmunology (PNI) and the mind–body connection, Norman Cousins, the well-known editor of *The Saturday Review*, deduced and effectively showed with his own painful, debilitating disease (ankylosing spondylitis) that laughter helps the body to heal (Cousins, 1976). Recently, Lee Berk, along with one of the fathers of PNI, Dr. David Felten, published research that confirms what Cousins had intuited ... that there is significant beneficial modulation of immune parameters with laughter (Berk et al., 2001). One hour of viewing a video that causes "mirthful laughter" is correlated to increases in natural killer cell activity; immunoglobulins G, A, and M (IgG, IgA, IgM); interferon-γ; leukocytes; and granulocytes. What is perhaps the most fascinating part of this research is that many of the increased immune parameters remained elevated (as compared with baseline levels) up to 12 hours later.

Realistically, humor and laughter are adjunct therapies, yet very powerful ones. In fact, they are therapeutically so effective that major hospitals in this country and around the world permit circus clowns to perform for children in cancer and burn wards. Patch Adams, the physician and professional clown (who Robin Williams so effectively portrayed in the movie of the same name) movingly conveys his feelings about humor: "I believe humor and love are at the core of good bedside manner, burnout prevention, and malpractice prevention, and for these alone, humor deserves a central place in a medical practice, but let us not deny its value in just raw fun. Despite my long, deep experiences with humor, I still can be brought to tears of joy over its power" (Micozzi, 2001).

LOVE

Dean Ornish is the physician who told heart patients all across America how to eat right, exercise, engage in social support groups, and meditate in order to reduce their likelihood of further heart disease. Health insurance companies recongnized the financial benefits of his program, and now over 40 insurance companies nationwide cover the program. In this book *Love and Survival*, Ornish then maintains that "the real epidemic in our culture is not only physical heart disease, but also what I call *emotional and spiritual heart disease*" (Ornish, 1998). Ornish reviews the extensive body of medical evidence showing that loneliness and isolation are detrimental to our health and increase the likelihood of premature death from *any* cause by two to five times. James Lynch, in his provocative book, *A Cry Unheard*, reviews similar issues and also some of the best studies on the startling impact of loneliness as a major hidden cause of heart disease, subsequent cardiac events (e.g., heart attack), and death from cardiac events (Lynch, 2000).

So, the hard scientific evidence is there: love or even meaningful social connections can keep us healthier (see Chapters 2 and 3). But, how can this happen; how can we use love and intimacy to increase our well-being? Ornish's book includes an account of his personal journey through terrors of loneliness. Through his determination to learn to be alone with himself, he discovered that he had to develop a strong sense of a separate self before being able to skillfully participate in intimate relationships. Yet, Ornish also strongly advocates group therapy for cardiac patients and others to learn to express feelings. These two seemingly disparate themes come together in an interview Ornish conducts with Jon Kabat-Zinn, Ph.D., the founder of the Stress Reduction Clinic at the University of Massachusetts Medical Center in Worcester. Kabat-Zinn speaks about finding an inner peace that is a total willingness to be at peace right now with things as they are. Think about that. It means that you can stop letting your boss get to you and perhaps even appreciate the lessons as to why he or she acts the way he or she does. It means that you can be more accepting and understanding of why your partner does not and perhaps cannot do things the way you would like them done. But, it also means that there is a deep acceptance of yourself. Kabat-Zinn concludes, "To me, that [inner peace] is synonymous with love, and synonymous with intimacy, and synonymous with the highest wisdom and courage."

Don Miguel Ruiz, a Toltec Indian from rural Mexico, has written a book called *The Mastery of Love*, which takes Ornish's discussion to a deeper level (Ruiz, 1999). Ruiz believes that mastery of self-love can transform one's life and create an awareness that allows people to open their hearts and be an expression of "Spirit, Love, and Life." He states, "The heart is in direct communication with the human soul, and when the heart speaks, even with the resistance of the head, something inside you changes; your heart opens another heart, and true love is possible." Ruiz's book is not a book of medical evidence; it is a beautiful, inspirational book about learning to love yourself as well as others so that each day can be a joyful expression of life.

Before taking a look at the healing modalities that fall into the NIH Category 5 of energy therapies (see first paragraph of this chapter), we will review the pineal gland in Chapter 6. The pineal is our master gland and the transducer and translator of external environmental information to the electrical and hormonal signals that the body is capable of reading.

REFERENCES

Achterberg, J., *Imagery in Healing: Shamanism and Modern Medicine*, Shambhala, Boston, 1985.

Achterberg, J., Imagery, ceremony, and healing rituals: interview by Bonnie Horrigan, *Alternative Ther. Health Med.*, 5 (5), 77–83, 1999.

Achterberg, J. and Lawlis, G.F., *Imagery of Cancer*, Institute for Personality and Ability Testing, Champaign, IL, 1978.

Achterberg, J., Kenner, C., and Cassey, D., Behavioral strategies for the reduction of pain and anxiety associated with orthopedic trauma, *Biofeedback Self Regul.*, 14 (2), 101–114, 1989.

Akduman, L. and Olk, R.J., Subthreshold (invisible) modified grid diode laser photocoagulation in diffuse diabetic macular edema (DDME), *Ophthalmic Surg. Lasers*, 30(9), 706–714, 1999.

Alimi, D., Rubino, C., Leandri, E.P., and Brule, S.F., Analgesic effects of auricular acupuncture for cancer pain, *J. Pain Symptom Manage.*, 19 (2), 81–82, 2000.

Asawanonda, P., Anderson, R.R., Chang, Y., and Taylor, C.R., 308-nm excimer laser for the treatment of psoriasis: a dose-response study, *Arch. Dermatol.*, 136 (5), 619–624, 2000.

Ashton, C. et al., Self-hypnosis reduces anxiety following coronary artery bypass surgery: a prospective, randomized trial, *J. Cardiovasc. Surg.*, 38 (1), 69–75, 1997.

Ashton, R.C. et al., The effects of self-hypnosis on quality of life following coronary artery bypass surgery: preliminary results of a prospective, randomized trial, *J. Alternative Complementary Med.*, 1 (3) 285–290, 1995.

Babak, O.I. and Honcharova, L.I., The microwave therapy of patients with duodenal peptic ulcer who took part in the cleanup of the aftermath of the accident at the Chernobyl Atomic Electric Power Station, *Likars'ka Sprava/Ministerstvo Okhorony Zdorov'ia Ukrainy*, (7–8), 51–53, 1995.

Balon, J. et al., A comparison of active and simulated chiropractic manipulation as adjunctive treatment for childhood asthma, *New England J. Med.*, 339 (15), 1013–1020, 1998.

Bandello, F., Lanzetta, P., and Menchini, U., When and how to do a grid laser for diabetic macular edema, *Documenta Ophthalmologica, Adv. Ophthalmol.*, 97 (3–4), 415–419, 1999.

Becker, R.O. and Selden, G., *The Body Electric*, William Morrow and Company, New York, 1985.

Berk, L.S., Felten, D.L., Tan, S.A., Bittman, B.B., and Westengard, J., Modulation of neuroimmune parameters during eustress of humor-associated mirthful laughter, *Alternative Ther. Health Med.*, 7 (2), 62–76, 2001.

Blumenthal, M., Ed., *The Complete German Commission E Monographs*, Integrative Medicine Communications, Boston, 1998.

Bove, G. and Nilsson, N., Spinal manipulation in the treatment of episodic tension-type headache: a randomized controlled trial, *JAMA: J. Am. Medical Assoc.*, 280 (18), 1576–1579, 1998.

Breiling, B.J., Ed., *Light Years Ahead: the Illustrated Guide to Full Spectrum and Color Light in Mindbody Healing*, Celestial Arts, Berkeley, CA, 1996.

Brockhaus, A. and Elger, C.E., Hypalgesic efficacy of acupuncture on experimental pain in man: comparison of laser acupuncture and needle acupuncture, *Pain*, 43 (2), 181–185, 1990.

Bronfort, G., Evans, R.L., Kubic, P., and Filkin, P., Chronic pediatric asthma and chiropractic spinal manipulation: a prospective clinical series and randomized clinical pilot study, *J. Manipulative Physiological Ther.*, 24 (6), 369–377, 2001a.

Bronfort, G., Evans, R., Nelson, B., Aker, P.D., Goldsmith, C.H., and Vernon, H., A randomized clinical trial of exercise and spinal manipulation for patients with chronic neck pain, *Spine*, 26 (7), 788–797, 2001b.

Brown, B.B., Specificity of EEG-photic flicker responses to color as related to visual imagery ability, *Psychophysiol.*, 2 (3), 197–207, 1966.

Brown, B.B., Recognition of aspects of consciousness through association with EEG alpha activity represented by a light signal, *Psychophysiology*, 6 (4), 442–452, 1970.

Brown, C.S., Parker, N., Ling, F., and Wan, J., Effect of magnets on chronic pelvic pain, *Obstet. Gynecol.*, 95 (4), S29, 2000.

Camillieri, G., Margheritini, F., Maresca, G., and Mariani, P.P., Postoperative bleeding following notchplasty in anterior cruciate ligament reconstruction: thermal radio frequency versus powered instrumentation, *Knee Surg., Sports Traumatol., Arthroscopy: Off. J. ESSKA*, 9 (1), 12–14, 2001.

Chen, H., Recent studies on auriculacupuncture and its mechanism, *J. Traditional Chin. Med.*, 13 (2), 129–143, 1993.

Chen, Z. and Chen, Z., 48 cases of anxiety syndrome treated by massage, *J. Traditional Chin. Med.*, 18 (4), 282–284, 1998.

Cherkin, D.C. et al., Randomized trial comparing traditional Chinese medical acupuncture, therapeutic massage, and self-care education for chronic low back pain, *Arch. Intern. Med.*, 161 (8), 1081–1088, 2001.

Childre, D.L., *Freeze Frame: One Minute Stress Management*, Planetary Publications, Boulder Creek, CO, 1994.

Childre, D.L., Martin, H., and Beech, D., *The HeartMath Solution: The Institute of HeartMath's Revolutionary Program for Engaging the Power of the Heart's Intelligence*, HarperCollins Publishers, San Francisco, 1999.

Conway, P.J., Chiropractic approach to running injuries, *Clinics Podiatric Med. Surg.*, 18 (2), 351–362, 2001.

Cousins, N., Anatomy of an illness (as perceived by the patient), *New England J. Med.*, 295 (26), 1463–1485, 1976.

Cowings, P.S. and Toscano, W.B., Autogenic-feedback training exercise is superior to promethazine for control of motion sickness symptoms, *J. Clinical Pharmacol.*, 40 (10), 1154–1165, 2000.

Defechereux, T., Meurisse, M., Hamoir, E., Gollogly, L., Joris, J., and Faymonville, M.E., Hypnoanesthesia for endocrine cervical surgery: a statement of practice, *J. Alternative Complementary Med.*, 5 (6), 509–520, 1999.

Dewhurst-Maddock, O., *The Book of Sound Therapy: Heal Yourself with Music and Voice*, Simon and Schuster, New York, 1993.

Dillbeck, M.C. and Bronson, E.C., Short-term longitudinal effects of the transcendental meditation technique on EEG power and coherence, *Int. J. Neurosci.*, 14 (3–4), 147–151, 1981.

Dodd, III, G.D. et al., Minimally invasive treatment of malignant hepatic tumors: at the threshold of a major breakthrough, *Radiographics*, 20 (1), 9–27, 2000.

Dossey, L., Hypnosis: a window into the soul of healing, *Alternative Ther. Health Med.*, 6 (2), 12–111, 2000.

Drobyshev, V.A., Filippova, G.N., Loseva, M.I., Shpagina, L.A., Shelepova, N.V., and Zhelezniak, M.S., The use of low-frequency magnetotherapy and EHF puncture in the combined treatment of arterial hypertension in vibration-induced disease, *Voprosy Kurortologii, Fizioterapii, i Lechebnoi Fizicheskoi Kultury*, 3, 9–11, 2000.

Dziublik, A.A., Mukhin, A.A., Ugarov, B.N., and Chechel, L.V., The use of microwave resonance therapy on patients with chronic nonspecific lung diseases, *Vrachebnoe Delo.*, 3, 55–56, 1989.

Eastman, C.I., Young, M.A., Fogg, L.F., Liu, L., and Meaden, P.M., Bright light treatment of winter depression: a placebo-controlled trial, *Arch. Gen. Psychiatry*, 55 (10), 883–889, 1998.

Edwards, C.L., Sudhakar, S., Scales, M.T., Applegate, K.L., Webster, W., and Dunn, R.H., Electromyographic (EMG) biofeedback in the comprehensive treatment of central pain and ataxic tremor following thalamic stroke, *Appl. Psychophysiol. Biofeedback*, 25 (4), 229–240, 2000.

Edwards, S., *The Emerging Field of BioAcoustics*, Sound Health, Athens, OH, 1997.

Ernst, E. and Kanji, N., Autogenic training for stress and anxiety: a systemic review, *Complementary Ther. Med.*, 8 (2), 106–110, 2000.

Falk, M.H. and Issels, R.D., Hyperthermia in oncology, *Int. J. Hyperthermia*, 17 (1), 1–18, 2001.

Fenn, A.J. and King, G.A., Adaptive radiofrequency hyperthermia-phased array system for improved cancer therapy: phantom target measurements, *Int. J. Hyperthermia*, 10 (2), 189–208, 1994.

Flores, R., Dance for health: improving fitness in African American and Hispanic adolescents, *Public Health Rep.*, 110 (2), 189–193, 1995.

Freeman, L.W. and Lawlis, G.F., Eds. *Mosby's Complementary and Alternative Medicine: A Research Based Approach*, Mosby, St. Louis, 2001.

George, M.S., Lisanby, S.H. and Sackeim, H.A., Transcranial magnetic stimulation: applications in neuropsychiatry, *Arch. Gen. Psychiatry*, 56 (4), 300–311, 1999.

Goats, G.C., Continuous short-wave (radio-frequency) diathermy, *Br. J. Sports Med.*, 23 (2), 123–127, 1989.

Green, C., Martin, C.W., Bassett, K., and Kazanjian, A., A systematic review of craniosacral therapy: biological plausibility, assessment reliability and clinical effectiveness, *Complementary Ther. Med.*, 7 (4), 201–207, 1999.

Green, E. and Green, A., *Beyond Biofeedback*, Delta, New York, 1977.

Hanten, W.P., Dawson, D.D., Iwata, M., Seiden, M., Whitten, F.G. and Zink, T., Craniosacral rhythm: reliability and relationships with cardiac and respiratory rates, *J. Orthopaedic Sports Phys. Ther.*, 27 (3), 213–218, 1998.

Hoffman, R.E., Boutros, N.N., Hu, S., Berman, R.M., Krystal, J.H., and Charney, D.S., Transcranial magnetic stimulation and auditory hallucinations in schizophrenia, *Lancet*, 355 (9209), 1073–1075, 2000.

Hurwitz, M.D., Kaplan, I.D., Svensson, G.K., Hynynen, K. and Hansen, M.S., Feasibility and patient tolerance of a novel transrectal ultrasound hyperthermia system for treatment of prostate cancer, *Int. J. Hyperthermia*, 17 (1), 31–37, 2001.

Institute of Medicine, *Dietary Reference Intakes for Calcium, Phosphorus, Magnesium, Vitamin D, and Fluoride*, National Academy Press, Washington, D.C., 1999.

Institute of Medicine, *Dietary Reference Intakes for Thiamin, Riboflavin, Niacin, Vitamin B₆, Folate, Vitamin B₁₂, Pantothenic Acid, Biotin, and Choline*, National Academy Press, Washington, D.C., 2000.

Ishikawa, M. et al., Intraoperative microwave coagulation therapy for large hepatic tumors, *J. Hepato-Biliary-Pancreatic Surg.*, 7 (6), 587–591, 2000.

Jacobs, K.W. and Suess, J.F., Effects of four psychological primary colors on anxiety state, *Perceptual Motor Skills*, 41 (1), 207–210, 1975.

Jarski, R.W. et al., The effectiveness of osteopathic manipulative treatment as complementary therapy following surgery: a prospective, match-controlled outcome study, *Alternative Ther. Health Med.*, 6 (5), 77–81, 2000.

Jermyn, R.T., A nonsurgical approach to low back pain, *J. Am. Osteopathic Assoc.*, 101 (4): S6–S11, 2001.

Jones, J.W. and Richman, B.W., Treatment of refractory angina pectoris by transmyocardial laser revascularization, *Mo. Med.*, 98 (4), 148–151, 2001.

Jordan, A., Bendix, T., Nielsen, H., Hansen, F.R., Host, D., and Winkel, A., Intensive training, physiotherapy, or manipulation for patients with chronic neck pain: a prospective, single-blinded, randomized clinical trial, *Spine*, 23 (3), 311–318, 1998.

Jovanović-Ignjatić, Z. and Raković, D., A review of current research in microwave resonance therapy: novel opportunities in medical treatment, *Acupuncture Electro-Ther. Res.*, 24 (2), 105–125, 1999.

Kahn, J., *Principles and Practices of Electrotherapy*, Churchill Livingstone, New York, 1994.

King, C.E., Clelland, J.A., Knowles, C.J., and Jackson, J.R., Effect of helium-neon laser auriculotherapy on experimental pain threshold, *Phys. Ther.*, 70 (1), 24–30, 1990.

Kirsch, D.L., *The Science behind Cranial Electrotherapy Stimulation*, Medical Scope Publishing, Edmonton, Alberta, 1999.

Klein, E. et al., Therapeutic efficacy of right prefrontal slow repetitive transcranial magnetic stimulation in major depression: a double-blind controlled study, *Arch. Gen. Psychiatry*, 56 (4), 315–320, 1999.

Kokura, S. et al., Anti-tumor effects of hyperthermia plus granulocyte colony-stimulating factor, *Jpn. J. Cancer Res.*, 87 (8), 862–866, 1996.

Krutmann, J., Phototherapy for atopic dermatitis, *Clinical Experimental Dermatol.*, 25 (7), 552–558, 2000.

Kuz'menko, V.M., The role of microwave resonance therapy in the combined treatment of patients with cerebral atherosclerosis, *Likars'ka Sprava/Ministerstvo Okhorony Zdorov'ia Ukrainy*, 7, 146–148, 1998.

Lam, R.W., Buchanan, A., Mador, J.A., Corral, M.R., and Remick, R.A., The effects of ultraviolet-A wavelengths in light therapy for seasonal depression, *J. Affective Disorders*, 24 (4), 237–243, 1992.

Lam, R.W., Tam, E.M., Shiah, I.S., Yatham, L.N., and Zis, A.P., Effects of light therapy on suicidal ideation in patients with winter depression, *J. Clinical Psychiatry*, 61 (1), 30–32, 2000.

Lam, R.W., Lee, S.K., Tam, E.M., Grewal, A., and Yatham, L.N., An open trial of light therapy for women with seasonal affective disorder and comorbid bulimia nervosa, *J. Clinical Psychiatry*, 62 (3), 164–168, 2001.

Lawrence, R., Rosch, P., and Plowden, J., *Magnet Therapy: The Pain Cure Alternative*, Prima Health, Rocklin, CA, 1998.

Lehmann, T.R. et al., Efficacy of electroacupuncture and TENS in the rehabilitation of chronic low back pain patients, *Pain*, 26 (3), 277–290, 1986.

Leste, A. and Rust, J., Effects of dance on anxiety, *Perceptual Motor Skills*, 58 (3), 767–772, 1984.

Lewis, S.M., Clelland, J.A., Knowles, C.J., Jackson, J.R., and Dimick, A.R., Effects of auricular acupuncture-like transcutaneous electrical nerve stimulation on pain levels following wound care in patients with burns: a pilot study, *J. Burn Care Rehabil.*, 11 (4), 322–329, 1990.

Lieberman, J., *Light Medicine of the Future: How We Can Use It to Heal Ourselves Now*, Bear & Co., Santa Fe, NM, 1991.

Liss, S. and Liss, B., Physiological and therapeutic effects of high frequency electrical pulses, *Integrative Physiological Behavioral Sci.*, 31 (2), 88–95, 1996.

Livraghi, T. et al., Hepatocellular carcinoma: radio-frequency ablation of medium and large lesions, *Radiology*, 214 (3), 761–768, 2000.

Lynch, J.J., *A Cry Unheard: New Insights into the Medical Consequences of Loneliness*, Bancroft Press, Baltimore, MD, 2000.

Magnus, W.W. and Gamber, R.G., Osteopathic manipulative treatment: student attitudes before and after intensive clinical exposure, *J. Am. Osteopathic Assoc.*, 97 (2), 109–113, 1997.

Magoun, H.I., *Osteopathy in the Cranial Field*, Journal Printing Co., Kirksville, MO, 1976.

Mavromatis, A., *Hypnagogia: the Unique State of Consciousness between Wakefulness and Sleep*, Routedge & Kegan Paul Ltd., London, 1987.

McDannold, N.J. and Jolesz, F.A., Magnetic resonance image-guided thermal ablations, *Top. Magnetic Resonance Imaging*, 11 (3), 191–202, 2000.

McDermott, J.H., Antioxidant nutrients: current dietary recommendations and research update, *J. Am. Pharm. Assoc.*, 40 (6), 785–799, 2000.

McKinney, C.H., Antoni, M.H., Kumar, M., Tims, F.C., and McCabe, P.M., Effects of guided imagery and music (GIM) therapy on mood and cortisol in healthy adults, *Health Psychol.*, 16 (4), 390–400, 1997.

McPartland, J.M. and Mein, E.A., Entrainment and the cranial rhythmic impulse, *Alternative Ther. Health Med.*, 3 (1), 40–45, 1997.

Meade, T.W., Dyer, S., Browne, W., Townsend, J., and Frank, A.O., Low back pain of mechanical origin: randomised comparison of chiropractic and hospital outpatient treatment, *Br. Medical J. (Clinical Res. Ed.)*, 300 (6737), 1431–1437, 1990.

Meesters, Y., Beersma, D.G., Bouhuys, A.L., and van den Hoofdakker, R.H., Prophylactic treatment of seasonal affective disorder (SAD) by using light visors: bright white or infrared light? *Biological Psychiatry*, 46 (2), 239–246, 1999.

Melzack, R. and Wall P., Pain mechanisms: a new theory, *Science*, 150 (699), 971–979, 1965.

Micozzi, M.S., Ed., *Fundamentals of Complementary and Alternative Medicine*, 2nd ed., Churchill Livingston, New York, 2001.

Miller, J.W. et al., Photodynamic therapy with verteporfin for choroidal neovascularization caused by age-related macular degeneration: results of a single treatment in a phase 1 and 2 study, *Arch. Ophthalmol.*, 117 (9), 1161–1173, 1999.

Morita, A., Kobayashi, K., Isomura, I., Tsuji, T., and Krutmann, J., Ultraviolet A1 (340–400 nm) phototherapy for scleroderma in systemic sclerosis, *J. Am. Acad. Dermatol.*, 43 (4), 670–674, 2000.

Moser, D.K., Dracup, K., Woo, M.A., and Stevenson, L.W., Voluntary control of vascular tone by using skin-temperature biofeedback-relaxation in patients with advanced heart failure, *Alternative Ther. Health Med.*, 3 (1), 18–21, 1997.

Murphy, M. and Donovan, S., *The Physical and Psychological Effects of Meditation*, Institute of Noetic Sciences, Sausalito, CA, 1997.

Murray, C.C. and Kitchen, S., Effect of pulse repetition rate on the perception of thermal sensation with pulsed shortwave diathermy, *Physiotherapy Res. Int.: J. Researchers Clinicians Phys. Ther.*, 5 (2), 73–84, 2000.

Nakao, M. et al., Clinical effects of blood pressure biofeedback treatment on hypertension by auto-shaping, *Psychosomatic Med.*, 59 (3), 331–338, 1997.

Nelson, C.F., Bronfort, G., Evans, R., Boline, P., Goldsmith, C., and Anderson, A.V., The efficacy of spinal manipulation, amitriptyline and the combination of both therapies for the prophylaxis of migraine headache, *J. Manipulative Physiological Ther.*, 21 (8), 511–519, 1998.

NLP Comprehensive, *A Pocket Guide to NLP*, NLP Comprehensive, Boulder, CO, 1991.

Nordenström, B.E.W., *Exploring BCEC-Systems (Biologically Closed Electric Circuits)*, Nordic Medical Publications, Stockholm, Sweden, 1998.

Noreau, L., Martineau, H., Roy, L., and Belzile, M., Effects of a modified dance-based exercise on cardiorespiratory fitness, psychological state and health status of persons with rheumatoid arthritis, *Am. J. Phys. Med. Rehabil.*, 74 (1), 19–27, 1995.

Ornish, D., *Love and Survival*, HarperCollins, New York, 1998.

Ozcan, C. et al., Long-term survival after ablation of the atrioventricular node and implantation of a permanent pacemaker in patients with atrial fibrillation, *New England J. Med.*, 344 (14), 1043–1051, 2001.

Pages, I.H., Jahr, S., Schaufele, M.K., and Conradi, E., Comparative analysis of biofeedback and physical therapy for treatment of urinary stress incontinence in women, *Am. J. Phys. Med. Rehabil.*, 80 (7), 494–502, 2001.

Patiakina, O.K., Antonian, R.G., and Zagorskaia, E.E., Treatment of subjective noise in the ear by impulse low-frequency electromagnetic field (preliminary results), *Vestnik Otorinolaringologii*, 1, 59–60, 1998.

Petrovic, V. and Bhisitkul, R.B., Lasers and diabetic retinopathy: the art of gentle destruction, *Diabetes Technol. Ther.*, 1 (2), 177–187, 1999.

Polderman, M.C., Huizinga, T.W., LeCessie, S., and Pavel, S., UVA-1 cold light treatment of SLE: a double blind, placebo controlled crossover trial, *Ann. Rheumatic Dis.*, 60 (2), 112–115, 2001.

Pratt-Harrington, D., Galbreath technique: a manipulative treatment for otitis media revisited, *J. Am. Osteopathic Assoc.*, 100 (10), 635–639, 2000.

Radmayr, C., Schlager, A., Studen, M., and Bartsch, G., Prospective randomized trial using laser acupuncture versus desmopressin in the treatment of nocturnal enuresis, *Eur. Urol.*, 40 (2), 201–205, 2001.

Reeves, R.A., Edmonds, E.M., and Transou, D.L., Effects of color and trait anxiety on state anxiety, *Perceptual Motor Skills*, 46 (3), 855–858, 1978.

Richards, D.G., Mein, E.A., and Nelson, C.D., Chiropractic manipulation for childhood asthma, *New England J. Med.*, 340 (5), 391–392, 1999.

Rogers, J.S., Witt, P.L., Gross, M.T., Hacke, J.D., and Genova, P.A., Simultaneous palpation of the craniosacral rate at the head and feet: intrarater and interrater reliability and rate comparisons, *Phys. Ther.*, 78 (11), 1175–1185, 1998.

Roider, J., Brinkmann, R., Wirbelauer, C., Laqua, H., and Birngruber, R., Retinal sparing by selective retinal pigment epithelial photocoagulation, *Arch. Ophthalmol.*, 117 (8), 1028–1034, 1999.

Rolf Institute of Structural Integration, *The Rolfing® Technique of Connective Tissue Manipulation*, Rolf Institute, Boulder, CO, 1976.

Rosch, P.J., Magnetotherapy for cancer, heart disease, pain and aging, *Health Stress: Newsl. Am. Inst. Stress*, 6, 1–8, 1997.

Rosenthal, N.E., Sack, D.A., Carpenter, C.J., Parry, B.L., Mendelson, W.B., and Wehr, T.A., Antidepressant effects of light in seasonal affective disorder, *Am. J. Psychiatry*, 142 (2), 163–170, 1985.

Rosenthal, N.E. et al., Seasonal affective disorder: a description of the syndrome and preliminary findings with light therapy, *Arch. Gen. Psychiatry*, 41 (1), 72–80, 1984.

Rossi, S. et al., Percutaneous radio-frequency thermal ablation of nonresectable hepatocellular carcinoma after occlusion of tumor blood supply, *Radiology*, 217 (1), 119–126, 2000.

Ruiz, D.M., *The Mastery of Love*, Amber-Allen, San Rafael, CA, 1999.

Sack, R.L., Lewy, A.J., White, D.M., Singer, C.M., Fireman, M.J., and Vandiver, R., Morning vs. evening light treatment for winter depression: evidence that the therapeutic effects of light are mediated by circadian phase shifts, *Arch. Gen. Psychiatry*, 47 (4), 342–351, 1990.

Salmore, R.G. and Nelson, J.P., The effect of preprocedure teaching, relaxation instruction, and music on anxiety as measured by blood pressures in an outpatient gastrointestinal endoscopy laboratory, *Gastroenterol. Nursing*, 23 (3), 102–10, 2000.

Sandyk, R., The influence of the pineal gland on migraine and cluster headaches and effects of treatment with picoTesla magnetic fields, *Int. J. Neurosci.*, 67 (1–4), 145–171, 1992.

Sandyk, R., Reversal of a visuoconstructional disorder by weak electromagnetic fields in a child with Tourette's syndrome, *Int. J. Neurosci.*, 90 (3–4), 159–167, 1997a.

Sandyk, R., Therapeutic effects of alternating current pulsed electromagnetic fields in multiple sclerosis, *J. Alternative Complementary Med.*, 3 (4), 365–386, 1997b.

Sandyk, R., Reversal of a body image disorder (macrosomatognosia) in Parkinson's disease by treatment with AC pulsed electromagnetic fields, *Int. J. Neurosci.*, 93 (1–2), 43–54, 1998.

Sandyk, R., Impairment of depth perception in multiple sclerosis is improved by treatment with AC pulsed electromagnetic fields, *Int. J. Neurosci.*, 98 (1–2), 83–94, 1999.

Sandyk, R., Anninos, R.A., and Tsagas, N., Magnetic fields and seasonality of affective illness: implications for therapy, *Int. J. Neurosci.*, 58 (3–4), 261–267, 1991.

Schlager, A., Offer, T., and Baldissera, I., Laser stimulation of acupuncture point P6 reduces postoperative vomiting in children undergoing strabismus surgery, *Br. J. Anaesthesia*, 81 (4), 529–532, 1998.

Shankar, A. et al., Neo-adjuvant therapy improves resectability rates for colorectal liver metastases, *Ann. R. Coll. Surgeons Engl.*, 83 (2), 85–88, 2001.

Shapiro, F., *Eye Movement Desensitization and Reprocessing: Basic Principles, Protocols, and Procedures*, Guilford, New York, 1995.

Shevchenko, A.I., The correction of the immune status at the postoperative rehabilitative stage in lung cancer patients by using millimeter-wave resonance therapy, *Likars'ka Sprava/Ministerstvo Okhorony Zdorovia Ukrainy*, 2, 95–97, 2000.

Shibata, T., Niinobu, T., Ogata, N., and Takami, M., Microwave coagulation therapy for multiple hepatic metastases from colorectal carcinoma, *Cancer*, 89 (2), 276–284, 2000.

Shimada, S. et al., Complications and management of microwave coagulation therapy for primary and metastatic liver tumors, *Surg. Today*, 28 (11), 1130–1137, 1998.

Siedentopf, C.M., Golaszewski, S.M., Mottaghy, F.M., Ruff, C.C., and Felber, S., Functional magnetic resonance imaging detects activation of the visual association cortex during laser acupuncture of the foot in humans, *Neurosci. Lett.*, 327 (1), 53–56, 2002.

Simonton, S.S. and Sherman, A.C., Psychological aspects of mind-body medicine: promises and pitfalls from research with cancer patients, *Alternative Ther.*, 4 (4), 50–67, 1998.

Spinhoven, P. and ter Kuile, M.M., Treatment outcome expectancies and hypnotic susceptibility as moderators of pain reduction in patients with chronic tension-type headache, *Int. J. Clinical Experimental Hypnosis*, 48 (3), 290–305, 2000.

Stevinson, C., Honan, W., Cooke, B., and Ernst, E., Neurological complications of cervical spine manipulation, *J. R. Soc. Med.*, 94 (3), 107–110, 2001.

Sullivan, D.M., Ben-Yosef, R., and Kapp, D.S., Stanford 3D hyperthermia treatment planning system: technical review and clinical summary, *Int. J. Hyperthermia*, 9 (5), 627–643, 1993.

Suomi, R. and Koceja, D.M., Effect of magnetic insoles on postural sway measures in men and women during a static balance test, *Perceptual Motor Skills*, 92 (2), 469–476, 2001.

Terman, M. and Terman, J.S., Bright light therapy: side effects and benefits across the symptom spectrum, *J. Clinical Psychiatry*, 60 (11), 799–808, 1999.

Terman, M., Terman, J.S., and Ross, D.C., A controlled trial of timed bright light and negative air ionization for treatment of winter depression, *Arch. Gen. Psychiatry*, 55 (10), 875–882, 1998.

Terman, J.S., Terman, M., Lo, E.S., and Cooper, T.B., Circadian time of morning light administration and therapeutic response in winter depression, *Arch. Gen. Psychiatry*, 58 (1), 69–75, 2001.

Tettambel, M.A., Osteopathic treatment considerations for rheumatic diseases, *J. Am. Osteopathic Assoc.*, 101 (4), S18–S20, 2001.

Tomatis, A., *The Ear and Language*, Moulin Publishing, Ontario, 1996.

Trager, M. and Hammond, C., *Movement as a Way to Agelessness: A Guide to Trager Mentastics*, Station Hill Press, Barrytown, NY, 1987.

Travis, F. and Wallace, R.K., Autonomic and EEG patterns during eyes-closed rest and transcendental meditation (TM) practice: the basis for a neural model of TM practice, *Consciousness Cognition*, 8 (3), 302–318, 1999.

Trock, D.H., Electromagnetic fields and magnets: investigational treatment for musculoskeletal disorders, *Rheumatic Dis. Clinics North America*, 26 (1), 51–62, 2000.

Trumbo, P., Yates, A.A., Schlicker, S., and Poos, M., Dietary reference intakes: vitamin A, vitamin K, arsenic, boron, chromium, copper, iodine, iron, manganese, molybdenum, nickel, silicon, vanadium, and zinc, *J. Am. Dietary Assoc.*, 101 (3), 294–301, 2001.

Tuchin, P.J., Pollard, H., and Bonello, R., A randomized controlled trial of chiropractic spinal manipulative therapy for migraine, *J. Manipulative Physiological Ther.*, 23 (2), 91–95, 2000.

Van Buskirk, R.L., A manipulative technique of Andrew Taylor Still as reported by Charles Hazzard, DO, in 1905, *J. Am. Osteopathic Assoc.*, 96 (10), 597–602, 1996.

Vicenzino, B., Collins, D., and Wright, A., The initial effects of a cervical spine manipulative physiotherapy treatment on the pain and dysfunction of lateral epicondylalgia, *Pain*, 68 (1), 69–74, 1996

Wallace, R.K., Silver, J., Mills, P.J., Dillbeck, M.C., and Wagoner, D.E., Systolic blood pressure and long-term practice of the Transcendental Meditation™ and TM–Sidhi program: effects of TM on systolic blood pressure, *Psychosomatic Med.*, 45 (1), 41–46, 1983.

Walleczek, J., Electromagnetic field effects on cells of the immune system: the role of calcium signaling, *FASEB J.: Off. Publ. Fed. Am. Soc. Experimental Biol.*, 6 (13), 3177–3185, 1992.

Walleczek, J. and Budinger, T.F., Pulsed magnetic field effects on calcium signaling in lymphocytes: dependence on cell status and field intensity, *FEBS Lett.*, 314 (3), 351–355, 1992.

Walther, M.C. et al., A phase 2 study of radio frequency interstitial tissue ablation of localized renal tumors, *J. Urol.*, 163 (5), 1424–1427, 2000.

Weaver, M.T. and McGrady, A., A provisional model to predict blood pressure response to biofeedback-assisted relaxation, *Biofeedback Self-Regul.*, 20 (3), 229–240, 1995.

Weintraub, M.I., Magnetic bio-stimulation in painful diabetic peripheral neuropathy: a novel intervention—a randomized, double-placebo crossover study, *Am. J. Pain Manage.*, 9 (1), 8–17, 1999.

Wenneberg, S.R. et al., A controlled study of the effects of the transcendental meditation program on cardiovascular reactivity and ambulatory blood pressure, *Int. J. Neurosci.*, 89 (1–2), 15–28, 1997.

Werner, O.R., Wallace, R.K., Charles, B., Janssen, G., Stryker, T., and Chalmers, R.A., Long-term endocrinologic changes in subjects practicing the transcendental meditation and TM–Sidhi program, *Psychosomatic Med.*, 48 (1–2), 59–66, 1986.

White, J.M., State of the science of music interventions: critical care and perioperative practice, *Crit. Care Nursing Units North America*, 12 (2), 219–225, 2000.

Wiesel, P.H. et al., Patient satisfaction after biofeedback for constipation and pelvic floor dyssynergia, *Swiss Medical Weekly*, 131 (11–12), 152–156, 2001.

Williams, N., Managing back pain in general practice—is osteopathy the new paradigm? *Br. J. Gen. Pract.: J. R. Coll. Gen. Pract.*, 47 (423), 653–655, 1997.

Wong, T.W. and Fung, K.P., Acupuncture from needle to laser, *Fam. Pract.*, 8 (2), 168–170, 1991.

Yamamoto, K. and Tanaka, Y., Radiofrequency capacitive hyperthermia for unresectable hepatic cancers, *J. Gastroenterol.*, 32 (3), 361–366, 1997.

Yamasaki, T., Kurokawa, F., Shirahashi, H., Kusano, N., Hironaka, K., and Okita, K., Percutaneous radiofrequency ablation therapy with combined angiography and computed tomography assistance for patients with hepatocellular carcinoma, *Cancer*, 91 (7), 1342–1348, 2001.

Zeitlin, D., Keller, S.E., Shiflett, S.C., Schleifer, S.J., and Bartlett, J.A., Immunological effects of massage therapy during academic stress, *Psychosomatic Med.*, 62 (1), 83–84, 2000.

ADDITIONAL RESOURCES

ACUPUNCTURE

American Academy of Medical Acupuncture (AAMA); 323-937-5514; available on-line at http://medicalacupuncture.org.

Benson, H. and Stark, M., *Timeless Healing: The Power and Biology of Belief*, Scribner, New York, 1996.

Bioacoustics, available on-line at www.soundhealthinc.com.

Bio-Electrography, available on-line at http://www.psy.aau.dk/bioelec/index.htm.

Council of Colleges of Acupuncture and Oriental Medicine (CCAOM); 301-313-0868; available on-line at http://www.ccaom.org/.

Educational Kinesiology Foundation of North America; 800-356-2109; available on-line at www.braingym.org.

National Certification Commission for Acupuncture and Oriental Medicine (NCCAOM); 703-548-9004; available on-line at http://www.nccaom.org/.

National Sports Acupuncture Association (NSAA); 206-374-2505; available on-line at http://www.sportsacupuncture.com/.

HOMEOPATHY

Benveniste, J., Meta-analysis of homoeopathy trials, *Lancet*, 351 (9099), 367, 1998.

Green, E.E. and Green, A.M., Biofeedback and states of consciousness, in *Handbook of States of Consciousness*, Wolman, B.B. and Ullman, M., Eds., Van Nostrand Reinhold, New York, 1986, pp. 553–589.

Hübner's Medical Resonance Therapy Music; available on-line at www.peterhuebner.com.

Jonas, W.B. and Levin, J.S., *Essentials of Complementary and Alternative Medicine*, Lippincott, Williams, & Wilkins, Baltimore, 1999.

Thomas, P., Homeopathy in the USA, *Br. Homeopathic J.*, 90 (2), 99–103, 2001.

QIGONG

National QiGong Association, USA, (888) 815-1893, P.O. Box 252, Lakeland, MN 55043; www.nqa.org.

Qigong Institute, 561 Berkeley Ave., Menlo Park, CA 94025; www.qigonginstitute.org.

SEASONAL AFFECTIVE DISORDER (SAD)

Bio-Brite, Inc., 4340 East–West Hwy., Suite 401, Bethesda, MD 20814; 800-621-5483.

Light Energy Company, 1056 NW 179th Place, Seattle, WA 98177; 800-544-4826; www.light-energycompany.com.

National Institute of Mental Health (NIMH) trial; available on-line at http://clinicaltrials.gov.

North American Philips, 200 Franklin Square Drive, Somerset, NJ 08873; 800-752-2852; www.lighting.philips.com/nam.

Ott-Light Systems, Inc., 28 Parker Way, Santa Barbara, CA 93101; 800-234-3724; www.ott-biolight.com.

Weese, J.L., Harbison, S.P., Stiller, G.D., Henry, D.H., and Fisher, S.A., Neoadjuvant chemotherapy, radical resection with intraoperative radiation therapy (IORT): improved treatment for gastric adenocarcinoma, *Surgery*, 128 (4), 564–571, 2000.

6 The Pineal Gland: Physiology Meets Energy

To everything there is a season and a time to every purpose under heaven ... a time to be born, and a time to die.

Ecclesiastes

CONTENTS

INTRODUCTION

The pineal gland is arguably both the most misunderstood and underrated endocrine gland in the human body. Until 40 years ago, almost nothing was known about the pineal; it was considered unimportant and physiologically useless. Yet, René Descartes stated that the pineal is the "seat of the soul," and Eastern religions have described the pineal as the mysterious "third eye," the seat of wisdom, or the source of inner light. Although these beliefs were based on some rudimentary knowledge of the pineal as being photosensitive, the alignment of the pineal with spirituality has, more likely than not, been a deterrent to serious scientific research, relegating the pineal to the realm of the unknowable (see Zrenner, 1985, for a history of the pineal gland).

Complicating matters further, Descartes's expression linking the pineal and the soul generally is misunderstood. The philosopher, who is undoubtedly even better known for his exclamation, "cogito ergo sum" (I think, therefore I am/exist), believed that the ability to think is irrefutable evidence that the mind exists. His dualistic philosophical system divides the universe into mutually exclusive but interacting elements of spirit/mind or God and matter. Descartes's "seat of the soul" expression stems from his belief that the pineal is the interface between the spiritual and the material worlds, which as we will explore in the final chapter of this book, may well be true.

It is my contention that the pineal is the master gland. I suspect that, by the time you finish reading this chapter, you are likely to agree with me. In this chapter and the following two chapters, we will travel full circle: beginning with the essential neuroendocrinological aspects of the pineal that makes it our master gland and then progressing to how it may interface with "spiritual" (which will be redefined as "subtle energy" in Chapter 8) experiences, which paradoxically bring us back to fundamental principles of pineal physiology.

OVERVIEW OF THE PINEAL GLAND

Only in the last 30 to 40 years has an accurate understanding of the functions of the pineal begun to emerge. Most of this understanding has stemmed from the isolation of melatonin (N-acetyl-5-methoxytryptamine), the major pineal hormone (Lerner et al., 1958). The pineal has the ability to transform neural input into endocrine output. It is the tiny but mighty gland that is our liaison to the world around us. It converts light, temperature, and magnetic environmental information into neuroendocrine signals that can change the course of the body's functioning, often via its primary hormone, melatonin. Numerous studies now have shown the pineal to be the regulator and orchestrator of many neuroendocrine- and neuroimmune-modulating functions in the body.

The pineal's most widely known function is its ability to use external light to generate an entrainment of the body to daily (circadian) and seasonal (circannual) rhythms of the sleep–wake cycle. The word *circadian* comes from two Latin words: *circa*, meaning around, and *dies*, meaning day. In addition to sleep–wake cycles, circadian rhythms are found in the body's metabolism, hormone levels, blood pressure, and core temperature, to name a few. The pineal and its major hormone melatonin are capable of activating and regulating major body systems, including the stress and immune systems (see Bubenik et al., 1998, for a review of clinical utilizations of melatonin). In the following pages, we cover the structure and functions of the pineal, demonstrating its role as the body's primary neuroendocrine regulator and systems integrator.

PHYSIOLOGICAL CHARACTERISTICS OF THE PINEAL GLAND

In humans, the pineal gland lies above the superior colliculi and below the splenium of the corpus callosum at the posterodorsal aspect of the third ventricle. Embryologically, it arises from the ependyma (the membrane that lines the ventricles of the brain) of the third ventricle. In some lower vertebrates, the pineal arises from the median of the dorsal wall of the thalamus. It weighs 50 to 150 milligrams in humans and is 7 millimeters in length and 5 millimeters in width…about the size of a pencil eraser. Its name derives from the Latin word *pinea*, or pinecone, because of its cone-shaped appearance. As mentioned in Chapter 1, 240 million years ago vertebrates literally had a third eye on the top of their head, and today some invertebrates, such as lampreys, still possess a third eye. The pineal gland in both vertebrates and invertebrates has retained its photosensitive qualities.

The pineal gland undergoes a gradual process of calcification throughout life. Calcification actually begins in childhood. By early adulthood, it can be seen on radiograph in about 53% of the population and is evident in approximately 80% of elderly individuals. Recent work comparing the degree of calcification, as measured by computed tomography, to urinary melatonin excretion shows an association between lower levels of melatonin and calcification (Kunz et al., 1999). Degree of calcification has also been correlated to daytime tiredness and sleep disturbance (Kunz et al., 1998). There is one remarkable study published by the *British Medical Journal* over 15 years ago that indicates a correlation between pineal calcification in humans and a poor sense of direction (Bayliss et al., 1985). This report is intriguing when compared with studies on homing pigeons, whose pineal gland is paramount to survival, indicated by a brain weight of 10% (compared with 1% for humans). When homing pigeons have extensive calcification, they too lose their sense of direction. Perhaps, researchers should begin to study the correlation between pineal calcification and senility.

Unlike other structures of the central nervous system (CNS), the pineal gland lacks a blood–brain barrier, permitting direct reception of exogenous substances and endogenous hormones or neurotransmitters via the peripheral circulation. In addition, the pineal gland's major hormone, melatonin, is highly lipophilic, which means that it easily passes out of the pineal via cell membranes, including the epithelial cells in the blood vessels, the lymph vessels, the serous cavities, and the cavities of the heart. Consequently, melatonin is found not only in the blood but also in an assortment of fluids, including the saliva, cerebral spinal fluid (CSF), male seminal fluid, amniotic fluid, and the fluid in the anterior chamber of the eye (Reiter, 1991b, 1993a). The lack of a blood–brain barrier and the lipophilic quality of melatonin places the pineal gland in the optimal position for its responsibilities as the primary endocrine transducer and regulator of hormonal signals (i.e., as the master gland).

NEURAL PATHWAY FROM THE ENVIRONMENT TO THE PINEAL: THE RETINOHYPOTHALAMIC–PINEAL SYSTEM

In 1960, Ariëns Kappers identified postganglionic sympathetic neurons as the main source of pineal innervation (Lewy, 1983). In addition, a neural pathway has been established from the eye to the pineal gland (illustrated in Figure 6.1). The pathway begins at the ganglion cells of the retina, which have axons that make up the retinohypothalamic tract. Electrical signals from the retinohypothalamic tract reach the suprachiasmatic nucleus (SCN), located in the hypothalamus. The SCN is our biological clock, which will be described in more detail later in this chapter. From the hypothalamus, long descending axons of hypothalamic neurons synapse on autonomic neurons of the intermediolateral cell column in the upper thoracic spinal cord. The signals continue via the paraventricular nuclei to the spinal cord, where preganglionic axons exit the spinal cord to terminate on neurons in the superior cervical ganglia. Postganglionic neurons from the superior cervical ganglia travel back up and terminate in the pineal gland. Unlike many invertebrates whose pineal glands are connected to the roof of the brain, in mammals these postganglionic neurons replace any direct nerve connection to the brain.

In the early 1960s, Richard Wurtman and his mentor Julius Axelrod determined that in periods of darkness, the postganglionic (sympathetic) fibers from the superior cervical ganglia release norepinephrine (the major hormonal input) into the synaptic cleft, activating the retinohypothalamic–pineal system (Wurtman et al., 1963a, 1963b, 1964). The pineal contains both neuroglial cells and pinealocytes. The pinealocytes are the all-important receptor cells within the pineal. Pinealocytes secrete various peptides and neurotransmitters (see next section) in addition to melatonin (the major hormonal output). When norepinephrine stimulates β-adrenergic receptor sites at night, melatonin is synthesized and secreted from the pinealocytes. The melatonin is quickly released into the CSF and venous circulation, probably by passive diffusion (Reiter, 1991b; Reiter et al., 1995).

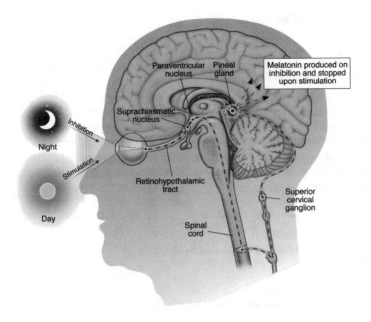

FIGURE 6.1 Neural pathway from the eye to the pineal. (See color insert following page 74.)

SECRETIONS OF THE PINEAL

NEUROPEPTIDES IN THE PINEAL

The pineal contains receptor cites for various neuropeptides, including those for norepinephrine (α- and β-adrenergic), serotonin, dopamine, glutamate, benzodiazepines, γ-aminobutyric acid (GABA), acetylcholine, and nicotine (Ebadi and Govitrapong, 1986). As just mentioned, norepinephrine is the primary pineal neurotransmitter. Recall that in the chapter on the relaxation system (Chapter 4), we learned that melatonin not only fits into its own receptor, but also into the benzodiazepine receptor (Marangos et al., 1981).

A group of researchers from Buenos Aires first showed that there are benzodiazepine receptors in the bovine pineal, and then a few years later they located them in the human pineal (Lowenstein and Cardinali, 1982; Lowenstein et al., 1984). Both benzodiazepines and melatonin reduce anxiety, alleviate depression, and aid insomnia. Melatonin, however, has fewer side effects (Garfinkel et al., 1999; Raghavendra et al., 2000). Recall that diazepan can suppress melatonin-binding sites, an action reversed by exogenous melatonin, and that peripheral benzodiazepine receptors can reverse the antidepressant action of melatonin (Atsmon et al., 1996; Raghavendra et al., 2000). In addition to the pineal, benzodiazepine receptors are present on platelets and monocytes, which implicates melatonin in the modulation of the cardiovascular and immune system—more on melatonin and the immune system will follow (Moingeon et al., 1984; Ruff et al., 1985). Clearly, a portrait emerges of a reciprocal and interactive relationship between these two molecules.

HORMONES IN THE PINEAL

The list of hormones found in the pineal is quite extensive (see Table 6.1 for a partial list). The pineal influences the secretion of these hormones, potentially resulting in significant functional and physiological changes. It is possible that some of the hormones are synthesized in the pineal and others arrive there via the circulation, but their presence still appears to have an impact on system function. For the most part, the pineal has an inhibitory impact on hormones and body function (e.g., it can reduce adrenal or gonadal weight), but there are some notable exceptions (e.g., it generally enhances the immune system). The extensive number of hormones found in the pineal, alone, is indicative of the broad influence of the pineal gland (Table 6.1) (Relkin, 1983; Vaughan, 1984).

TABLE 6.1
Hormones Found in the Pineal

Melatonin
Serotonin
N-acetyl-serotonin (NAS)
Cortisol
Corticotropin-releasing hormone (CRH)
Aldosterone
Insulin
Thyrotropin-releasing hormone (TRH)
Growth hormone (GH)
Gonadotropin-releasing hormone (GnRH)
Follicle-stimulating hormone (FSH)
Luteinizing hormone (LH)
Prolactin
Adrenocorticotropic hormone (ACTH)
Oxytocin
Somatostatin
Antidiuretic hormone
Prostaglandins
Melanocyte-stimulating hormone (MSH)

MELATONIN—THE MAJOR PINEAL HORMONE

Melatonin is the hormone that regulates our circadian, or sleep–wake, cycle. In 1958, melatonin (N-acetyl-5-methyoxytryptamine) was first isolated by Aaron Lerner, an American dermatologist (Lerner et al., 1958). Lerner isolated the melatonin, which was known to lighten skin melanocytes of amphibians and fish, from 250,000 bovine pineal glands (Binkley, 1988). Curiously, melatonin also is found in plants, particularly of the rice family, and some researchers claim that it can enter the blood and bind to melatonin receptor cites when ingested (Hattori et al., 1995; Reiter et al., 2001). However, in a personal communication, Richard Wurtman at Massachusetts Institute of Technology (MIT) said, "At present, there is no evidence that any food, eaten in any quantity, significantly elevates plasma melatonin levels." In so many words, conclusive evidence simply has not been established. It is, however, an intriguing line of research, which in my opinion, warrants further study.

Endogenous circadian rhythms of not only melatonin, but also of core body temperature and cortisol, average 24.18 hours in both young and elderly humans (Czeisler et al., 1999). Daytime administration of small doses of melatonin increases fatigue, decreases oral temperature, and impairs vigilance tasks (Arendt et al., 1984, 1985; Dollins et al., 1994). An 80-mg dose of melatonin can raise normal nighttime concentrations by 350 to 10,000 times (Waldhauser et al., 1984).

As any new parent might guess infants under 3 months of age secrete very little melatonin. Fortunately, this trend soon changes as humans reach peak concentration levels in the first to third years of life (Brzezinski, 1997). As mentioned, melatonin production progressively declines throughout life, showing considerable depletion with age: 250 pg/ml at ages 1 to 3; 120 pg/ml at ages 8 to 15; and declining gradually to 20 pg/ml by age 50 to 70 (Utiger, 1992).

MELATONIN DOSING AND SIDE EFFECTS

The side effects of melatonin, as reported in research studies, are remarkably low and mainly concern headache and fatigue. Because melatonin is not regulated by the Food and Drug Administration (it is categorized as a supplement because it is naturally found in foods), it is possible that there are detrimental effects that are not generally known. Important research shows that an optimal dose of melatonin for those individuals whose levels are subnormal seems to be 0.3 mg, although it is presently sold in tablets many times greater than is needed for this therapeutic effect (Zhdanova et al., 2001). At the relatively safe dose of 0.3 mg, the areas for physician-guided administration that appear to be the most promising include its use for perimenopausal women, the blind or elderly patient who suffers from insomnia, and possibly for some cancer (e.g., there have been encouraging results from some studies on estrogen-dependent breast cancer) and AIDS patients.

MEASURING MELATONIN

As stated, melatonin concentrations can be measured from plasma, saliva, the CSF, or urine. Melatonin synthesis occurs in the retina, Harderian gland, lymphocytes, monocytes, bone marrow cells, ovary, and the gut (Arendt, 1988; Reiter et al., 2000). Animal studies show that the increased level of pineal melatonin production during darkness is paralleled by an increased level of melatonin in the blood (Rollag et al., 1978). Although melatonin can be synthesized in areas other than the pineal, it is generally thought that the contribution of melatonin measured in blood plasma is solely of pineal origin because pinealectomized animals had no detectable plasma melatonin (Cogburn et al., 1987; Foa et al., 1992; Lewy et al., 1980b). However, other research on animals shows that at least some of the plasma melatonin loss from pinealectomy is regained if the animal is retested several weeks later (Osol et al., 1985; Vakkuri et al., 1985). A case study published in the *New England Journal of Medicine* reported that the removal of a cancerous pineal gland from a patient resulted in the disappearance of plasma melatonin, although the diseased gland had been capable of normal melatonin secretion and circadian rhythm (Neuwelt, et al. 1983). The researchers concluded that the pineal is the sole source of plasma melatonin in humans. In support of this concept is the knowledge that pineal gland removal in humans is accompanied by chronic and severe insomnia, which can in turn be ameliorated by melatonin administration (Etzioni et al., 1996; Jan et al., 2001; Vorkapic et al., 1987).

While concentrations of urinary and salivary melatonin are not identical to plasma melatonin levels, there is a consistently parallel relationship. For example, levels of a major melatonin urinary metabolite closely correlate to plasma melatonin levels, and saliva concentrations of melatonin maintain a correlation that is approximately 70% lower than those in the blood (Arendt, 1988; Kennaway and Voultsios, 1998; Lynch et al., 1975; Waldhauser et al., 1984). The Kennaway study found that there is a highly significant correlation between the ratio of free plasma to total plasma melatonin and in the saliva melatonin to total plasma melatonin ratio. These results were the first solid confirmation of an association between salivary and circulating melatonin levels.

MELATONIN SYNTHESIS

The process of melatonin synthesis (see Figure 6.2) was investigated and resolved in the 1960s, largely by Julius Axelrod, Richard Wurtman, and David Klein (Wurtman, 1963b, 1964). When norepinephrine stimulates the β-adrenergic receptor sites in the pineal, melatonin is not directly secreted from the pinealocytes, but rather it triggers a series of intracellular responses by which the pineal metabolizes the amino acid, tryptophan, into melatonin (Arendt, 1988; Wurtman and Moskowitz, 1977a). Tryptophan is taken up by the pineal from the circulating blood and converted to 5-hydroxytryptophan (5-HTP) by tryptophan 5-hydroxylase, a process that occurs more actively at night. Greater quantities of 5-HTP are stored in the pineal than anywhere else in the CNS. The decarboxylation of 5-HTP by the enzyme, aromatic L-amino acid decarboxylase, results in the production of serotonin, which also is found in large quantities in the pineal. The enzyme serotonin N-acetyltransferase (NAT) then N-acetylates serotonin to N-acetyl-serotonin (NAS). At night, when norepinephrine stimulates the β-adrenergic receptors, it causes the stimulation of the nucleotide cyclic adenosine monophosphate (cAMP), which serves as a second messenger. A cAMP-dependent protein kinase and a transcription of messenger RNA are fundamental to the activation of the NAT enzyme. Finally, the enzyme hydroxyindole-O-methyltransferase (HIOMT) O-methylates NAS, resulting in melatonin (Reiter, 1991a, 1991b, 1993a). Over 40 years ago, two prominent researchers, Julius Axelrod and Herbert Weissbach, at the National Institutes of Health (NIH) determined that the two enzymes NAT and HIOMT were essential to the synthesis of melatonin (Axelrod and Weissbach, 1960; Weissbach et al., 1960).

A great deal of research has been performed to determine the importance of the role of each of the precursors of melatonin. For example, because levels of NAT increase 25 to 100 times within a few minutes of darkness, it is presumed that NAT is the rate-limiting enzyme in melatonin synthesis (Maestroni and Conti, 1991a). Results of a study performed on mice showed that autocrine and paracrine actions

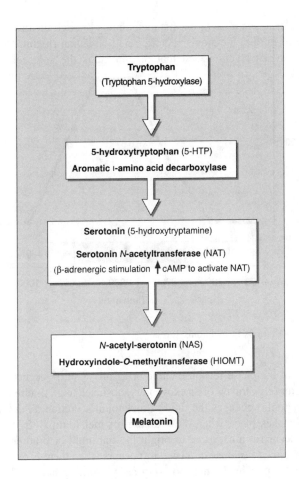

FIGURE 6.2 Synthesis of melatonin.

of 5-HTP in the pineal may be involved in the regulation of the secretion of melatonin (Reiter et al., 1990). Furthermore, levels of both 5-HTP and NAS decline after midnight (Oxenkrug et al., 1990). These fluctuations correspond to the research on melatonin phase shifts and light suppression, which are described in the following section.

MELATONIN PHASE-RESPONSE CURVE AND SUPPRESSION BY LIGHT

Normally, melatonin follows a reliable bell-shaped pattern of peaking at night and returning to lower levels by morning (see Figure 6.3). This phase-response curve may vary significantly even among healthy individuals (up to 30 ng per 8-hour interval), but it maintains a fairly consistent pattern for any particular person, allowing for the gradual and steady changes that correlate to shifts in season (Wurtman and Moskowitz, 1977b). Light does not actually cause the response curve (the SCN does), but rather entrains or alters it.

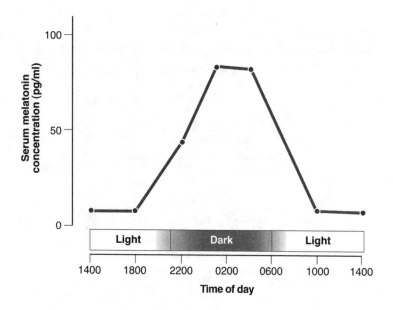

FIGURE 6.3 Variations in melatonin levels.

A "reset" of the phase-response curve or a "phase shift" occurs when an environmental factor (e.g., travel) or an exogenous substance (e.g., β-adrenergic blocking agents or melatonin) changes the time of melatonin secretion. A *delayed response* or phase shift takes place when the secretion of melatonin shifts to a later time, which could occur from exposure to bright light at night or β-adrenergic blocking agents. An *advanced response* or phase shift occurs when there is exposure to bright light in the latter part of the night or very early morning hours. This results in a phase shift that causes melatonin to secrete earlier in the night.

Virtually all investigations into the function of melatonin utilized the experimental setup of determining whether a phase shift has occurred. Hundreds of studies that have been performed on plants, insects, and mammals, including humans, confirm the fact that exposure to bright light at night causes a phase delay, and exposure to bright light in the very early morning hours results in a phase advance (Czeisler et al., 1989; Jewett et al., 1991; Lynch et al., 1978). The optimal time of melatonin administration to shift the cycle to an earlier time of day is between 8 hours before and 4 hours after the increase in endogenous plasma melatonin production. The optimal time of melatonin administration to shift the cycle to a later time of day is between 8 and 16 hours after the increase in endogenous plasma melatonin production (Sack et al., 2000). This information is crucial to the effective clinical administration of melatonin and to achieving experimental results that are not needlessly spurious. In humans, gender does not appear in any way to affect light-induced melatonin suppression (Nathan et al., 2000). Table 6.2 shows the illumination levels associated with commonly encountered environmental situations.

TABLE 6.2
Illumination Levels Associated with Environmental Situations

Event	Illumination Level (lux)
Noontime, summer solstice, 35° N latitude	113,284
Noontime, winter solstice, 35° N latitude	58,895
Most extreme black storm cloud conditions	7,000–11,000
Twilight begins	8,200
Full moon	0.37 (max)
Typical school classroom (general lighting)	400–700
General office lighting (typing)	500–750

Source: Hughes, P.C., et al., *Pineal Res.*, 5, 1–67, 1987.

As long ago as the early 1960s, researchers recognized that the enzyme HIOMT (the last catalyst in melatonin production) is suppressed when animals are exposed to continuous light (Wurtman et al., 1964). However, in a landmark experiment in 1980, Alfred Lewy and colleagues discovered, contrary to previous trials, that light does suppress human melatonin levels. The salient variable was that it took an intensity of light higher than ordinary room light to achieve the suppression (Lewy et al., 1980a). By the end of that decade, the dose-dependent relationship between light intensity and the associated degree of melatonin suppression had been established. The suppression levels at intensities of 3000, 1000, 500, 350, and 200 lux were 71%, 67%, 44%, 38%, and 16%, respectively (McIntyre et al., 1989a). The different light intensities produced discrete suppression of melatonin within 1 hour of light exposure at midnight, regardless of the intensity. A light intensity of 1000 lux is sufficient to suppress melatonin to near daytime levels (McIntyre et al., 1989a). However, light intensity of 200 lux does not produce statistically significant melatonin suppression when compared with control samples (McIntyre et al., 1989b). Interestingly, Charles Czeisler, at Harvard Medicine School, has now shown that the pineal is most susceptible to the influence of light when core body temperature is lowest, that is, around 4 A.M. to 5 A.M. (Boivin and Czeisler, 1998).

CLINICAL APPLICATIONS FOR MELATONIN

Insomnia and Jet Lag

Melatonin, perhaps, is best known for its ability to alleviate insomnia and jet lag. An understanding of phase shifts provides a medical framework by which melatonin is used to ameliorate insomnia and to speed the adjustment to a new time zone. Its use for the elderly with subnormal levels and for blind people with free-running rhythms indicates that there is an enormous improvement in quality of life for many of these individuals. However, the research is mixed on both efficacy and safety for long-term use in individuals with inherently normal levels. While melatonin may be effective in some people to reduce jet lag, there are serious questions about what effects its use might have on the other hormones of the body (Arendt and Marks, 1982; Arendt, 1988).

Nighttime Work, Mental Disorders, Anti-Aging

Charles Czeisler and colleagues at Harvard performed research that shows precisely what environment factors must be maintained in order to provide a reasonable adjustment to nighttime work (Czeisler et al., 1990). The researchers explain that thousands of U.S. employees are required to work at night, significantly increasing their risk of sleep disorders and possibly adversely affecting cardiovascular disease, gastrointestinal illness, and reproductive dysfunction in women. They found that conditions of intensely bright light (7000 to 12,000 lux) during the nighttime working hours and complete darkness during the daytime sleeping hours (in spite of exposure to outdoor lighting during a morning commute) causes a complete circadian adaptation to the night work schedule after 4 days. Concomitant shifts of plasma cortisol levels and urinary excretion rates plus higher alertness and cognitive performance assessments indicated that the subjects adapted significantly better than did controls.

Abnormal levels of melatonin also have been associated with some mental disorders, particularly depression. Its use as a therapeutic agent has not been well established for mental illness, but the use of light therapy has been shown to relieve depression, particularly with seasonally related depression (see Chapter 5).

Data on melatonin's role as an anti-aging substance is controversial, but intriguing. Researchers have hypothesized that the pineal is the gland that defines aging—as it involutes and melatonin production decreases, the signs of aging increase (Cardarelli, 1990; Nair et al., 1986; Rozencwaig et al., 1987). Other researchers speculate that as we age, our melatonin levels decrease, and therefore, the body's ability to protect itself against oxidative damage, and thus cancer, is diminished (Reiter, 1993a). Although it has not been substantiated in humans, chronic evening administration of melatonin to rodents has been shown to lengthen life. Nineteen-month-old mice that were administered melatonin in drinking water had a mean survival time of 931 days compared with 752 for the controls, approximately a 20% longer life span (Maestroni et al., 1988a). There appeared to be quality-of-life factors present as well, with the experimental mice retaining greater weight, better quality of fur, and superior all-around vigor.

Whether or not scientists are ever able to establish a correlation between the pineal and the aging process remains to be seen, but research has already shown that there is a significant correlation between aging and peak levels of plasma melatonin (Nair et al., 1986). In the early 1990s, Richard Wurtman and his colleagues at MIT showed that physiological doses of melatonin (which raise blood levels to those occurring normally at nighttime) promote sleep onset. Ten years later, they showed that the reason many people over 50 have insomnia is because their nocturnal melatonin secretion is below normal. Administration of a physiological dose of melatonin largely cures their insomnia (Zhdanova et al., 2001).

MELATONIN RECEPTORS

There are melatonin receptors not only in the brain, but also in various tissues throughout the body. The neural receptors found in the SCN are involved in circadian rhythms. The non-neural, membrane-signaling receptors are largely involved in reproductive regulation, including seasonal breeding. The receptors in the peripheral tissues are as yet a mystery and may be involved in a variety of interactions, including the regulation of body temperature and functions relating to the vascular system and the heart.

Membrane-Signaling Pathway

Recent work has determined that melatonin function is dependent upon high-affinity G protein-coupled seven-transmembrane receptors, called *ML1* and *ML2*. These membrane receptors, or binding sites, have been cloned in humans and are called *Mel$_{1a}$* and *Mel$_{1b}$* (Reppert et al., 1995; Slaugenhaupt et al., 1995). Mel$_{1a}$ receptors are far more numerous than Mel$_{1b}$ receptors. Mel$_{1b}$ receptors are predominantly found in the retina and are possibly involved in melatonin phase-shifting functions (Carlberg, 2000). Mel$_{1a}$ is found predominantly in the SCN and the pars tuberalis (Carlberg, 2000; Stankov and Reiter, 1990). The receptors are also expressed in the pars distalis (also located in the anterior portion of the pituitary), but only during the fetal and perinatal stages of life, and these may be instrumental in the light-induced development of the gonadotropic axis (Hazlerigg, 2001). Mel$_{1a}$ receptors are possibly the melatonin receptors involved in limiting the action of the SCN, our biological clocks, and binding sites appear to be different for daily circadian cycles than for longer photoperiodic melatonin variations (Schuster et al., 2001).

Nuclear-Signaling Pathway

There is also a nuclear-signaling pathway for melatonin, but it does not appear to be as sensitive as the membrane-signaling pathways. Nuclear receptors in humans include RZR/RORα and RZRβ (Wiesenberg et al., 1995). The RZR/RORα receptors are found both in the brain and the peripheral nervous system (Wiesenberg et al., 1995). There is evidence that these are the receptors predominantly involved in immune modulation. However, Mel$_{1a}$ receptors also have been found on lymphocytes, so obviously membrane receptors are involved in the peripheral system as well (Carlberg, 2000). When melatonin appears in concentrations higher than that provided by membrane or nuclear binding, it has a free radical scavenging function. We will review this and other immune-related topics in the chapter section entitled "Melatonin and the Immune and Stress Systems."

OUR WAKE–SLEEP SWITCH

In 1998, two studies were published attesting to the existence of novel neuropeptide proteins found in the hypothalamus. One group of researchers called the proteins *hypocretins* (HCRT-1 and HCRT-2) and determined that they were excitatory CNS neurotransmitters (de Lecea et al., 1998). The other group called them *orexin* (OR-R1 and OR-R2) and reported that the proteins were important to the control of feeding and to energy homeostasis (Sakurai et al., 1998). Hypocretin and orexin are two names for an identical molecule; therefore, we have chosen to use the name *orexin* for the rest of our discussion. A few years later, some of the same researchers determined that these neuropeptides were located in the pineal gland and that they had the ability to limit norepinephrine stimulation (Mikkelsen et al., 2001). This was big news because norepinephrine is the neurotransmitter, you will recall, that stimulates melatonin synthesis. A group at Harvard determined that there is actually an on–off switch that controls our movement between sleep and wakefulness states (Saper et al., 2001). In short, two opposing sets of neurons create a mechanism akin to a flip-flop switch in which there is great internal resistance to the switch being flipped. It is infrequent but rapid, and it is triggered by orexin. It moves us from being asleep to being awake and vice versa. While, as we are about to learn, the SCN is the location of the on–off switch, orexin actually flips the switch.

CLOCKWORKS—THE SUPRACHIASMATIC NUCLEUS (SCN)

The SCN is our biological clock and it, not light, ultimately is the location of the on–off switch for melatonin synthesis (Stetson and Watson-Whitmyre, 1976; Weaver, 1998). However, light both entrains and suppresses the levels of melatonin via the SCN. The SCN is located in the hypothalamus and receives environmental input via the retinohypothalamic tract. A measurement of melatonin is the most effective way to track a change in the circadian rhythm of the SCN. The SCN is fundamental to each of three major components of the circadian system: entrainment pathways, pacemakers, and output pathways to effector systems (Moore, 1995a). It modulates our neuroendocrine systems according to the current light pattern by regulating the secretion of melatonin and other hormones of the pineal. Clearly, the biological clock is indispensable to the basic functioning of the human body. But how is light information conveyed from the environment to this tiny SCN nucleus? What do the clock parts look like? And what resets the clock when the days start getting longer in the spring and shorter in the fall and winter?

We know that light somehow travels to the SCN via retinal projections in the retinohypothalamic tract that arise from discrete retinal ganglion cells (Moore 1995a, 1995b). The portion of retinohypothalamic tract that carries the transduced light impulse to the SCN also ends at the anterior hypothalamus (Leak and Moore, 1997). This is significant because lesions to the anterior hypothalamus result in impaired immune function. As we will see in the chapter section entitled "Melatonin and the Immune and Stress Systems," the SCN and melatonin production are closely related to immune performance.

The SCN is a paired structure with two subdivisions: a ventral core, which is located above the optic chiasm and receives transduced photic input, and a dorsal shell, which surrounds the core and receives input from nonvisual sources. Research has shown that the core and shell differ in their functioning in several respects (Leak and Moore, 2001). Efferent fibers project from both the core and the shell to similar areas on the other side of the SCN, and messages that travel via efferent projections to the periphery vary, depending on whether they originated from the core or the shell (Leak et al., 1999; Leak and Moore, 2001). Similarly, afferent neuronal messages going to the SCN contain functionally discrete messages that differ, depending upon whether they are being sent to the core or the shell. It may be that the projections from the SCN to the posterior hypothalamus mediate the arousal function of the circadian timing system (Abrahamson et al., 2001).

Local connections as well as afferent and efferent patterns offer insights into the pacemaker functions of the SCN. Circadian rhythm is determined by light via neural inputs and other information that flows through and out of the SCN. The rhythmic beating of these tiny nuclei is the timepiece of our lives. The physiological setup gives rise to strong speculation that the rhythm is the result of individual SCN neurons that are coupled (either between the core and shell or between the nuclei on each side, or both) to produce the circadian message (Leak et al., 1999). In fact, there is evidence to support the theory that the SCN is functionally organized into two left- and right-side oscillatory components that cycle in antiphase (see Figure 6.4), with efferent projections to brain regions outside of the SCN that maintain the rhythm (de la Iglesia et al., 2000).

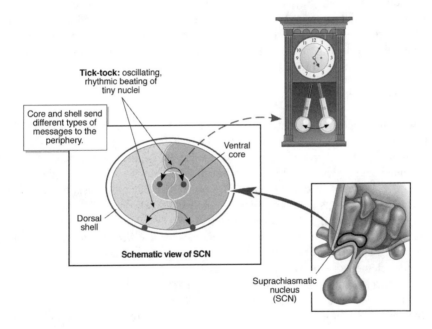

FIGURE 6.4 Oscillating patterns within the SCN. (See color insert following page 74.)

Keep in mind a portrait of a timekeeper whose task it is to harmonize not only our daily cadence but our lifetime rhythms as well. Then, mentally step back and try to hold the image of this internal timekeeper in harmonic resonance with the physical earth as well as with seen and unseen energy. We will speak more about this notion at the end of the chapter.

CLOCK COMPONENTS

Single-Cell Oscillators

What are the clock components? Recall the fascinating experiment reviewed in Chapter 1 in which nuclei from the SCN placed in a petri dish continued an electrical firing that maintained a 24-hour circadian rhythm (Hastings, 1998; Welsh et al., 1995). The neurons in the petri dishes did not synchronize to one another, however, which meant that they fired off independently, without any oscillating pattern (Welsh et al., 1995). The SCN is composed of many of these autonomous single-cell oscillators, which when coordinated or synchronized generate a circadian output that affects our body rhythms, as we know them (Reppert and Weaver, 2001).

In this section, we will look at some of the factors that produce synchronization among the autonomous circadian oscillators and how the synchronization influences the body rhythms (see Ishida et al., 1999; Jin et al., 1999; Miller, 1998, for a review). Interesting research shows that circadian oscillators reside in peripheral tissues as well as in the SCN of the pineal, but the SCN also controls the rhythm of the peripheral oscillators (Balsalobre et al., 2000; Reppert, 2000; Reppert and Weaver, 2001). As a result of this synchronization, the body maintains circadian rhythms for not only the sleep–wake cycle but for temperature, blood pressure, immune-cell count, and hormones that impact entire body systems, such as cortisol (stress) and prolactin (immune and reproduction).

Gene-Driven Feedback Loops

How do the opposing oscillations within the clock, for instance, for day and night rhythms, stay in sync? The entrainment of the SCN is triggered by a complex process (involving genes and proteins encoded to regulate numerous physiological processes) and then calibrated and reset by contact with light (Morris et al., 1998; Vitaterna et al., 2001). Circadian oscillator genes have transcriptional and translational autoregulated feedback loops with both negative and positive elements (Allada et al., 2001; King and Takahashi, 2000; Shearman et al., 2000). Various components of the negative feedback loop were first and more easily identified, but recently progress has been made in identifying the components of positive feedback loops, which are the core elements to circadian rhythmicity.

To understand the functions of a gene, researchers find genetic mutations of the wild-type or normal genes (which also provide an opportunity to clone the gene). They then insert or breed this mutation into test subjects (e.g., mice, fruit flies). How the mutation changes normal performance (e.g., causes phase advances, phase delays, or arrhythmic patterns) provides information regarding its inherent functioning. The research on clock genes began with two proteins from fruit flies (*Drosophila*) and one from a bread mold (*Neurospora*). The genes from the fruit flies are period (*per*) and timeless (*tim*), and the clock gene discovered from the bread mold is called *frequency* (*frq*) (Konopka and Benzer, 1971; Sehgal et al., 1991). The two fruit-fly genes were eventually located in the mouse (Ishida et al., 1991; Sangoram et al., 1998; Zylka et al., 1998). Two proteins involved in restarting the SCN clock genes, Clock and BMAL1, also have been located in both the fruit fly and mouse (Antoch et al., 1997; Darlington et al., 1998; King and Takahashi, 1997). The clock gene is an activator of the circadian system.

Joseph Takahashi and colleagues at Northwestern University were the first to identify the circadian clock gene in humans, which is expressed particularly in the SCN and cerebellum (Steeves et al., 1999). It appears that the clock gene in humans (as in mice) is required to maintain a rhythmicity in individual SCN neurons, but that a separate (but still unknown) mechanism within the SCN is synchronizing all of these neurons (Herzog et al., 1998). Think about it: your biological clock just keeps going … tick, tick, tick. These genes and proteins may well be the power source to the incessant, rhythmic ticking.

OCULAR PHOTOTRANSDUCTION: RESEARCH ON INDIVIDUALS WHO ARE BLIND

Photoreceptors receive the information to reset and adjust our biological clocks via the entrainment of light. We digress a moment before a discussion of photoreceptors to examine research performed on blind people, which gives important insight into ocular phototransduction. The majority of individuals who are blind have either an unusual circadian rhythm or a free-running rhythm (approximately 50% of those examined), but they show no impairment in the synthesis of melatonin. Free-running rhythms are characterized by a consistent delay in the circadian rhythm of about 60 to 70 minutes a day. Therefore, these people spend about half a month with their melatonin level telling them to sleep during the day and the other half of the month in a normal sleep–wake cycle (Lewy and Newsome, 1983; Sack et al., 1992).

In 1995, Charles Czeisler and several of his colleagues at Harvard performed some very interesting research on 11 blind subjects who had no conscious perception of light (Czeisler et al., 1995). They used the classic experiment of exposing the subject and controls to bright light at night to assess whether the normally higher nighttime melatonin levels would decrease. In 3 of the 11 blind subjects exposed to light, the melatonin levels decreased at essentially the same percentage as it did for the sighted controls. Curiously, it was only these three subjects who had reported no prior sleeping difficulties, while the remaining eight subjects reported a history of insomnia. These results strongly suggest that there is some photic function retained in the subjects whose melatonin is suppressed by light, despite the presence of damage that has eliminated the pupillary reflex and any perception of light. The researchers reasoned that the photoreceptive system that mediates melatonin expression must be distinctly different from the photoreceptive system that governs light perception "either quantitatively (i.e., in requiring only a few conventional receptors) or qualitatively (i.e., in using a novel phototransductive system with a distinct subgroup of retinal ganglion cells)."

Studies on the ocular photoreceptive system in blind people appropriately led to the therapeutic use of melatonin to entrain their circadian rhythms. Research now shows that melatonin, given at a dose of 10 mg per day, can appropriately phase-advance the circadian cycle for blind people, alleviating the burden of insomnia (Sack et al., 2000). It also appears that the dose of melatonin can be reduced to 5 mg once the individual is entrained to a nighttime sleep cycle. Research to determine whether the dose could be further lowered is warranted in light of the work by Zhdanova et al., who demonstrated that a dose of 0.3 mg was optimal in those individuals whose levels are subnormal (Zhdanova et al., 2001). Furthermore, researchers encourage a comprehensive evaluation of the circadian system before bilateral enucleation (i.e., removal of eyes damaged from disease or injury) is performed (Czeisler et al., 1995).

How Is the Clock Set? Capturing and Sending Light to the SCN

As we have indicated, light has something to do with how our biological clock adjusts itself, that is, how it makes the necessary corrections as days lengthen or shorten with seasonal changes. So, naturally, scientists want to locate the photoreceptors that pass this information from the environment to the SCN. The obvious place to look would be the light-sensitive rods and cones in the retina that provide us with our visual information. However, research on people who are blind gives us cause to question the role of rods and cones as primary phototransducers. Corroborating this supposition is a study that found that cone degeneration in aged mice did not render them incapable of circadian phase shifts and that their responses to light were similar to that of controls (Provencio et al., 1994). Following this study, two experiments established that mutant mice, lacking both rods and cones, still exhibited melatonin suppression when exposed to light (Freedman et al., 1999; Lucas et al., 1999). This finding conclusively demonstrates that something other than rods and cones are conveying the light information; in other words, they are not the sought-after photoreceptors. Research on humans is similar and shows that there is a unique short-wavelength–sensitive photopigment involved in light-induced melatonin suppression, providing the first direct evidence of a nonrod, noncone photoreceptive system in humans (Thapan et al., 2001). So if not rods and cones, what might these photoreceptors be?

One possibility is cryptochrome, the vitamin B-based, light-absorbing protein pigment in the eye and SCN, which is sensitive to blue light (Ivanchenko et al., 2001). It is found both in the retinal ganglion and the inner retina (Sancar, 2000). Cryptochrome was discovered in plants and identified as the protein that allows plants to bend toward light. Other possible photoreceptors are the nonrod, noncone vitamin A-based opsin photopigments, such as melanopsin (Provencio et al., 1998). The retinal distribution of melanopsin cells bears a striking resemblance to the retinal cells known to connect to the SCN in rodents. The inner retina seems to be the only mammalian site at which melanopsin is expressed, suggesting a role in nonvisual photoreceptive tasks (Provencio et al., 2000). So, in the end, melanopsin and cryptochrome are viable, but unconfirmed, photoreceptor candidates of the mammalian clock.

There are those working on finding the receptors who are convinced that multiple photoreceptors will be identified, which is a feasible conclusion given the complex interactions of the clock components (Lucas et al., 2001). It also is known that nonmammalian vertebrates possess multiple photoreceptors (Foster and Soni, 1998). There are, however, others who have done work showing that a single photopigment may be responsible for photo entrainment, suggesting that it may involve a novel opsin (Brainard et al., 2001). Scientists know that the photoreceptors for melatonin synthesis have a spectral sensitivity (i.e., the range most sensitive to stimulating melatonin release) between 400 and 650 nm. This helps to limit the choices but, unfortunately, a definitive mammalian photoreceptor has not yet been established.

MELATONIN AND THE IMMUNE AND STRESS SYSTEMS

As discussed in the chapter on the relaxation system (Chapter 4), melatonin is an important immune modulator of both the innate and acquired immune systems (Jankovic et al., 1970; Maestroni et al., 1989). However, melatonin may most effectively support the immune system by reducing the effects of stress (Maestroni and Conti, 1991a). Immune system suppression caused by corticosterone is reversed by melatonin, and its stress-ameliorating qualities appear to occur via melatonin's immune-enhancing capability (Khan et al., 1990; Maestroni et al., 1986; Maestroni et al., 1987a). The benzodiazepine receptors present on platelets and monocytes may be the avenue through which melatonin modulates the immune system (Moingeon et al., 1984; Ruff et al., 1985). Evidence also exists that melatonin is involved in an integrative systemic response designed to increase immune resiliency during the winter months (Nelson and Drazen, 2000). Because immune suppression is a major consequence of chronic stress, it is possible that melatonin's stabilizing properties promote equilibrium and ease the body back from stress to homeostasis by invigorating the immune system. Further research needs to be performed in order to understand this relationship more fully.

MELATONIN'S HUMORAL IMMUNE RESPONSES

Melatonin is involved in both humoral and cell-mediated immune responses, and pinealectomy or other means of blocking melatonin are correlated with distinct immune depression (Maestroni and Conti, 1991a). Furthermore, melatonin produces antistress and immune-enhancing effects in rodents in a circadian-dependent manner, that is the effects are dependent upon evening administration (Maestroni and Conti, 1989a). Researchers tested the immune-enhancing effects of melatonin in mice by giving them exogenous melatonin and then exposing them to an immunosuppressant—sheep red blood cells (SRBC). They found that melatonin administered in the evening enhances the antibody response in a dose-dependent manner, beginning at the low dose of 10 µg/kg of body weight, and results in reversal of the humoral suppression (Maestroni et al., 1986). The work of untangling the mechanisms of action for these functions is ongoing. However, it is known that melatonin, at least in part, stimulates humoral immune responses by increasing the survival rate of B-lymphocyte precursor cells found in the bone marrow (Yu et al., 2000).

MELATONIN'S CELL-MEDIATED IMMUNE RESPONSES

Melatonin stimulates cell-mediated immune responses by inhibiting apoptosis of T lymphocytes in the thymus and by enhancing T lymphocyte cytokine and opioid release (Maestroni, 1993; Maestroni, 1999; Yu et al., 2000). In other words, it allows more T lymphocytes to mature and to function more effectively. In addition, melatonin increases the proliferation of cells, such as monocytes, natural killer (NK) cells, and pre-B lymphocytes, during red blood cell formation (Maestroni and Conti, 1996; Maestroni, 1999, 2001b). Activation of the melatonin receptors results in an enhanced release of T helper cell cytokines, including γ-interferon, IL-1, IL-2, and others (Guerrero et al., 2000; Maestroni and Conti, 1996; Maestroni, 1999, 2001b). Monocytes at certain states of maturation actually express melatonin receptors (Maestroni, 2001a). Furthermore, melatonin is capable of enhancing immunological memory to a primary specific T-cell-dependent antigen during immunization (Maestroni et al., 1988b; Maestroni et al., 1989). All of these findings point to the fact that melatonin plays a significant role in cell-mediated immune responses.

MELATONIN'S NONRECEPTOR IMMUNE ACTIONS: FREE RADICAL SCAVENGER

Research on the immune system has established that melatonin also has non-receptor immune actions, particularly its ability to be a powerful free radical scavenger (Poeggeler et al., 1993; Tan et al., 1993). As mentioned, melatonin is highly lipophilic, allowing it to easily enter any cell in the body and permitting it to be an effective free radical scavenger (Reiter et al., 1996, 2000). When presented to the hydroxyl radical, the most toxic of the oxygen-based radicals, melatonin has been shown to be a more effective antioxidant than the better-known glutathione or vitamin E (Reiter et al., 1995)! Other work being done by Reiter's team purports to have demonstrated that melatonin also can scavenge hydrogen peroxide (Tan et al., 2000). Melatonin is capable of interacting with many of the inflammatory cytokines involved in immune responses and, consequently, reduces the potential damage of some of the powerful chemicals used in chemotherapy that destroy healthy tissue (Reiter, 1993a; Reiter et al., 1996; Reiter et al., 2000). Tests on rats using a carcinogen, safrole, showed that melatonin protects against DNA-associated damage (Tan et al., 1993). Furthermore, melatonin significantly augments the immune response to IL-2 in advanced cancer patients (Lissoni et al., 1992, 1994).

Melatonin is found in higher levels in human estrogen receptor-positive breast cancer cells than in the blood (Reiter et al., 2000). Pretreatment of human breast cancer cells with melatonin prior to administration of the chemotherapeutic agent tamoxifen renders the tamoxifen a hundred times more powerful an inhibitor of breast cancer cell growth (Wilson et al., 1992). Melatonin and tamoxifen are both free radical scavengers that, when used together, are more able to prevent the membrane rigidity that occurs from free radical attack than either alone (Garcia et al., 1998). The obvious next step would be to test these findings on human breast cancer patients. Our search turned up studies from only one lab—Paolo Lissoni and his group in Milan, Italy. The results of Lissoni's phase II trials indicate that in about 28% of metastatic cancer patients, concomitant use of melatonin and tamoxifen (or other appropriate chemotherapy) resulted in some positive therapeutic response, whether or not the primary tumor was breast cancer (Lissoni et al., 1995, 1996). Similar enhancement of therapeutic response of melatonin in combination with chemotherapeutic agents has been confirmed in studies published more recently (Cerea et al., 2003; Lissoni et al., 2003). Lissoni's research also showed that the combination of melatonin and chemotherapy significantly reduces side effects of chemotherapy, including malaise and weakness (Lissoni et al., 1997).

While research in this area appears to be progressing at a snail's pace, the results of epidemiological studies actually warrant further investigation into the correlation between melatonin and breast cancer. Disturbing findings from two separate labs show a correlation between increased rates of breast cancer in women who work night shifts. While the increased risk is moderate in the beginning, the more years that their nighttime melatonin levels are disturbed by night work, the greater the risk women have of developing breast cancer. One study reported that a daily average of 5.7 hours of night work over 10 years doubled a woman's chance of developing breast cancer (Davis et al., 2001b). In another study, 30 years of some night shift work placed the women at a 36% higher risk of developing breast cancer (Schernhammer et al., 2001). The beguiling aspect of the study is that the greater number of years of night work, the higher is the rate of cancer. Can low levels of melatonin (for a whole host of reasons, including stress) over many years influence a person's health? There is now some research to support this speculation.

Opioid Peptides, Melatonin, and Immunity

Interactions between melatonin and the immune system are mediated by endogenous opioid peptides (secreted either from the immune cells themselves or from the neuroendocrine system) and require a primed immune cell to be activated (Lissoni et al., 1994; Maestroni et al., 1987a; Maestroni et al., 1987b; Maestroni, 1989; Maestroni and Conti, 1991a). The fact that an opioid antagonist (naltrexone) completely abolishes melatonin's immune-enhancing role and that melatonin is completely ineffective when used for *in vitro* experiments confirms the crucial role of opioids in the proper functioning of melatonin (Lissoni et al., 1986; Maestroni et al., 1988a). Activated, circulating T lymphocytes and T helper cells are stimulated by melatonin, likely in a paracrine or autocrine manner, and then release endogenous opioids. This process results in immune-enhancing and stress-reducing responses (Maestroni and Conti, 1991a). In humans, melatonin is elevated during the night, and β-endorphin secretion is low; the opposite holds true during the day. Intriguingly, the thymus (the site of T-lymphocyte maturation) is one of the main targets of melatonin. The presence of both melatonin and opioid receptors in the thymus strongly suggests a role for melatonin in immune recovery following elevated corticosteroid levels, such as occurs with stress or disease (Maestroni and Conti, 1991b, 1991c).

Melatonin and Hematopoiesis

Hematopoiesis is the production of the formed blood elements, which occurs primarily via the bone marrow stromal cells and, secondarily, in the liver. The blood cells include erythrocytes, platelets, polymorphonuclear neutrophil leukocytes, and B lymphocytes. Like the immune system, hematopoiesis is influenced by both neural and endocrine factors. The multifaceted regulation of hematopoiesis involves a variety of circulating and membrane-based cytokines, growth factors, and antigens that are presented to B and T cells. Recently, work has been done to identify new entities, such as neuropeptides or neurotransmitters, involved in hematopoiesis. Melatonin has been identified as one of these new factors that performs a crucial function in the hematopoietic process. It appears that melatonin has roles both in acute immune conditions as well as in general immune homeostasis or maintenance via the hematopoietic system.

It is already known that bone marrow contains high concentrations of melatonin as well as both the NAT and HIOMT enzymes needed for its synthesis (Conti et al., 2000). Levels of bone marrow melatonin in pinealectomized animals remain high, which indicates that melatonin most likely is synthesized in the bone marrow itself or at least is concentrated there (Conti et al., 2000; Tan et al., 1999). Amazingly, levels of melatonin in bone marrow are three orders of magnitude greater than those measured in the blood at night—even for pinealectomized animals (Maestroni, 2000; Reiter et al., 2000).

Fascinating studies by Georges Maestroni in Switzerland indicate that bone marrow from mice not only has high levels of melatonin, but also contains a substantial amount of catecholamines—with both factors being involved in hemato-poiesis (Maestroni et al., 1997, 1998; Maestroni, 2000). Melatonin's role as a regulatory hormone in the hematopoietic process, like the catecholamines, is pre-dominantly related to immune function. Maestroni and colleagues determined that the activation of melatonin receptors causes an increase in the secretion of T helper cytokines, such as γ-interferon, IL-2, various opioid cytokines, and possibly several others. The opioids induced by melatonin receptor activation subsequently bind to κ-opioid receptors that are present on stromal bone marrow macrophages (Maestroni, 1999). It is these melatonin-induced opioids that actually are capable of influencing the hematopoietic process.

This newly identified immune–hematopoietic network receives messages from the environment via the brain, conveyed, at least in part, by catecholamines and melatonin. Maestroni points out that we now have two (i.e., the catecholamines and melatonin) intriguing and unsuspected factors that are capable of transducing envi-ronmental information into the process of blood and immune cell formation. Mae-stroni explains, "This subtle environmental influence of the blood-forming system might be even more fundamental than that exerted by the cytokine network" (Mae-stroni, 2000). Catecholamines transduce aspects of the rest–activity rhythm, and melatonin conveys circadian information. Maestroni appropriately wonders if there could, therefore, be a neural regulation of the hematopoietic process that might influence a disease such as leukemia, acute infection, or stress (Maestroni, 2000). In other words, this is clearly an avenue by which our general level of well-being or heightened state of stress is conveyed to our blood-forming mechanisms, and thus to our immune system. This is but one more major example of both whole systems integration and an environmentally based feedback loop between the endocrine, the immune, and now, the hematopoietic system.

MELATONIN AND PROLACTIN

The influence of the pineal on the immune system is complex and varied. For example, the pineal helps regulate the secretion of prolactin from the anterior pitu-itary (Lissoni et al., 1990). In humans, prolactin is dependent on both light and melatonin for its synthesis. Like melatonin, prolactin is a modulator of the immune system. It stimulates lymphocytes to secrete cytokines, is secreted by lymphocytes, and inhibits natural killer (NK) cell activity (Bernton et al., 1991; Hiestand et al., 1986; Matera et al., 1990; Reichlin, 1993). New research indicates that prolactin actually is produced within the thymus (as mentioned, a major target site for melatonin) and has paracrine and autocrine actions, which serve to regulate thymic action (Savino et al., 1998).

SUMMARY: MELATONIN AND THE IMMUNE SYSTEM

Just as melatonin boasts discrete immune-enhancing characteristics, certain immune products (e.g., γ-interferon, colony-stimulating factors, and IL-2), in turn, are capable of modulating the synthesis of melatonin in the pineal (Maestroni, 1993). Here again we have one of those remarkable instances of systems interacting in a bidirectional manner, reminiscent of the systems integration paradigms reviewed in Chapter 2 (Maestroni, 1999). What can be culled from the various studies cited in this section? Similar to the picture that emerged with the systems integration paradigms, we see that melatonin has a variety of major endocrine actions. However, it also has autocrine or paracrine actions that enable interactive and integrative mechanisms to occur in a cumulative manner, which can result in outcomes just as significant as the more forcefully acting hormones and neurotransmitters. Melatonin potentially could allow the body to remember not only chemical information, but it could also help to retain a memory of the environmental factors contributing to or just simply present at the time of illness or stress. All of these issues provide more evidence that the pineal is our master gland.

MELATONIN AND THE REPRODUCTIVE SYSTEM

Although it is known that melatonin is involved in the reproductive patterns of seasonal breeders, such as animals and birds (the darker times of year increase melatonin production and decrease reproductive hormones), its significance in human reproduction has remained controversial. In animals, melatonin limits the pituitary release of GnRH and regulates LH, FSH, and prolactin (Reiter, 1980). Historically, evidence supporting a relationship between melatonin and the reproductive hormones in humans was based on findings of reproductive disorders associated with diseases (e.g., tumors) of the pineal gland. For example, in 1898 Heubner described a boy with a pineal tumor who exhibited precocious puberty (the thinking being that melatonin was not available to suppress the sexual development). Then in 1954, when Kitay showed that destructive tumors were associated with precocious puberty and that hyperactive tumors were associated with delayed puberty, much research energy was invested in trying to determine a functional relationship between melatonin and the sex hormones (reviewed in Lewy, 1983, and Tamarkin et al., 1985). Because there are melatonin receptors in both the brain and the reproductive organs and because there are reproductive hormone receptors in the pineal gland, it is very tempting to speculate that there must be a causal relationship (Luboshitzky and Lavie, 1999). However, whether or not a correlation exists in humans remains ambiguous.

ANIMAL STUDIES

In 1963, Richard Wurtman and coworkers were the first to show that exogenous melatonin negatively impacts mammalian reproductive functions (Wurtman et al., 1963a). Russel Reiter and his colleagues in Texas have been instrumental in determining the various effects of melatonin on the reproductive system (Reiter and Johnson, 1974a, 1974b; Reiter, 1980). Reiter worked with hamsters to assess correlations between the size of the reproductive organs and exposure to light, dark, and/or melatonin. One significant finding was that the constant administration of melatonin caused a "functional pinealectomy" in both the male and female hamsters (Reiter et al., 1981).

However, there were seemingly conflicting results from his studies. The discovery in 1976 that antigonadotropic effects are influenced by the time of day in which exogenous melatonin is administered provided the first piece to unraveling the puzzle of why the research had yielded conflicting findings (Tamarkin et al., 1976). If melatonin is administered in the afternoon or evening, it combines with the endogenous melatonin and results in the dramatic gonadal degeneration seen in the earlier studies. However, morning administration of melatonin does not exhibit these effects. Reiter put these findings together with his knowledge that various hormones are capable of inhibiting their own actions (recall the role that cortisol plays in the stress response), desensitizing or down-regulating their own effects. He deduced that morning administration falls on already saturated melatonin receptors and creates a state of chronic down-regulation, which therefore prevents antigonadotropic effects (Reiter et al., 1981). Such information about the effects of melatonin on animals opened the way to a better understanding of its impact on humans.

HUMAN STUDIES

In humans, as already mentioned, absolute concentrations of plasma melatonin peak somewhere between the ages of 2 and 5 years and then proceed to decline throughout life (Wurtman, 2000). At the turn of the last century, Marburg posed the theory that the pineal regulates the onset of puberty, and researchers have been trying to prove him right (or wrong) ever since. By the 1990s, researchers began to realize that the decrease in melatonin levels was not so much linked to the child's age as to the child's level of sexual maturation. Russel Reiter and Franz Halberg, for example, both determined that the Tanner stages 1 to 5 of sexual maturation (which is a method to classify pubertal development) are correlated to significant decreases in nocturnal melatonin (Reiter, 1998; Salti et al., 2000; Tanner and Whitehouse, 1976). However, these studies still do not establish a causal relationship. Furthermore, other research shows that prepubertal children, who have a higher melatonin secretion rate, may simply metabolize melatonin faster than adults (Carvallo and Ritschel, 1996). Clearly, there is a correlation between a decrease in melatonin and the onset of puberty, but why this is so still remains an enigma.

Although it has not been established that melatonin regulates gonadotropic hormones in men, a correlation between melatonin and these hormones has frequently been reported, particularly because of abnormalities in hormone levels. Low

GnRH levels, for instance, are correlated to increased melatonin, while elevated gonadotropin levels are correlated to low melatonin (Luboshitzky et al., 1996). But, once again, a cause-and-effect relationship remains questionable because long-term administration of melatonin does not alter the secretions of the major reproductive hormones (e.g., LH, testosterone, and FSH), although evening administration of melatonin to normal males does result in a next-day reduction of LH (Luboshitzky et al., 1999; Luboshitzky et al., 2000). In spite of melatonin's apparent antigonadotropic properties, a functional relationship has not yet been definitively established.

Research on the correlation between women's menstrual cycles and melatonin levels suggests that melatonin is not a factor in the cyclical menstrual phases (Berga and Yen, 1990; Brzezinski et al., 1988). However, elevated melatonin levels have been observed in amenorrheic women and decreased levels with premenstrual depression (Berga et al., 1988; Brzezinski et al., 1987, 1988; Parry et al., 1990). As stated, levels of melatonin decrease with age, and Russel Reiter and others have established that there are significant decreases in nocturnal melatonin during menopause (Reiter, 1998). Researchers in Finland determined that urinary melatonin excretion declined by 41% in women 40 to 44 years of age and that there was then a second significant decline of 35% in women between the age groups of 50 to 55 and 55 to 59 (Vakkuri et al., 1996). These decreases occurred in inverse relationship to FSH, whose levels are known to increase with age. The fact that the largest decline in melatonin occurs before the onset of menopause is intriguing, yet once again, it does not establish a causal relationship. Nonetheless, the correlation is pronounced, with research showing that healthy menopausal women who were given melatonin for up to 6 months exhibited an increase in thyroid hormone levels. In addition, a decrease in the pituitary hormones LH and FSH (both increase with age) was observed for younger menopausal women and those with low levels of melatonin before treatment initiation (Bellipanni et al., 2001).

Recall that, in the sections on the SCN, we proposed that its rhythmic beating is not only the timepiece of our daily cycles, but also of the totality of our lives, cradle to grave. The physiological and scientific correlations between melatonin and its impact on our reproductive development and denouement are examples of the role that the SCN plays in configuring the larger rhythmic patterns of life. The SCN and melatonin are integral to lifelong personal patterns, potentially in a harmonic resonance with the environment around us.

CHRONOBIOLOGY

Chronobiology involves the science of our biological clock (i.e., the SCN) as it is expressed in our personal physiological rhythm (e.g., am I a morning or an evening person?). However, chronobiology also concerns the science of how our biological clocks are disrupted by or determine the daily rhythms of a particular illness and even the time of optimal medication administration. Franz Halberg, who some called the father of chronobiology, initiated the study of body rhythms in the late 1950s and continues to provide valuable research to the field (Halberg, 1983; Halberg et al., 2001). Halberg ascertained literally dozens of circadian patterns present in humans and other species, including thyroid function in Peking ducks; rhythms of susceptibility to an insecticide (pyrethrum) in cockroaches and houseflies; and the peak times of the day that symptoms of asthma, schizophrenia, and narcolepsy are expressed in humans (Astier and Bayle, 1970; Halberg et al., 1968; Passouant et al., 1969; Reinberg et al., 1970; Reindl et al., 1969; Sullivan et al., 1970).

In the intervening years, we have learned much about body rhythms and how they relate to particular diseases. These findings interface with our knowledge of the pineal and circadian hormonal secretions. For instance, the morning surge in sympathetic activity (e.g., increased epinephrine and norepinephrine secretion, higher blood pressure and heart rate levels) and increase in cortisol levels correlate to cardiovascular disease, including ischemia, myocardial infarction, stroke, and sudden death (Muller et al., 1987; Muller et al., 1989; Panza et al., 1991; Pepine, 1991; Quyyumi, 1990). The fact is that humans tend to have a heart attack in the morning—generally between about 6 A.M. and noon—when the sympathetic system is fully active and our stress hormone system is at its peak.

Similarly, the progression of disease and the intensity of side effects for patients with colorectal cancer are enormously influenced by the time of day that chemotherapeutic drugs are administered and their correlation to concurrent radiation therapy (Bressolle et al., 1999; Hrushesky, 1985, 2001; Peters et al., 1987; Thrall et al., 2000). Regrettably, these factors have been brought to the attention of few physicians in the United States. Research stemming from a laboratory in Villejuif, France, has actually shown that lack of a distinct circadian rest–activity rhythm in cancer patients is a novel independent prognostic factor for survival (Levi, 2000; Mormont et al., 2000). The researchers encourage chronotherapeutic adjustments as part of these patients' overall cancer treatment, that is protocols designed to adjust their circadian rhythms more in line with usual patterns and with normal levels of melatonin expression.

From a broader perspective, chronobiology is expressed in the patterns of both human and animal nervous, stress, immune, and reproductive systems. We have discrete daily, yearly, and lifetime biochemical patterns and rhythms. In the following section, we will begin to consider how the articulation of our internal hormonal energy is reflected in and reflective of energetic variations that surround us.

ELECTROMAGNETIC ENERGY AND THE PINEAL: A LINK TO EASTERN ENERGY CONCEPTS

Light can be described as the visible portion of the electromagnetic spectrum (see Figure 6.5). We have already explained how light can modify our internal clocks, causing phase advances or delays. Is it possible that other portions of the electromagnetic spectrum can also entrain our biological clocks? An increasingly large body of research seems to support this hypothesis (see Wilson et al., 1989, for a review of earlier studies). Russel Reiter and his colleagues, for example, have performed numerous experiments showing that the nonvisible portion of the electromagnetic spectrum decreases melatonin levels, just as visible light does. Reiter has shown that nighttime exposure of animals and humans to pulsed static and very low-frequency magnetic fields reduces melatonin production and plasma levels in a

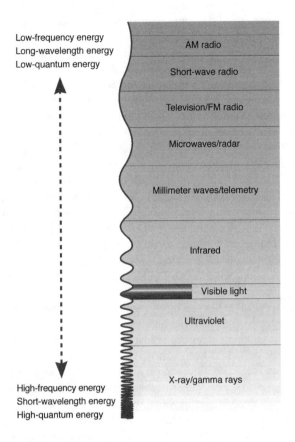

FIGURE 6.5 Electromagnetic spectrum.

manner very akin to nighttime exposure to light, although it is not known whether the mechanism of action is the same (Reiter, 1992; Reiter and Richardon, 1992; Reiter, 1993a, 1993b, 1994).

Reiter's research is significant because of the ongoing, and often heated, debate as to whether these low-frequency magnetic fields are detrimental to our health. Studies on humans show that nighttime residential exposure to 60 Hz lowers urinary melatonin levels, particularly in winter and especially in women taking various medications, including calcium-channel blockers and beta blockers as well as psychotropic medications (Davis et al., 2001a). A study performed at the Lawrence Berkeley National Laboratory and then replicated by the U.S. Environmental Protection Agency established that 60 Hz reduced the ability of both melatonin and of tamoxifen to effectively inhibit human breast cancer cells *in vitro* (Blackman et al., 2001; Harland and Liburdy, 1997). Although I have yet to see comparable *in vivo* experiments, I find this research disconcerting, particularly when juxtaposed with the previously mentioned research on women who work night shifts and have increased rates of breast cancer (Davis et al., 2001b; Schernhammer et al., 2001).

While the researchers from the night shift studies speculate that the cause may be increased release of estrogen induced by decreased melatonin, there is also the possibility that the increased incidence of breast cancer is simply related to the role that melatonin plays as an effective free radical scavenger (Reiter, 1994). Furthermore, it is plausible that similar amounts of melatonin are synthesized but that tissue that is exposed to larger amounts of free radicals from the electromagnetic exposure may be using the circulating melatonin at augmented rates (Reiter, 1998).

Duration of exposure to electromagnetic fields may be a key variable. While it is known that electromagnetic exposure in the 50- to 60-Hz range can suppress melatonin levels, there may be a set, but unknown, length of time before the suppression occurs (Brendel et al., 2000; Rosen et al., 1998). Most of the experiments (that we have found) showing a correlation between exposure to electromagnetic fields and reduced melatonin levels indicate an effect only when they are carried out for weeks and not days (Graham et al., 2000; Grota et al., 1994; Selmaoui and Touitou, 1999). However, contrary to this trend, researchers at the NIH exposed pinealocytes from rodents to low-frequency electromagnetic fields and found an average melatonin suppression of 46% after only 12 hours (Rosen et al., 1998).

In the mid-1990s, Ewa Lindstrom and her colleagues at Umea University in Sweden did a series of experiments on magnetic fields and lymphocytes. In one experiment, she found that cells (called *Jurkat cells*) from a leukemia cell line, subjected to low-frequency magnetic fields, responded in a manner similar to what would occur if the cells had been exposed to antibodies (Lindstrom et al., 1993, 1995a, 1995b). Lindstrom continues to perform research in support of these findings (Lindstrom et al., 2001). She suggests that her original findings may buttress the speculative, but provocative, findings of Liboff and colleagues, who are also doing research on electromagnetic fields and cell membranes.

Liboff claims to have shown that certain resonance frequencies (which Libof refers to as *cyclotron resonance*) exist for several biologically important ions, including calcium (which is required for proper nerve function, among other things). The resonance frequency, ostensibly, only exists if the magnetic field is within the earth's amplitude range (Liboff and McLeod, 1988; Liboff, 1997; Smith et al., 1987). This research is profoundly controversial because it indicates that electromagnetic energy (not peptides, neurotransmitters, etc.) is the cause of the change in membrane gradient. The notion that a calcium ion could pass through a cell's membrane without the interaction of some ligand goes against all that is understood about ion channels. The research indicates that there may be "receptors" for electromagnetic energy— just as there are receptors for numerous hormones or neurotransmitters. We found one researcher who purports to have disproved both Lindstrom and Liboff's findings (Coulton and Barker, 1993). Liboff's research may not be well known and, therefore, few scientists would be trying to replicate it or to determine why Coulton was unable to replicate it.

If Liboff's research is not spurious, then we are looking at a physiological receptor, located on a given cell membrane, whose function is to receive electromagnetic energy. If there is an electromagnetic signature on the receptor identical to the one on the molecule, there is a match—an electromagnetic match. It is current knowledge that all known receptors interact with their endogenous ligands through mechanisms that include electromagnetic properties. However, Liboff's work is the first research purporting to show a discrete electromagnetic receptor.

CONCLUDING THOUGHTS

Let us quickly review the information presented in this chapter. The pineal is the central component to an amazing tract of electromagnetic information, which is dependent on light impingement. Special phototransducing receptors convert light information to electrical signals, which then travel through our biological clock or circadian pacemaker (i.e., the SCN) to set and adjust our inner rhythms. The electrical signals continue their journey, checking in with the hypothalamus, in case there is any input there, traveling down the brainstem, and finally traversing to the pineal. The power of the pineal is in its ability to then interpret and decipher the already decoded environmental input and disseminate it, via a neuroendocrine response, to all of the body systems. As we have reviewed, the pineal affects endocrine, autonomic, hypothalamic, and immune responses. The pineal is our all-purpose, comprehensive regulatory gland. It is primarily inhibitory but plays the crucial role of facilitating the translation of environmental messages (i.e., energy) into neuroendocrine signals that can be dispersed throughout the body. Ergo, scientifically, I would call the pineal our master gland.

It is my contention that our inner rhythms, which are influenced by environmental light, electricity, and magnetism, are a reflection of, or complement to, the sun-center geophysical signatures of our physical universe. The pineal gland senses magnetic alterations in the environment. The oscillating neurons of the SCN entrain the endocrine and nervous systems according to the cues received by the external environment. This occurs daily, but it also occurs in longer pacemaker rhythms, called *ultradian cycles*, such as puberty or menopause for women. Consequently, there is circadian and ultradian rhythmicity to each of our internal body systems. Ultimately, this interaction allows for something like a harmonic resonance between our internal rhythm (both circadian and ultradian) and the subtle energies, which are also called *spiritual energy* or referred to as *Qi* in the Chinese system of medicine. This harmonic resonance is perpetually present, but it is more accessible to our personal experience when we entrain our body and mind to a subtler energy frequency. It is why music can be so calming to our souls—it restores the endocrine symphony when we are distressed or stressed. The musical harmonics are entrained by the SCN and modulated by the pineal.

The pineal is the cornerstone of the biochemical interface with our environment *and* with the subtle energy that both supports and transcends our sense perceptions and sustains our body as much as any nourishment we consume (see Chapter 8 for a discussion of subtle energy). While the pineal is the energy transducer that sends hormonal and electrical messages throughout the body, the chakras, as described in Eastern religious and medical systems, are the energy transducers for subtle energy. Chakras, speculatively, are energetic portals that permit a subtler, but profoundly sustaining, energy to enter the body. Chakras, speculatively, open and connect into the ANS, interacting richly with the endocrine system. We will cover this topic in some detail in the final chapter of the book (Chapter 8).

However, for now I would like to deliver the caveat that the seventh chakra, which is located at the crown of the head, is in physiological terms associated with the pineal and the CNS. The seventh chakra would theoretically connect, via the CNS, to the autonomic nervous system and then to interact richly with the endocrine system. This construct allows for a systemic coherence of our internal and external environments. Hold these thoughts and we will revisit this topic again in the last chapter of the book.

Our understanding of time is based on scientific constructs that bundle up traversing energy in a linear fashion, yet mystics through the ages have made statements to the effect that "all things are one." If we have the courage to alter our belief systems a bit, we can begin to see that all things are part of a tapestry—the body, the mind, the spirit. So perhaps the pineal, as Descartes declared, is indeed the "seat of the soul," because it may well be the interface between our body and our soul—that is, the corridor by which we can experience our spirituality.

Next, we will take a look at the healing modalities that fall into the NIH Category 5 (as described in Chapter 5), which encompasses energy therapies. We will describe how energy-medicine modalities can help us live healthier lives.

REFERENCES

Abrahamson, E.E., Leak, R.K., and Moore, R.Y., The suprachiasmatic nucleus projects to posterior hypothalamic arousal systems, *Neuroreport*, 12 (2), 435–440, 2001.

Allada, R., Emery, P., Takahashi, J.S., and Rosbash, M., Stopping time: the genetics of fly and mouse circadian clocks, *Ann. Rev. Neurosci.*, 24, 1091–1119, 2001.

Antoch, M.P. et al., Functional identification of the mouse circadian clock gene by transgenic BAC rescue, *Cell.*, 89 (4), 655–667, 1997.

Arendt, J., Melatonin, *Clinical Endocrinol.*, 29 (2), 205–229, 1988.

Arendt, J. and Marks, V., Physiological changes underlying jet lag, *Br. Medical J.*, 284 (6310), 144–146, 1982.

Arendt, J., Borbely, A.A., Franey, C., and Wright, J., The effects of chronic, small doses of melatonin given in the late afternoon on fatigue in man: a preliminary study, *Neurosci. Lett.*, 45 (3), 317–321, 1984.

Arendt, J. et al., Some effects of melatonin and the control of its secretion in humans, *Ciba Found. Symp.*, 117, 266–283, 1985.

Astier, H. and Bayle, J.D., Plasma clearing of 125I-L-thyroxine after hypophysectomy and hypophyseal autograft in ducks, *J. Physiol.*, 62 (Suppl. 2), 237, 1970.

Atsmon, J. et al., Reciprocal effects of chronic diazepam and melatonin on brain melatonin and benzodiazepine binding sites, *J. Pineal Res.*, 20 (2), 65–71, 1996.

Axelrod, J. and Weissbach, H., Enzymatic O-methylation of N-acetylserotonin to melatonin, *Science*, 131 (3409), 1312, 1960.

Balsalobre, A., Brown, S.A., Marcacci, L., Reichardt, H.M., Schutz, G., and Schibler, U., Resetting of circadian time in peripheral tissues by glucocorticoid signaling, *Science*, 289 (5488), 2344–2347, 2000.

Bayliss, C.R., Bishop, N.L., and Fowler, R.C., Pineal gland calcification and defective sense of direction, *Br. Medical J. (Clinical Res. Ed.)*, 291 (6511), 1758–1759, 1985.

Bellipanni, G., Bianchi, P., Pierpaoli, W., Bulian, D., and Ilyia, E., Effects of melatonin in perimenopausal women: a randomized and placebo controlled study, *Exper. Gerontol.*, 36 (2), 297–310, 2001.

Berga, S.L. and Yen, S.S., Circadian pattern of plasma melatonin concentrations during four phases of the human menstrual cycle, *Neuroendocrinology*, 51 (5), 606–612, 1990.

Berga, S.L., Mortola, J.F., and Yen, S.S.C., Amplification of nocturnal melatonin secretion in women with functional hypothalamic amenorrhea, *J. Clinical Endocrinol. Metab.*, 66 (1), 242–244, 1988.

Bernton, E.W., Bryant, H.U., and Holaday, J.W., Prolactin and immune function, in *Psychoneuroimmunology*, 2nd ed., Ader, R., Felten, D.L., and Cohen, N., Eds., Academic Press, New York, 1991, pp. 403–428.

Binkley, S., *The Pineal: Endocrine and Neuroendocrine Function*, Prentice Hall, Englewood Cliffs, NJ, 1988.

Blackman, C.F., Benane, S.G., and House, D.E., The influence of 1.2 microT, 60 Hz magnetic fields on melatonin- and tamoxifen-induced inhibition of MCF-7 cell growth, *Bioelectromagnetics*, 22 (2), 122–128, 2001.

Boivin, D.B. and Czeisler, C.A., Resetting of circadian melatonin and cortisol rhythms in humans by ordinary room light, *Neuroreport*, 9 (5), 779–782, 1998.

Brainard, G.C. et al., Action spectrum for melatonin regulation in humans: evidence for a novel circadian photoreceptor, *J. Neurosci.: Off. J. Soc. Neurosci.*, 21 (16), 6405–6412, 2001.

Brendel, H., Niehaus, M., and Lerchl, A., Direct suppressive effects of weak magnetic fields (50 Hz and 16 2/3 Hz) on melatonin synthesis in the pineal gland of Djungarian hamsters (*Phodopus sungorus*), *J. Pineal Res.*, 29 (4), 228–233, 2000.

Bressolle, F. et al., Circadian rhythm of 5-fluorouracil population pharmacokinetics in patients with metastatic colorectal cancer, *Cancer Chemother. Pharmacol.*, 44 (4), 295–302, 1999.

Brzezinski, A., Melatonin in humans, *New England J. Med.*, 336 (3), 186–195, 1997.

Brzezinski, A., Seibel, M.M., Lynch, H.J., Deng, M.H., and Wurtman, R.J., Melatonin in human preovulatory follicular fluid, *J. Clinical Endocrinol. Metab.*, 64 (4), 865–867, 1987.

Brzezinski, A., Lynch, H.J., Seibel, M.M., Deng, M.H., Nader, T.M., and Wurtman, R.J., The circadian rhythm of plasma melatonin during the normal menstrual cycle and in amenorrheic women, *J. Clinical Endocrinol. Metab.*, 66 (5), 891–895, 1988.

Bubenik, G.A. et al., Prospects of the clinical utilization of melatonin, *Biological Signals Receptors*, 7 (4), 195–219, 1998.

Cardarelli, N.F., The role of a thymus-pineal axis in an immune mechanism of aging, *J. Theoretical Biol.*, 145 (3), 397–405, 1990.

Carlberg, C., Gene regulation by melatonin, in Neuroimmunomodulation: Perspectives at the New Millennium, *Annals of the New York Academy of Sciences*, Vol. 917, Conti, A., Maestroni, G.J.M., McCann, S.M., Sternberg, E.M., Lipton, J.M., and Smith, C.C., Eds., New York Academy of Sciences, New York, 2000, pp. 387–396.

Carvallo, A. and Ritschel, W.A., Pharmacokinetics of melatonin in human sexual maturation, *J. Clinical Endocrinol. Metabol.*, 81 (5), 1882–1886, 1996.

Cerea, G. et al., Biomodulation of cancer chemotherapy for metastatic colorectal cancer: a randomized study of weekly low-dose irinotecan alone versus irinotecan plus the oncostatic pineal hormone melatonin in metastatic colorectal cancer patients progressing on 5-fluorouracil-containing combinations, *Anticancer Res.*, 23 (2C), 1951–1954, 2003.

Cogburn, L.A., Wilson-Placentra, S., and Letcher, L.R., Influence of pinealectomy on plasma and extrapineal melatonin rhythms in young chickens (*Gallus domesticus*), *Gen. Comp. Endocrinol.*, 68 (3), 343–356, 1987.

Conti, A., Conconi, S., Hertens, E., Skwarlo-Sonta, K., Markowska, M., and Maestroni, J.M., Evidence for melatonin synthesis in mouse and human bone marrow cells, *J. Pineal Res.*, 28 (4), 193–202, 2000.

Coulton, L.A. and Barker, A.T., Magnetic fields and intracellular calcium: effects on lymphocytes exposed to conditions for "cyclotron resonance," *Phys. Med. Biol.*, 38 (3), 347–360, 1993.

Czeisler, C.A., Johnson, M.P., Duffy, J.F., Brown, E.N., Ronda, J.M., and Kronauer, R.E., Exposure to bright light and darkness to treat physiologic maladaptation to night work, *New England J. Med.*, 322 (18), 1253–1259, 1990.

Czeisler, C.A. et al., Bright light induction of strong (type 0) resetting of the human circadian pacemaker, *Science*, 244 (4910), 1328–1333, 1989.

Czeisler, C.A. et al., Suppression of melatonin secretion in some blind patients by exposure to bright light, *New England J. Med.*, 332 (1), 6–11, 1995.

Czeisler, C.A. et al., Stability, precision, and near-24-hour period of the human circadian pacemaker, *Science*, 284 (5423), 2177–2181, 1999.

Darlington, T.K. et al., Closing the circadian loop: clock-induced transcription of its own inhibitors *per* and *tim*, *Science*, 280 (5369), 1599–1603, 1998.

Davis, S., Kaune, W.T., Mirick, D.K., Chen, C., and Stevens, R.G., Residential magnetic fields, light-at-night, and nocturnal urinary 6-sulfatoxymelatonin concentration in women, *Am. J. Epidemiol.*, 154 (7), 591–600, 2001a.

Davis, S., Mirick, D.K., and Stevens, R.G., Night shift work, light at night, and risk of breast cancer, *J. Natl. Cancer Inst.*, 93 (20), 1557–1562, 2001b.

de la Iglesia, H.O., Meyer, J., Carpino, A., and Schwartz, W.J., Antiphase oscillation of the left and right suprachiasmatic nuclei, *Science*, 290 (5492), 799–801, 2000.

de Lecea, L., Kilduff, T.S., Peyron, C., Gao, X., Foye, P.E., Danielson, P.E., Fukuhara, C., Battenberg, E.L., Gautvik, V.T., Bartlett, II, F.S., Frankel, W.N., van den Pol, A.N., Bloom, F.E., Gautvik, K.M., and Sutcliffe, J.G., The hypocretins: hypothalamus-specific peptides with neuroexcitatory activity, *Proc. Natl. Acad. Sci. U.S.A.*, 95 (1), 322–327, 1998.

Dollins, A.B., Zhdanova, I.V., Wurtman, R.J., Lynch, H.J., and Deng, M.H., Effect of inducing nocturnal serum melatonin concentrations in daytime on sleep, mood, body temperature, and performance, *Proc. Natl. Acad. Sci. U.S.A.*, 9 (5), 1824–1828, 1994.

Ebadi, M. and Govitrapong, P., Orphan transmitters and their receptor sites in the pineal gland, in *Pineal Research Reviews*, Vol. 4, Reiter, R.J., Ed., Alan R. Liss, New York, 1986, pp. 1–54.

Etzioni, A., Luboshitzky, R., Tiosano, D., Ben-Harush, M., Goldsher, D., and Lavie, P., Melatonin replacement corrects sleep disturbances in a child with pineal tumor, *Neurology*, 46 (1), 261–263, 1996.

Foa, A., Janik, D., and Minutini, L., Circadian rhythms of plasma melatonin in the ruin lizard *Podarcis sicula*: effects of pinealectomy, *J. Pineal Res.*, 12 (3), 109–113, 1992.

Foster, R.G. and Soni, B.G., Extraretinal photoreceptors and their regulation of temporal physiology, *Rev. Reprod.*, 3 (3), 145–150, 1998.

Freedman, M.S. et al., Regulation of mammalian circadian behavior by non-rod, non-cone, ocular photoreceptors, *Science*, 284 (5413), 502–504, 1999.

Garcia, J.J. et al., Melatonin enhances tamoxifen's ability to prevent the reduction in microsomal membrane fluidity induced by lipid peroxidation, *J. Membrane Biol.*, 162 (1), 59–65, 1998.

Garfinkel, D., Zisapel, N., Wainstein, J., and Laudon, M., Facilitation of benzodiazepine discontinuation by melatonin: a new clinical approach, *Arch. Intern. Med.*, 159 (20), 2456–2460, 1999.

Graham, C., Cook, M.R., Sastre, A., Riffle, D.W., and Gerkovich, M.M., Multi-night exposure to 60-Hz magnetic fields: effects on melatonin and its enzymatic metabolite, *J. Pineal Res.*, 28 (1), 1–8, 2000.

Grota, L.J., Reiter, R.J., Keng, P., and Michaelson, S., Electric field exposure alters serum melatonin but not pineal melatonin synthesis in male rats, *Bioelectromagnetics*, 15 (5), 427–437, 1994.

Guerrero, J.M., Pozo, D., García-Mauriño, S., Osuna, C., Molinero, P., and Calvo, J.R., Involvement of nuclear receptors in the enhanced IL-2 production by melatonin in Jurkat cells, in Neuroimmunomodulation: Perspectives at the New Millennium, *Annals of the New York Academy of Sciences*, Vol. 917, Conti, A., Maestroni, G.J.M., McCann, S.M., Sternberg, E.M., Lipton, J.M., and Smith, C.C., Eds., New York Academy of Sciences, New York, 2000, pp. 397–403.

Halberg, F., Quo vadis basic and clinical chronobiology: promise for health maintenance, *Am. J. Anat.*, 168 (4), 543–594, 1983.

Halberg, F., Vestergaard, P., and Sakai, M., Rhythmometry on urinary 17-ketosteroid excretion by healthy men and women and patients with chronic schizophrenia; possible chronopathology in depressive illness, *Archives d'anatomie, d'histologie, d'embryologie normales experimentales*, 51 (1), 299–311, 1968.

Halberg, F.E., Cornelissen, G., Otsuka, K., Schwartzkopff, O., Halberg, J., and Bakken, E.E., Chronomics, *Biomed. Pharmacother.*, 55 (Suppl. 1), 153S–190S, 2001

Harland, J.D. and Liburdy, R.P., Environmental magnetic fields inhibit the antiproliferative action of tamoxifen and melatonin in a human breast cancer cell line, *Bioelectromagnetics*, 18 (8), 555–562, 1997.

Hastings, M., The brain, circadian rhythms, and clock genes, *Br. Medical J.*, 317 (7174), 1704–1707, 1998.

Hattori, A. et al., Identification of melatonin in plants and its effects on plasma melatonin levels and binding to melatonin receptors in vertebrates, *Biochem. Molecular Biol. Int.*, 35 (3), 627–634, 1995.

Hazlerigg, D.G., What is the role of melatonin within the anterior pituitary? *J. Endocrinol.*, 170 (3), 493–501, 2001.

Herzog, E.D., Takahashi, J.S., and Block, G.D., Clock controls of circadian period in isolated suprachiasmatic nucleus neurons, *Nat. Neurosci.*, 1 (8), 708–713, 1998.

Hiestand, P.C., Mekler, P., Nordmann, R., Grieder, A., and Permmongkol, C., Prolactin as a modulator of lymphocyte responsiveness provides a possible mechanism of action for cyclosporine, *Proc. Natl. Acad. Sci. U.S.A.*, 83 (8), 2599–2603, 1986.

Hrushesky, W.J., Circadian timing of cancer chemotherapy, *Science*, 228 (4695), 73–75, 1985.

Hrushesky, W.J., Tumor chronobiology, *J. Controlled Release: Off. J. Controlled Release Soc.*, 74 (1–3), 27–30, 2001.

Hughes, P.C. et al., Optic radiation, *Pineal Res.*, 5, 1–67, 1987.

Ishida, N., Kaneko, M., and Allada, R., Biological clocks, *Proc. Natl. Acad. Sci. U.S.A.*, 96 (16), 8819–8820, 1999.

Ishida, N. et al., Diurnal regulation of per repeat mRNA in the suprachiasmatic nucleus in rat brain, *Neurosci. Lett.*, 122 (1), 113–116, 1991.

Ivanchenko, M., Stanewsky, R., and Giebultowicz, J.M., Circadian photoreception in *Drosophila*: functions of cryptochrome in peripheral and central clocks, *J. Biological Rhythms*, 16 (3), 205–215, 2001.

Jan, J.E., Tai, J., Hahn, G., and Rothstein, R.R., Melatonin replacement therapy in a child with a pineal tumor, *J. Child Neurol.*, 16 (2), 139–140, 2001.

Jankovic, B.D., Isakovic, K., and Petrovic, S., Effect of pinealectomy on immune reactions in the rat, *Immunology*, 18 (1), 1–6, 1970.

Jewett, M.E., Kronauer, R.E., and Czeisler, C.A., Light-induced suppression of endogenous circadian amplitude in humans, *Nature*, 350 (6313), 59–62, 1991.

Jin, X., Shearman, L.P., Weaver, D.R., Zylka, M.J., de Vries, G.J., and Reppert, S.M., A molecular mechanism regulating rhythmic output from the suprachiasmatic circadian clock, *Cell*, 96 (1), 57–68, 1999.

Kennaway, D.J. and Voultsios, A., Circadian rhythm of free melatonin in human plasma, *J. Clinical Endocrinol. Metab.*, 83 (3), 1013–1015, 1998.

Khan, R., Daya, S., and Potgieter, B., Evidence for a modulation of the stress response by the pineal gland, *Experientia*, 46 (8), 860–862, 1990.

King, D.P. and Takahashi, J.S., Molecular genetics of circadian rhythms in mammals, *Ann. Rev. Neurosci.*, 23, 713–742, 2000.

King, D.P. et al., Positional cloning of the mouse circadian clock gene, *Cell*, 89 (4), 641–653, 1997.

Konopka, R.J. and Benzer, S., Clock mutants of *Drosophila melanogaster*, *Proc. Natl. Acad. Sci. U.S.A.*, 68 (9), 2112–2116, 1971.

Kunz, D., Bes, F., Schlattmann, P., and Herrmann, W.M., On pineal calcification and its relation to subjective sleep perception: a hypothesis-driven pilot study, *Psychiatry Res.*, 82 (3), 187–191, 1998.

Kunz, D. et al., A new concept for melatonin deficit: on pineal calcification and melatonin excretion, *Neuropsychopharmacology*, 21 (6), 765–772, 1999.

Leak, R.K. and Moore, R.Y., Identification of retinal ganglion cells projecting to the lateral hypothalamic area of the rat, *Brain Res.*, 770 (1–2), 105–114, 1997.

Leak, R.K. and Moore, R.Y., Topographic organization of suprachiasmatic nucleus projection neurons, *J. Comp. Neurol.*, 433 (3), 312–334, 2001.

Leak, R.K., Card, J.P., and Moore, R.Y., Suprachiasmatic pacemaker organization analyzed by viral transynaptic transport, *Brain Res.*, 819 (1–2), 23–32, 1999.

Lerner, A.B., Case, J.D., Takahashi, Y., Lee, T.H., and Mori, W., Isolation of melatonin, the pineal gland factor that lightens melanocytes, *J. Am. Chemical Soc.*, 80, 2587–2592, 1958.

Levi, F., Therapeutic implications of circadian rhythms in cancer patients, *Novartis Found. Symp.*, 227, 119–136, 2000.

Lewy, A.J., Biochemistry and regulation of mammalian melatonin production, in *The Pineal Gland*, Relkin, R., Ed., Elsevier, 1983b, pp. 77–128.

Lewy, A.J. and Newsome, D.A., Different types of melatonin circadian secretory rhythms in some blind subjects, *J. Clinical Endocrinol. Metab.*, 56 (6), 1103–1107, 1983.

Lewy, A.J., Wehr, T.A., Goodwin, F.K., Newsome, D.A., and Markey, S.P., Light suppresses melatonin secretion in humans, *Science*, 210 (4475), 1267–1269, 1980a.

Lewy, A.J., Tetsuo, M., Markey, S.P., Goodwin, F.K., and Kopin, I.J., Pinealectomy abolishes plasma melatonin in the rat, *J. Clinical Endocrinol. Metab.*, 50 (1), 204–205, 1980b.

Liboff, A.R., Electric-field ion cyclotron resonance, *Bioelectromagnetics*, 18 (1), 85–87, 1997.

Liboff, A.R. and McLeod, B.R., Kinetics of channelized membrane ions in magnetic fields, *Bioelectromagnetics*, 9 (1), 39–51, 1988.

Lindstrom, E., Lindstrom, P., Berglund, A., Mild, K.H., and Lundgren, E., Intracellular calcium oscillations induced in a T-cell line by a weak 50 Hz magnetic field, *J. Cell. Physiol.*, 156 (2), 395–398, 1993.

Lindstrom, E., Berglund, A., Mild, K.H., Lindstrom, P., and Lundgren, E., CD45 phosphates in Jurkat cells is necessary for response to applied ELF magnetic fields, *FEBS Lett.*, 370 (1–2), 118–122, 1995a.

Lindstrom, E., Lindstrom, P., Berglund, A., Lundgren, E., and Mild, K.H., Intracellular calcium oscillations in a T-cell line after exposure to extremely-low-frequency magnetic fields with variable frequencies and flux densities, *Bioelectromagnetics*, 16 (1), 41–47, 1995b.

Lindstrom, E., Still, M., Mattsson, M.O., Mild, K.H., and Luben, R.A., ELF magnetic fields initiate protein tyrosine phosphorylation of the T cell receptor complex, *Bioelectrochemistry*, 53 (1), 73–78, 2001.

Lissoni, P., Barni, S., Tancini, G., Fossati, V., and Frigerio, F., Pineal-opioid system interactions in the control of immunoinflammatory responses, in Neuroimmunomodulation: the State of the Art, *Annals of the New York Academy of Sciences,* Vol. 741, Fabris, N., Markovic, B.M., Spector, N.H., and Jankovic, B.D., Eds., New York Academy of Sciences, New York, 1994, pp. 191–196.

Lissoni, P., Chilelli, M., Villa, S., Cerizza, L., and Tancini, G., Five years survival in metastatic non-small cell lung cancer patients treated with chemotherapy alone or chemotherapy and melatonin: a randomized trial, *J. Pineal Res.*, 14 (1), 1–10, 2003.

Lissoni, P., Mainini, E., Mazzi, C., Cattaneo, G., and Barni, S., A study of pineal–prolactin interaction: prolactin response to an acute melatonin injection in patients with hyperprolactinemia, *J. Endocrinological Invest.*, 13 (2), 85–89, 1990.

Lissoni, P. et al., A clinical study on the relationship between the pineal gland and the opioid system, *J. Neural Transmission*, 65 (1), 63–73, 1986.

Lissoni, P. et al., Immunological effects of a single evening subcutaneous injection of low-dose interleukin-2 in association with the pineal hormone melatonin in advanced cancer patients, *J. Biological Regulators Homeostatic Agents*, 6 (4), 132–136, 1992.

Lissoni, P. et al., Modulation of cancer endocrine therapy by melatonin: a phase II study of tamoxifen plus melatonin in metastatic breast cancer patients progressing under tamoxifen alone, *Br. J. Cancer*, 71 (4), 854–856, 1995.

Lissoni, P. et al., A phase II study of tamoxifen plus melatonin in metastatic solid tumour patients, *Br. J. Cancer*, 74 (9), 1446–1448, 1996.

Lissoni, P. et al., Treatment of cancer chemotherapy-induced toxicity with the pineal hormone melatonin, *Supportive Care Cancer: Off. J. Multinatl. Assoc. Supportive Care Cancer*, 5 (2), 126–129, 1997.

Lowenstein, P.R. and Cardinali, D.P., Benzodiazepine receptor sites in bovine pineal, *Eur. J. Pharmacol.*, 86 (2), 287–289, 1982.

Lowenstein, P.R., Rosenstein, R., Caputti, E., and Cardinali, D.P., Benzodiazepine binding sites in human pineal gland, *Eur. J. Pharmacol.*, 106 (2), 399–403, 1984.

Luboshitzky, R. and Lavie, P., Melatonin and sex hormone interrelationships—a review, *J. Pediatric Endocrinol. Metab.: JPEM*, 12 (3), 355–362, 1999.

Luboshitzky, R., Levi, M., Shen-Orr, Z., Blumenfeld, Z., Herer, P., and Lavie, P., Long-term melatonin administration does not alter pituitary-gonadal hormone secretion in normal men, *Hum. Reprod. (Oxford, Engl.)*, 15 (1), 60–65, 2000.

Luboshitzky, R., Shen-Orr, Z., Shochat, T., Herer, P., and Lavie, P., Melatonin administered in the afternoon decreases next-day luteinizing hormone levels in men: lack of antagonism by flumazenil, *J. Molecular Neurosci.: MN*, 12 (1), 75–80, 1999.

Luboshitzky, R., Wagner, O., Lavi, S., Herer, P., and Lavie, P., Abnormal melatonin secretion in male patients with hypogonadism, *J. Molecular Neurosci.: MN*, 7 (2), 91–98, 1996.

Lucas, R.J., Freedman, M.S., Munoz, M., Garcia-Fernandez, J.M., and Foster, R.G., Regulation of the mammalian pineal by non-rod, non-cone, ocular photoreceptors, *Science*, 284 (5413), 505–507, 1999.

Lucas, R.J., Freedman, M.S., Lupi, D., Munoz, M., David-Gray, Z.K., and Foster, R.G., Identifying the photoreceptive inputs to the mammalian circadian system using transgenic and retinally degenerate mice, *Behavioural Brain Res.*, 125 (1–2), 97–102, 2001.

Lynch, H.J., Wurtman, R.J., Moskowitz, M.A., Archer, M.C., and Ho, M.H., Daily rhythm in human urinary melatonin, *Science*, 187 (4172), 169–171, 1975.

Lynch, H.J., Jimerson, D.C., Ozaki, Y., Post, R.M., Bunney, Jr., W.E., and Wurtman, R.J., Entrainment of rhythmic melatonin secretion in man to a 12-hour phase shift in the light/dark cycle, *Life Sci.*, 23 (15), 1557–1563, 1978.

Maestroni, G.J., The immunoneuroendocrine role of melatonin, *J. Pineal Res.*, 14 (1), 1–10, 1993.

Maestroni, G.J., MLT and the immune-hematopoietic system, *Adv. Experimental Med. Biol.*, 460, 395–405, 1999.

Maestroni, G.J.M., Neurohormones and catecholamines as functional components of the bone marrow microenvironment, in Neuroimmunomodulation: Perspectives at the New Millennium, *Annals of the New York Academy of Sciences*, Vol. 917, Conti, A., Maestroni, G.J.M., McCann, S.M., Sternberg, E.M., Lipton, J.M., and Smith, C.C., Eds., New York Academy of Sciences, New York, 2000, pp. 29–37.

Maestroni, G.J.M., Melatonin and immune function, in *Psychoneuroimmunology*, 3rd ed., Ader, R., Felten, D.L., and Cohen, N., Eds., Academic Press, San Diego, CA, 2001a, pp. 433–443.

Maestroni, G.J., The immunotherapeutic potential of melatonin, *Expert Opinion Investigational Drugs*, 10 (3), 467–476, 2001b.

Maestroni, G.J. and Conti, A., Beta-endorphin and dynorphin mimic the circadian immunoenhancing and anti-stress effects of melatonin, *Int. J. Immunopharmacol.*, 11 (4), 333–340, 1989a.

Maestroni, G.J.M. and Conti, A., Role of the pineal neurohormone melatonin in the psychoneuroendocrine-immune network, in *Psychoneuroimmunology*, 2nd ed., Ader, R., Felten, D.L., and Cohen, N., Eds., Academic Press, San Diego, CA, 1991a, pp. 495–513.

Maestroni, G.J. and Conti, A., Anti-stress role of the melatonin-immuno-opioid network: evidence for a physiological mechanism involving T cell-derived, immunoreactive beta-endorphin and MET-enkephalin binding to thymic opioid receptors, *Int. J. Neurosci.*, 61 (3–4), 289–298, 1991b.

Maestroni, G.J. and Conti, A., Immuno-derived opioids as mediators of the immuno-enhancing and anti-stress action of melatonin, *Acta Neurologica*, 13 (4), 356–360, 1991c.

Maestroni, G.J. and Conti, A., Melatonin and the immune-hematopoietic system therapeutic and adverse pharmacological correlates, *Neuroimmunomodulation*, 3 (6), 325–332, 1996.

Maestroni, G.J., Conti, A., and Pierpaoli, W., Role of the pineal gland in immunity: circadian synthesis and release of melatonin modulates the antibody response and antagonizes the immunosuppressive effect of corticosterone, *J. Neuroimmunol.*, 13 (1), 19–30, 1986.

Maestroni, G.J.M., Conti, A., and Pierpaoli, W., The pineal gland and the circadian, opiatergic, immunoregulatory role of melatonin, in Neuroimmune Interactions: Proceedings of the Second International Workshop on Neuroimmunomodulation, *Annals of the New York Academy of Sciences,* Vol. 496, Jankovic, B.D., Markovic, B.M., and Spector, N.H., Eds., New York Academy of Sciences, New York, 1987a, pp. 67–77.

Maestroni, G.J., Conti, A., and Pierpaoli, W., Role of the pineal gland in immunity: II, melatonin enhances the antibody response via an opiatergic mechanism, *Clinical Experimental Immunol.,* 68 (2), 384–391, 1987b.

Maestroni, G.J.M., Conti, A., and Pierpaoli, W., Pineal melatonin, its fundamental immuno-regulatory role in aging and cancer, in Neuroimmunomodulation: Interventions in Aging and Cancer, *Annals of the New York Academy of Sciences,* Vol. 521, Pierpaoli, W. and Spector, N.H., Eds., New York Academy of Sciences, New York, 1988a, pp. 140–148.

Maestroni, G.J., Conti, A., and Pierpaoli, W., Role of the pineal gland in immunity: III, melatonin antagonizes the immunosuppressive effect of acute stress via an opiatergic mechanism, *Immunology,* 63 (3), 465–469, 1988b.

Maestroni, G.J.M., Conti, A., and Pierpaoli, W., Melatonin, stress, and the immune system, in Reiter, R.J., Ed., *Pineal Research Reviews,* Vol. 7, Alan R. Liss, New York, 1989, pp. 203–226.

Maestroni, G.J., Togni, M., and Covacci, V., Norepinephrine protects mice from acute lethal doses of carboplatin, *Experimental Hematol.,* 25 (6), 491–494, 1997.

Maestroni, G.J. et al., Neural and endogenous catecholamines in the bone marrow, Circadian association of norepinephrine with hematopoiesis, *Experimental Hematol.,* 26 (12), 1172–1177, 1998.

Marangos, P.J. et al., Inhibition of diazepam binding by tryptophan derivatives including melatonin and its brain metabolite *N*-acetyl-5-methoxy kynurenamine, *Life Sci.,* 29 (3), 259–267, 1981.

Matera, L., Cesano, A., Veglia, F., and Muccioli, G., Effect of prolactin on natural killer activity, in Neuropeptides and Immunopeptides: Messengers in a Neuroimmune Axis, *Annals of the New York Academy of Sciences,* Vol. 594, O'Dorisio, M.S. and Panerai, A., Eds., New York Academy of Sciences, New York, 1990, pp. 396–398.

McIntyre, I.M., Norman, T.R., Burrows, G.D., and Armstrong, S.M., Human melatonin suppression by light is intensity dependent, *J. Pineal Res.,* 6 (2), 149–156, 1989a.

McIntyre, I.M., Norman, T.R., Burrows, G.D., and Armstrong, S.M., Quantal melatonin suppression by exposure to low intensity light in man, *Life Sci.,* 45 (4), 327–332, 1989b.

Mikkelsen, J.D. et al., Hypocretin (orexin) in the rat pineal gland: a central transmitter with effects on noradrenaline-induced release of melatonin, *Eur. J. Neurosci.,* 14 (3), 419–425, 2001.

Miller, J.D., The SCN is comprised of a population of couple oscillators, *Chronobiol. Int.,* 15 (5), 489–511, 1998.

Moingeon, P. et al., Benzodiazepine receptors on human blood platelets, *Life Sci.,* 35 (20), 2003–2009, 1984.

Moore, R.Y., Organization of the mammalian circadian system, *Ciba Found. Symp.,* 183, 88–99, 1995a.

Moore, R.Y., The retinohypothalamic tract originates from a distinct subset of retinal ganglion cells, *J. Comp. Neurol.,* 352 (3), 351–366, 1995b.

Mormont, M.C. et al., Marked 24-h rest/activity rhythms are associated with better quality of life, better response, and longer survival in patients with metastatic colorectal cancer and good performance status, *Clinical Cancer Res.: Off. J. Am. Assoc. Cancer Res.*, 6 (8), 3038–3045, 2000.

Morris, M.E., Viswanathan, N., Kuhlman, S., Davis, F.C., and Weitz, C.J., A screen for genes induced in the suprachiasmatic nucleus by light, *Science*, 279 (5356), 1544–1547, 1998.

Muller, J.E., Tofler, G.H., Willich, S.N., and Stone, P.H., Circadian variation of cardiovascular disease and sympathetic activity, *J. Cardiovasc. Pharmacol.*, 10 (Suppl. 2), S104–111, 1987.

Muller, J.E., Tofler, G.H., and Stone, P.H., Circadian variation and triggers of onset of acute cardiovascular disease, *Circulation*, 79 (4), 733–743, 1989.

Nair, N.P.V., Hara Hariharasubramaniank, P.C., Isaac, I., and Thavundayil, J.X., Plasma melatonin—an index of brain aging in humans, *Biological Psychiatry*, 21 (2), 141–150, 1986.

Nathan, P.J., Wyndham, E.L., Burrows, G.D., and Norman, T.R., The effect of gender on the melatonin suppression by light: a dose response relationship, *J. Neural Transmission*, 107 (3), 271–279, 2000.

Nelson, R.J. and Drazen, D.L., Melatonin mediates seasonal changes in immune function, in Neuroimmunomodulation: Perspectives at the New Millennium, *Annals of the New York Academy of Sciences*, Vol. 917, Conti, A., Maestroni, G.J.M., McCann, S.M., Sternberg, E.M., Lipton, J.M., and Smith, C.C., Eds., New York Academy of Sciences, New York, 2000, pp. 404–415.

Neuwelt, E.A. and Lewy, A.J., Disappearance of plasma melatonin after removal of a neoplastic pineal gland, *New England J. Med.*, 308 (19), 1132–1135, 1983.

Osol, G., Schwartz, B., and Foss, D.C., Effects of time, photoperiod, and pinealectomy on ocular and plasma melatonin concentrations in the chick, *Gen. Comp. Endocrinol.*, 58 (3), 415–420, 1985.

Oxenkrug, G.F., Anderson, G.F., Dragovic, L., Blaivas, M., and Riederer, P., Circadian rhythms of human pineal melatonin, related indoles, and beta adrenoreceptors: post-mortem evaluation, *J. Pineal Res.*, 9 (1), 1–11, 1990.

Panza, J.P., Epstein, S.E., and Quyyumi, A.A., Circadian variation in vascular tone and its relation to α-sympathetic vasoconstrictor activity, *New England J. Med.*, 325 (14), 986–990, 1991.

Parry, B.L. et al., Altered waveform of plasma nocturnal melatonin secretion in premenstrual depression, *Arch. Gen. Psychiatry*, 47 (12), 1139–1146, 1990.

Passouant, P., Halberg, F., Genicot, R., Popoviciu, L., and Baldy-Moulinier, M., Periodicity of narcoleptic attacks and the circadian rhythm of rapid sleep, *Revue Neurologique*, 121 (2), 155–164, 1969.

Pepine, C.J., Circadian variations in myocardial ischemia, implications for management, *JAMA: J. Am. Medical Assoc.*, 265 (3), 386–390, 1991.

Peters, G.J., Van Dijk, J., Nadal, J.C., Van Groeningen, C.J., Lankelma, J., and Pinedo, H.M., Diurnal variation in the therapeutic efficacy of 5-fluorouracil against murine colon cancer, *In Vivo*, 1 (2), 113–117, 1987.

Poeggeler, B., Reiter, R.J., Tan, D.X., Chen, L.D., and Manchester, L.C., Melatonin, hydroxyl radical-mediated oxidative damage, and aging: a hypothesis, *J. Pineal Res.*, 14 (4), 151–168, 1993.

Provencio, I., Wong, S., Lederman, A.B., Argamaso, S.M., and Foster, R.G., Visual and circadian responses to light in aged retinally degenerate mice, *Vision Res.*, 34 (14), 1799–1806, 1994.

Provencio, I., Jiang, G., De Grip, W.J., Hayes, W.P., and Rollag, M.D., Melanopsin: an opsin in melanophores, brain, and eye, *Proc. Natl. Acad. Sci. U.S.A.*, 95 (1), 340–345, 1998.

Provencio, I., Rodriguez, I.R., Jiang, G., Hayes, W.P., Moreira, E.F., and Rollag, M.D., A novel human opsin in the inner retina, *J. Neurosci.*, 20 (2), 600–605, 2000.

Quyyumi, A.A., Circadian rhythms in cardiovascular disease, *Am. Heart J.*, 120 (3), 726–733, 1990.

Raghavendra, V., Kaur, G., and Kulkarni, S.K., Anti-depressant action of melatonin in chronic forced swimming-induced behavioral despair in mice, role of peripheral benzodiazepine receptor modulation, *Eur. Neuropsychopharmacol.: J. Eur. Coll. Neuropsychopharmacol.*, 10 (6), 473–481, 2000.

Reichlin, S., Neuroendocrine-immune interactions, *New England J. Med.*, 329 (17), 1246–1253, 1993.

Reinberg, A. et al., Circadian rhythm of respiratory functions and temperature in asthmatic patients staying in hypoallergenic environment, *Presse Medicale*, 78 (42), 1817–1821, 1970.

Reindl, K., Falliers, C., Halberg, F., Chai, H., Hillman, D., and Nelson, W., Circadian acrophase in peak expiratory flow rate and urinary electrolyte excretion of asthmatic children: phase shifting of rhythms by prednisone given in different circadian system phases, *Rassegna di neurologia vegeta*, 23 (1), 5–26, 1969.

Reiter, R.J., The pineal gland and its hormones in the control of reproduction in mammals, *Endocrine Rev.*, 1 (2), 109–130, 1980.

Reiter, R.J., Pineal melatonin: cell biology of its synthesis and of its physiological interactions, *Endocrine Rev.*, 12 (2), 151–180, 1991a.

Reiter, R.J., Pineal gland: interface between the photoperiodic environment and endocrine system, *Trends Endocrinol. Metab.*, 91, 13–19, 1991b.

Reiter, R.J., Alterations of the circadian melatonin rhythm by the electromagnetic spectrum: a study in environmental toxicology, *Regulatory Toxicol. Pharmacol.: RTP*, 15 (3), 226–244, 1992.

Reiter, R.J., The pineal gland: from last to first, *Endocrinologist*, 3 (6), 425–431, 1993a.

Reiter, R.J., Electromagnetic fields and melatonin production, *Biomed. Pharmacother.*, 47 (10), 439–444, 1993b.

Reiter, R.J., Melatonin suppression by static and extremely low frequency electromagnetic fields: relationship to the reported increased incidence of cancer, *Rev. Environ. Health*, 10 (3–4), 171–186, 1994.

Reiter, R.J., Melatonin and human reproduction, *Ann. Med.*, 30 (1), 103–108, 1998.

Reiter, R.J. and Johnson, L.Y., Depressant action of the pineal gland on pituitary luteinizing hormone and prolactin in male hamsters, *Hormone Res.*, 5 (5), 311–320, 1974a.

Reiter, R.J. and Johnson, L.Y., Pineal regulation of immunoreactive luteinizing hormone and prolactin in light-deprived female hamsters, *Fertil. Steril.*, 25 (11), 958–964, 1974b.

Reiter, R.J. and Richardson, B.A., Magnetic field effects on pineal indoleamine metabolism and possible biological consequences, *FASEB J.: Off. Publ. Fed. Am. Soc. Experimental Biol.*, 6 (6), 2283–2287, 1992.

Reiter, R.J., Calvo, J.R., Karbownik, M., Qi, W., and Tan, D.X., Melatonin and its relation to the immune system and inflammation, in Neuroimmunomodulation: Perspectives at the New Millennium, *Annals of the New York Academy of Sciences*, Vol. 917, Conti, A., Maestroni, G.J.M., McCann, S.M., Sternberg, E.M., Lipton, J.M., and Smith, C.C., Eds., New York Academy of Sciences, New York, 2000, pp. 376–386.

Reiter, R.J., Johnson, L.Y., Vaughan, M.K., and Richardson, B.A., Pineal constituents and reproductive physiology, *Progr. Clinical Biological Res.*, 74, 163–178, 1981.

Reiter, R.J., King, T.S., Steinlechner, S., Steger, R.W., and Richardson, B.A., Tryptophan administration inhibits nocturnal N-acetyltransferase activity and melatonin content in the rat pineal gland, *Neuroendocrinology*, 52, 291–296, 1990.

Reiter, R.J., Oh, C.-S., and Fujimori, O., Melatonin: its intracellular and genomic actions, *Trends Endocrinol. Metab.: TEM*, 7 (1), 22–27, 1996.

Reiter, R.J., Tan, D.X., Burkhardt, S., and Manchester, L.C., Melatonin in plants, *Nutrition Rev.*, 59 (9), 286–290, 2001.

Reiter, R.J. et al., A review of the evidence supporting melatonin's role as an antioxidant, *J. Pineal Res.*, 18 (1), 1–11, 1995.

Relkin, R., Pineal–hormonal interactions, in *The Pineal Gland*, Relkin, R., Ed., Elsevier, New York, 1983, pp. 77–128.

Reppert, S.M., Cellular and molecular basis of circadian timing in mammals, *Seminars Perinatol.*, 24 (4), 243–246, 2000.

Reppert, S.M. and Weaver, D.R., Molecular analysis of mammalian circadian rhythms, *Ann. Rev. Physiol.*, 63, 647–676, 2001.

Reppert, S.M., Godson, C., Mahle, C.D., Weaver, D.R., Slaugenhaupt, S.A., and Gusella, J.F., Molecular characterization of a second melatonin receptor expressed in human retina and brain: the Mel1b melatonin receptor, *Proc. Natl. Acad. Sci. U.S.A.*, 92 (19), 8734–8738, 1995.

Rollag, M.D., O'Callaghan, P.L., and Niswender, G.D., Serum melatonin concentrations during different stages of the annual reproductive cycle in ewes, *Biol. Reprod.*, 18 (2), 279–285, 1978.

Rosen, L.A., Barber, I., and Lyle, D.B., A 0.5 G, 60 Hz magnetic field suppresses melatonin production in pinealocytes, *Bioelectromagnetics*, 19 (2), 123–127, 1998.

Rozencwaig, R., Grad, B.R., and Ochoa, J., The role of melatonin and serotonin in aging, *Medical Hypotheses*, 23 (4), 337–352, 1987.

Ruff, M.R., Pert, C.B., Weber, R.J., Wahl, L.M., Wahl, S.M., and Paul, S.M., Benzodiazepine receptor-mediated chemotaxis of human monocytes, *Science*, 229 (4719), 1281–1283, 1985.

Sack, R.L., Lewy, A.J., Blood, M.L., Keith, L.D., and Nakagawa, H., Circadian rhythm abnormalities in totally blind people: incidence and clinical significance, *J. Clin. Endocrinol Metab.*, 75 (1), 127–134, 1992.

Sack, R.L., Brandes, R.W., Kendall, A.R., and Lewy, A.J., Entrainment of free-running circadian rhythms by melatonin in blind people, *New England J. Med.*, 343 (15), 1070–1077, 2000.

Sakurai, T. et al., Orexins and orexin receptors: a family of hypothalamic neuropeptides and G protein-coupled receptors that regulate feeding behavior, *Cell*, 92 (4), 573–585, 1998.

Salti, R. et al., Nocturnal melatonin patterns in children, *J. Clin. Endocrinol. Metab.*, 85 (6), 2137–2144, 2000.

Sancar, A., Cryptochrome: the second photoactive pigment in the eye and its role in circadian photoreception, *Ann. Rev. Biochem.*, 69, 31–67, 2000.

Sangoram, A.M. et al., Mammalian circadian autoregulatory loop: a timeless ortholog and mPer1 interact and negatively regulate Clock-BMAL1-induced transcription, *Neuron*, 21 (5), 1101–1113, 1998.

Saper, C.B., Chou, T.C., and Scammell, T.E., The sleep switch: hypothalamic control of sleep and wakefulness, *Trends Neurosci.*, 24 (12), 726–731, 2001.

Savino, W., Villa-Verde, D.M.S., Alves, L.A., and Dardenne, M., Neuroendocrine control of the thymus, in Neuroimmunomodulation Molecular Aspects, Integrative Systems, and Clinical Advances, *Annals of the New York Academy of Sciences*, Vol. 840, McCann, S.M., Sternberg, E.M., Lipton, J.M., Chrousos, G.P., Gold, P.W., and Smith, C.G., Eds., New York Academy of Sciences, New York, 1998, pp. 470–477.

Schernhammer, E.S. et al., Rotating night shifts and risk of breast cancer in women participating in the nurses' health study, *J. Natl. Cancer Inst.*, 93 (20), 1563–1568, 2001.

Schuster, C., Gauer, F., Malan, A., Recio, J., Pevet, P., and Masson-Pevet, M., The circadian clock, light/dark cycle and melatonin are differentially involved in the expression of daily and photoperiodic variations in mt(1) melatonin receptors in the Siberian and Syrian hamsters, *Neuroendocrinology*, 74 (1), 55–68, 2001.

Sehgal, A., Man, B., Price, J.L., Vosshall, L.B., and Young, M.W., New clock mutations in *Drosophila*, *Ann. New York Acad. Sci.*, 618, 1–10, 1991.

Selmaoui, B. and Touitou, Y., Age-related differences in serum melatonin and pineal NAT activity and in the response of rat pineal to a 50-Hz magnetic field, *Life Sci.*, 64 (24), 2291–2297, 1999.

Shearman, L.P. et al., Interacting molecular loops in the mammalian circadian clock, *Science*, 288 (5468), 1013–1019, 2000.

Slaugenhaupt, S.A., Roca, A.L., Liebert, C.B., Altherr, M.R., Gusella, J.F., and Reppert, S.M., Mapping of the gene for the Mel1a-melatonin receptor to human chromosome 4 (MTNR1A) and mouse chromosome 8 (Mtnr1a), *Genomics*, 27 (2), 355–357, 1995.

Smith, S.D., McLeod, B.R., Liboff, A.R., and Cooksey, K., Calcium cyclotron resonance and diatom mobility, *Bioelectromagnetics*, 8 (3), 215–227, 1987.

Stankov, B. and Reiter, R.J., Melatonin receptors: current status, facts and hypotheses, *Life Sci.*, 46 (14), 971–982, 1990.

Steeves, T.D. et al., Molecular cloning and characterization of the human clock gene: expression in the suprachiasmatic nuclei, *Genomics*, 57 (2), 189–200, 1999.

Stetson, M.H. and Watson-Whitmyre, M., Nucleus suprachiasmaticus: the biological clock in hamsters, *Science*, 191 (4223), 197–199, 1976.

Sullivan, W.N., Cawley, B., Hayes, D.K., Rosenthal, J., and Halberg, F., Circadian rhythm in susceptibility of house flies and Madeira cockroaches to pyrethrum, *J. Econ. Entomol.*, 63 (1), 159–163, 1970.

Tamarkin, L., Westrom, W.K., Hamill, A.I., and Goldman, B.D., Effect of melatonin on the reproductive systems of male and female Syrian hamsters: a diurnal rhythm in sensitivity to melatonin, *Endocrinology*, 99 (6), 1534–1541, 1976.

Tamarkin, L., Baird, C.J., and Almeida, O.F.X., Melatonin: a coordinating signal for mammalian reproduction? *Science*, 227 (4688), 714–720, 1985.

Tan, D.X. et al., The pineal hormone melatonin inhibits DNA-adduct formation induced by the chemical carcinogen safrole *in vivo*, *Cancer Lett.*, 70 (1–2), 65–71, 1993.

Tan, D.X. et al., Identification of highly elevated levels of melatonin in bone marrow: its origin and significance, *Biochimica Biophysica Acta.*, 1472 (1–2), 206–214, 1999.

Tan, D.X. et al., Melatonin directly scavenges hydrogen peroxide: a potentially new metabolic pathway of melatonin biotransformation, *Free Radical Biol. Med.*, 29 (11), 1177–1185, 2000.

Tanner, J.M. and Whitehouse, R.H., Clinical longitudinal standards for height, weight, height velocity, weight velocity, and stages of puberty, *Arch. Dis. Childhood*, 51 (3), 170–179, 1976.

Thapan, K., Arendt, J., and Skene, D.J., An action spectrum for melatonin suppression: evidence for a novel non-rod, non-cone photoreceptor system in humans, *J. Physiol.*, 535 (1), 261–267, 2001.

Thrall, M.M., Wood, P., King, V., Rivera, W., and Hrushesky, W., Investigation of the comparative toxicity of 5-FU bolus versus 5-FU continuous infusion circadian chemotherapy with concurrent radiation therapy in locally advanced rectal cancer, *Int. J. Radiat. Oncol., Biol., Phys.*, 46 (4), 873–881, 2000.

Utiger, R.D., Melatonin—the hormone of darkness, *New England J. Med.*, 327 (19), 1377–1379, 1992.

Vakkuri, O., Rintamaki, H., and Leppaluoto, J., Plasma and tissue concentrations of melatonin after midnight light exposure and pinealectomy in the pigeon, *J. Endocrinol.*, 105 (2), 263–268, 1985.

Vakkuri, O., Kivela, A., Leppaluoto, J., Valtonen, M., and Kauppila, A., Decrease in melatonin precedes follicle-stimulating hormone increase during perimenopause, *Eur. J. Endocrinol.*, 135 (2), 188–192, 1996.

Vaughan, M.K., Pineal peptides: an overview, in *The Pineal Gland*, Reiter, R.J., Ed., Raven Press Books, New York, 1984, pp. 39–81.

Vitaterna, M.H., Takahashi, J.S., and Turek, F.W., Overview of circadian rhythms, *Alcohol Res. Health: J. Natl. Inst. Alcohol Abuse Alcoholism*, 25 (2), 85–93, 2001.

Vitaterna, M.H. et al., Differential regulation of mammalian *Period* genes and circadian rhythmicity by cryptochromes 1 and 2, *Proc. Natl. Acad. Sci. U.S.A.*, 96 (21), 12114–12119, 1999.

Vorkapic, P., Waldhauser, F., Bruckner, R., Biegelmayer, C., Schmidbauer, M., and Pendl, G., Serum melatonin levels: a new neurodiagnostic tool in pineal region tumors? *Neurosurgery*, 21 (6), 817–824, 1987.

Waldhauser, F., Waldhauser, M., Lieberman, H.R., Deng, M.H., Lynch, H.J., and Wurtman, R.J., Bioavailability of oral melatonin in humans, *Neuroendocrinology*, 39 (4), 307–313, 1984.

Weaver, D.R., The suprachiasmatic nucleus: a 25-year retrospective, *J. Biological Rhythms*, 13 (2), 100–112, 1998.

Wiesenberg, I., Missbach, M., Kahlen, J.P., Schrader, M., and Carlberg, C., Transcriptional activation of the nuclear receptor RZR alpha by the pineal gland hormone melatonin and identification of CGP 52608 as a synthetic fluid, *Nucleic Acids Res.*, 23 (3), 327–333, 1995.

Weissbach, H., Redfield, B.G., and Axelrod, J., Biosynthesis of melatonin: enzymic conversion of serotonin to *N*-acetylserotonin, *Biochimica Biophysica Acta*, 43, 352–353, 1960.

Welsh, D.K., Logothetis, D.E., Meister, M., and Reppert, S.M., Individual neurons dissociated from rat suprachiasmatic nucleus express independently phased circadian firing rhythms, *Neuron*, 14 (4), 697–706, 1995.

Wilson, B.W., Stevens, R.G., and Anderson, L.E., Neuroendocrine mediated effects of electromagnetic-field exposure: possible role of the pineal gland, *Life Sci.*, 45 (15), 1319–1332, 1989.

Wilson, S.T., Blask, D.E., and Lemus-Wilson, A.M., Melatonin augments the sensitivity of MCF-7 human breast cancer cells to tamoxifen *in vitro*, *J. Clinical Endocrinol. Metab.*, 75 (2), 669–670, 1992.

Wurtman, R.J., Age-related decreases in melatonin secretion—clinical consequences, *J. Clinical Endocrinol. Metab.*, 85 (6), 2135–2136, 2000.

Wurtman, R.J. and Moskowitz, M.A., The pineal organ (first of two parts), *New England J. Med.*, 296 (23), 1329–1333, 1977a.

Wurtman, R.J. and Moskowitz, M.A., The pineal organ (second of two parts), *New England J. Med.*, 296 (24), 1383–1386, 1977b.

Wurtman, R.J., Axelrod, J., and Chu, E.W., Melatonin, a pineal substance: effect on the rat ovary, *Science*, 141 (3577), 277–278, 1963a.

Wurtman, R.J., Axelrod, J., and Phillips, L., Melatonin synthesis in the pineal gland: control by light, *Science*, 142 (3595), 1071–1073, 1963b.

Wurtman, R.J., Axelrod, J., and Fischer, J.E., Melatonin synthesis in the pineal gland: effect of light mediated by the sympathetic nervous system, *Science*, 143 (3612), 1328–1330, 1964.

Yu, Q., Miller, S.C., and Osmond, D.G., Melatonin inhibits apoptosis during early B-cell development in mouse bone marrow, *J. Pineal Res.*, 29 (2), 86–93, 2000.

Zhdanova, I.V., Wurtman, R.J., Regan, M.M., Taylor, J.A., Shi, J.P., and Leclair, O.U., Melatonin treatment for age-related insomnia, *J. Clinical Endocrinol. Metab.*, 86 (10), 4727–4730, 2001.

Zrenner, C., Theories of pineal function from classical antiquity to 1900: a history, in *Pineal Research Reviews*, Vol. 3, Reiter, R.J., Ed., Alan R. Liss, New York, 1985, pp. 1–40.

Zylka, M.J., Shearman, L.P., Levine, J.D., Jin, X., Weaver, D.R., and Reppert, S.M., Molecular analysis of mammalian timeless, *Neuron*, 21 (5), 1115–1122, 1998.

ADDITIONAL RESOURCES

Brzezinski, A. and Wurtman, R., The pineal gland: its possible roles in human reproduction, *Obstetrical Gynecological Surv.*, 43 (4), 197–207, 1988.

Burch, J.B., Reif, J.S., Yost, M.G., Keefe, T.J., and Pitrat, C.A., Reduced excretion of a melatonin metabolite in workers exposed to 60 Hz magnetic fields, *Am. J. Epidemiol.*, 150 (1), 27–36, 1999.

Lissoni, P. et al., Relation between lymphocyte subpopulations and pineal function in patients with early or metastatic cancer, in Neuroimmunomodulation: Interventions in Aging and Cancer, *Annals of the New York Academy of Sciences*, Vol. 521, Pierpaoli, W. and Spector, N.H., Eds., New York Academy of Sciences, New York, 1988, pp. 290–299.

O'Hara, B.F. et al., Developmental changes in nicotinic receptor mRNAs and responses to nicotine in the suprachiasmatic nucleus and other brain regions, *Brain Res.: Molecular Brain Res.*, 66 (1–2), 71–82, 1999.

Reiter, R.J., Tan, D.X., Poeggeler, B., and Kavet, R., Inconsistent suppression of nocturnal pineal melatonin synthesis and serum melatonin levels in rats exposed to pulsed DC magnetic fields, *Bioelectromagnetics*, 19 (5), 318–329, 1998.

Sehgal, A., Price, J.L., Man, B., and Young, M.W., Loss of circadian behavioral rhythms and *per* RNA oscillations in the *Drosophila* mutant *timeless*, *Science*, 263 (5153), 1603–1606, 1994.

Selby, C.P., Thompson, C., Schmitz, T.M., Van Gelder, R.N., and Sancar, A., Functional redundancy of cryptochromes and classical photoreceptors for nonvisual ocular photoreception in mice, *Proc. Natl. Acad. Sci. U.S.A.*, 97 (26), 14697–14702, 2000.

7 Energy Medicine: Cutting Edge Modalities

Does an organized energetic system that has clinical applications exist in the human body? Although biochemical and physiologic studies have provided insight into some of the biologic effects of acupuncture, acupuncture practice is based on a very different model of energy balance. This theory might or might not provide new insights to medical research, but it deserves further attention because of its potential for elucidating the basis for acupuncture.

National Institutes of Health (NIH) Consensus Statement on Acupuncture
November 1997

CONTENTS

In the previous chapters, we proceeded from learning about the wondrous, if not enigmatic, integration of the body's internal systems to understanding the profound role that the pineal gland plays in the conversion of external energy into the chemical or electrical energy of our internal physiology. These measurable paradigms are part of what has been called the *human energy field*. It is experienced by the body via hormones and peptides, but it interacts with other ambient fields, such as light, sound, electricity, and that of all living organisms. Research shows that our bodies are absorptive, reflective, and generative of informational energy fields. We absorb light and heat from the sun, but we also produce our own internal energy fields. Electromagnetic forces are evidenced both in Earth's atmosphere and in the binding of a discrete hormone to its appropriate receptor. Both internal and external aspects of our existence are part of the human energy field. In pondering this phenomenon, you will eventually recognize that the integration of complex systems that exist within your body is a reflection of the integration that exists between the body and all that is outside itself.

Undoubtedly, traditional Western medicine must expand its concept of healing to incorporate a human energy field, which is the foundation of Eastern medical systems, such as acupuncture. Knowledge of the existence and effects of the human energy field is the first stepping-stone on the path to understanding *integral physiology*, which is a new medical paradigm of integral medicine that unites the enormous contribution of Western medicine with the profound insights of Eastern systems of human energy and health. This is described in some detail in the last chapter. Ultimately, it is my personal belief that the physical body is a biofeedback machine for the soul; a fact that I believe will eventually be borne out by reliable scientific findings.

Currently, scientists are able to measure some types of energy that the eye cannot see. Conventional medicine commonly utilizes these types of energy in its diagnostic procedures, such as sonograms, x-rays, magnetic resonance imaging (MRIs), electrocardiograms (EKG), electroencephalograms (EEGs), and the positron emission tomography (PET) scans involved in nuclear medicine. There are various unconventional diagnostic devices that are being used to measure or evaluate subtle energy. This is an important frontier in science today, as it could finally confirm what healers and other intuitives have long experienced and known. The Motoyama machine for measuring flow in the meridians is popular in Japan. Another procedure, bioelectrography, can visualize the corona discharge of any living object. It is obtained by exposure to a high-frequency, high-voltage electromagnetic field. The image is then recorded on photographic paper or by modern video-recording equipment. The gas-discharge visualization (GDV) device and software, invented by the Russian scientist, Konstantin Korotkov (Korotkov, 2001, 2002), is currently one of the most technologically advanced bioelectrography devices. It takes Kirlian photography, technologically, a step further. The device is a fast, inexpensive, and relatively noninvasive means for the diagnostic evaluation of physiological and psychological states. Both basic and clinical research on GDV is currently being conducted in several countries, including the United States A two-day symposium in April 2002 at the NIH concluded that GDV bioelectrography is a promising technique that warrants further study (Francomano and Jones, 2003). Being a scientifically oriented physician, I would like to see studies performed that might reveal the potential applications of GDV (as well as other devices now being utilized in other parts of the world) for practical clinical use (see, for example, the section entitled "Brain Scans of Spiritual Experiences" in Chapter 8).

The energy that is referred to as a human energy field is also typically called *subtle energy*. To avoid semantic gyrations in defining terms, I simply think of subtle energy as energy that, for the typical person, is outside of the awareness provided by the five senses. Subtle energy has to do with healing energy, divine energy, or the Chinese concept of Qi, which is described as the fundamental energy of life. However, this effect is beginning to be recorded and measured. For example, it has been proposed that cells actually have receptor sites for subtle energy signals, and therefore the "noise" recorded from brain waves on an EEG may in fact be the sounds of signals being transmitted to specific receptor sites (Rosch, 1994). As we will review in this chapter and the final chapter, we may look very solid, but if medicine followed the tenets of modern physics, we would realize that we are composed of informational energy fields interacting with other energy fields, some more dense, some less dense. However, subtle energies may profoundly impact our physical and emotional health.

Following is a review of various healing modalities that can be considered to be subtle energy medicine. The bibliography provides you with a variety of resources if you are interested in more information about a particular technique.

MODALITIES OF SUBTLE ENERGY MEDICINE

The solution to the riddle of space and time lies outside of space and time.

Ludwig Wittgenstein, 1974

ACUPUNCTURE

In November 1997, a panel under the auspices of the NIH convened to formulate the first consensus statement on acupuncture. The NIH consensus panel was comprised of 12 experts from various health-related fields who met for 2½ days to assess the use and effectiveness of acupuncture for a variety of medical conditions. I am honored to have served as a panelist. The panel members spent months reading hundreds of scientific articles and abstracts before attending to the conference. At the conference, we listened to numerous presentations, discussed the studies that we had read, and then determined which research studies were worthy of further deliberation. The group of studies we selected as most relevant was then put to the scrutiny of the strictest scientific analysis to determine which of them were effective (NIH, 1997). The consensus statement describes promising results in the areas of adult postoperative and chemotherapy nausea and vomiting as well as for postoperative dental pain. In addition, there were several conditions for which the panel felt that acupuncture might be used as an adjunct treatment or as part of a comprehensive treatment plan, including addiction, stroke rehabilitation, headache, menstrual cramps, tennis elbow, fibromyalgia, myofascial pain, carpal tunnel syndrome, and asthma (NIH, 1997). The World Health Organization has a much longer list of recognized conditions that can be effectively treated with acupuncture. It includes the treatment of respiratory conditions, gastrointestinal illnesses, neurological and muscular disorders, as well as urinary and gynecological problems.

Acupuncture is a treatment based on traditional Chinese medicine, a system of healing that dates back thousands of years. In Chinese medicine, there is a central concept of a vital energy or life force, which is called *Qi*. Meridians are the names given to the complex pathways within our bodies along which Qi (a subtle energy) flows. Acupuncture points are specific points along the meridians at which Qi can be accessed and rebalanced. The homeostasis or balance of Qi is much like that of allostatic load in stress medicine (discussed in Chapter 3). If Qi becomes depleted or imbalanced, then physical, mental, and emotional dysfunction can occur. When there is too little or too much Qi in a given meridian or when the Qi stagnates or is blocked, physical disease can result. In the most basic terms, an acupuncture treatment consists of inserting ultrathin needles at various points on the body, known as gateways, to unblock or rebalance the flow of Qi. In fact, acupuncture techniques can encompass a very broad range of techniques for stimulating Qi, including moxibustion (the burning of the powdered leaves of mugwort [*Artemisia vulgaris*] to deliver gentle warmth), laser light, electromagnetic fields, and electrical current. Research in the 1970s and 1980s linked acupuncture analgesia to endogenous opioid peptide elaboration, particularly the endorphins. In 1995, acupuncture needles were no longer classified as "experimental" by the FDA.

Dick Larson, who holds a Ph.D. in acupuncture, has speculated convincingly that the myofascial tissue is the site of the elusive meridians of traditional acupuncture. Larson also effectively expresses how intertwined these meridians are with the myofascial tissue: "A disruption of the energy flow will manifest in the tissues. Conversely, a disruption in the order and balance of the tissues will ultimately manifest in the energy flow. The imbalance can start at either end of the spectrum. Eventually the physical and the energetic will reflect each other, because they are each other" (Larson, 1990).

QiGong

QiGong, which is translated as *chi*, cultivation or *chi* function, is a healing technique that has been practiced for thousands of years in China. *Qi* and *chi* are two spellings for the same word, meaning vital force or life energy force. We have chosen to use the spelling *Qi*. QiGong is an aspect of the practice of Chinese medicine. Like acupuncture, it can restore disturbances in Qi. In some traditions, QiGong is solely a meditative practice, although it is best known for the exercises created by physicians of the ancient martial arts traditions of China. There is, in addition, a breathing component to the practice of QiGong, which is intended to vitalize organs and increase one's energy level. Although many techniques that involve the cultivation of Qi emphasize an underlying goal of spiritual growth, the practice of medical QiGong begins with a positive and sometimes profound impact on physical health, but can expand into mental, emotional, and spiritual development as well. It is an evolving discipline that begins with daily calisthenics and breathing exercises, resulting in comprehensive healthcare and then a refined level of personal development. QiGong has recently been the focus of reports concerning its association with the alleviation of symptoms associated with cancer and other disease, and this is the aspect of the technique that is more popularly known (Lei et al., 1991; Sancier, 1999; Wu et al., 1999). Since the 1950s, China has established "hospitals" exclusively for the treatment of disease by QiGong.

QiGong masters have been tested in Western-style scientific protocols to assess their ability to facilitate healing in people. Currently available scientific equipment (e.g., the SQUID, which can measure the extremely sensitive magnetic field of the brain) measures forms of infrared, magnetic, and acoustical energy emitted from the hands of QiGong masters while practicing the technique. When a QiGong master is emitting Qi, a consistent shifting of EEG brain-wave patterns to the alpha state (7 to 14 Hz) occurs in the human or animal to which the Qi is being directed. In contrast, "fake" QiGong masters (who are actually experimental controls) are incapable of creating this change (Lee, 1999). Other research carried out in Austria illustrated that when an extremely well-trained QiGong master underwent neuromonitoring while practicing the technique, reproducible changes in transcranial Doppler sonography (e.g., stimulus-induced 40-Hz oscillations) and near-infrared spectroscopy were recorded (Litscher et al., 2001).

The QiGong healer diagnoses by passing a hand over the patient's body to scan the patient's energy field and by using acupressure to determine Qi disturbances (Jahnke, 1997). According to Richard Lee, a researcher on the effects of QiGong, QiGong masters emit infrasonic waves (a sound wave that cannot be detected by the human ear) at a range of about 70 dB (a wave intensity that is about 100 times more amplified than the infrasonic waves of a normal person) and at a frequency of 8 to 13.5 hertz, which is within the alpha range. In order for the QiGong master to be helpful, he or she must be able to produce an infrasonic amplitude and frequency of Qi that can be absorbed by the patient and, therefore, one that is biologically similar to the waveform of the patient. Infrasonic waves are acoustically the wavelength that is the most suitable resonant frequency for human tissue, and it is known that the human body can both emit and receive infrasonic waves.

QiGong typically is practiced in three phases. In preparation, the QiGong master quiets the mind. First, the QiGong master adds Qi to the patient, which can, in the receptive patient, increase his or her energy. This procedure generates what is described as a type of energetic chaos in the patient, which allows the possibility of reordering the mind and body. I believe this experience is akin to the concept that emotional trials can potentially bring self-evaluation and growth. The shift we must make to let go of tightly held but unhelpful habits can feel chaotic as we pass through that phase. Second, the "bad" or "pervasive" Qi is swept out of the body. Finally, the QiGong master helps reorder the "chaos" by performing a technique called *smoothing the Qi*. The patient is taught movement sequences that can be independently practiced to ameliorate a specific condition or to promote general health. The technique that involves the QiGong master sending Qi is called *external QiGong*, while the practice of the patient independently performing movement sequences or breathing exercises is called *internal QiGong*.

In the United States, various research projects are being carried out on the efficacy of QiGong. An interdisciplinary team funded by the NIH is conducting a large-sample clinical study on QiGong. The study is focusing on the difficulties and unique issues that must be taken into consideration in designing a clinical trial on energy medicine. Their main objective appears to be the promotion of more scholarly and accurate information on energy healing and on QiGong in particular (Ai et al., 2001). In addition, the Dana Farber Cancer Institute's Zakim Center for Integrated Therapies in Boston, Massachusetts, is running a trial on the efficacy of QiGong (compared with aerobic exercise) as an adjunct therapy for cancer patients.

Applied Kinesiology

Applied kinesiology uses the testing of muscle strength as a diagnostic procedure to indicate the health of various bodily functions. It uses the body's subtle energy system to reveal a correlation between weaknesses in muscle groups and imbalance or disease in the body. In other words, muscle strength is used as a tool to assess the functioning of the body, not the strength of the muscles per se. Points on the body, which correspond to acupuncture points, are treated with pressure to alleviate physical ailments. George J. Goodheart, Jr., a doctor of chiropractic medicine, happened upon the finding in the mid-1960s and developed the technique by progressively identifying associations between known disease or organ impairment (i.e., from an x-ray or some other conventionally accepted test) and specific muscle weakness. He performed cranial, sacral, or muscle adjustments that he claimed relieved the patient of the conventionally identified malady. There were several specific techniques he developed to carry out this procedure. Little scientific research has been performed on the technique. Touch for Health is an offshoot of applied kinesiology. The International College for Applied Kinesiology only admits licensed doctors, while Touch for Health can be studied and practiced by anyone choosing to take the training. It has more emphasis on strengthening and balancing muscles than does applied kinesiology. Educational kinesiology is an outgrowth of applied kinesiology that seeks to improve attention, memory, and learning.

Thought Field Therapy™ (TFT)

TFT, developed by Roger J. Callahan in the early 1980s, is also an offshoot of applied kinesiology (Callahan, 1985, 1995). An energy-based psychotherapy, TFT utilizes a unique interface between the techniques of applied kinesiology and the acupuncture meridian system to treat phobias, depression, and traumatic psychological problems, including highly successful outcomes with posttraumatic stress disorder. TFT is more effective for anxiety-related problems than for psychoses and has an accelerated rate of response for anxiety-related problems compared with traditional psychological therapies. Callahan felt that traumatic memories are energetically encoded within what he called *thought fields*, which can set off neurological and hormonal patterns of reaction. The technique uses self-applied percussion at acupuncture points (diagnosed by the therapist) and is performed in a sequence specific to the particular condition. While the patient performs the series of taps, an assessment of one's emotional or traumatic issue (what Callahan would call a perturbation in the thought field) is also performed. The tapping helps facilitate an attunement to the traumatic thought, thus allowing it to become conscious. The technique is designed to decode and release negative and bound-up energy from the thought field both by attuning to the thought field and by performing the percussive tapping. Verbal affirmations are utilized to reverse long-held psychological issues. A self-evaluation of one's current level of stress regarding the traumatic or negative issue that is being treated is used to assess treatment progress (Gallo, 1999).

THERAPEUTIC TOUCH (TT)

Therapeutic Touch was developed in the early 1970s by Dolores Krieger, Ph.D., R.N. (who was then a professor of nursing at New York University) and her long-time friend and mentor, Dora Kunz, a well-respected and highly developed clair-voyant healer (Krieger, 1979). More than 20 years before the first publications on TT, Krieger had participated in a meditation group at Kunz's home at Pumpkin Hollow Farm in the Berkshires of upstate New York (now the site of many TT retreats). In 1968, Kunz introduced Krieger to Oskar Estebany, a Hungarian citizen who was renowned as a gifted hands-on healer. As a result of this encounter, the two women decided to study healers and develop a technique of therapeutic touch to facilitate healing as an art that almost anyone could learn. Krieger did postdoctoral research on the healing technique (Krieger, 1975, 1976). Early studies showing increased hemoglobin levels in patients treated with TT convinced Krieger to dis-seminate the concept of TT and to train nurses and others in the technique. Today TT is a widely practiced form of therapy in hospitals and other health centers (Herdtner, 2000).

TT is a contemporary healing technique of laying on of hands (although most practitioners do not actually touch the patient's body) that is based on ancient principles of Indian or Chinese concepts of life force (prana and Qi, respectively). Krieger feels that healing is based on a transfer of this life energy, which is present in all living organisms (Quinn, 1989). The practitioner is trained both in intent and methodology. A quality of openness and willingness (i.e., intent) to heal is key to the efficacy of treatment (Heidt, 1990). After a period of centering, the practitioner places his or her hands slightly above the patient and energetically mobilizes areas of blocked energy. TT elicits a relaxation response and has been shown to be effective for degenerative arthritis, for increasing a sense of well-being and decreasing symp-toms of distress in cancer patients, and for decreasing stress in hospitalized children and adults as well as in the bereaved (Eckes Peck, 1997; Giasson and Bouchard, 1998; Kramer, 1990; Lafreniere et al., 1999; Quinn, 1993). A landmark study performed on 44 male college students showed faster wound healing from skin-punch biopsy (an intentionally administered skin wound used for tissue biopsy) in subjects receiving TT compared with those who did not. Although no subject (or the administering physician) knew that TT was being performed, 13 of 23 subjects who received TT had completely healed wounds by day 16 of the study, compared with none of the control subjects (Wirth, 1992). The study was disturbing to physi-cians skeptical of the efficacy of TT because it was impossible to explain away the effect on methodological grounds.

A heated controversy was initiated a few years later when the *Journal of the American Medical Association* (*JAMA*) published a study run by a 9-year-old girl and her mother, a nurse who is outspoken in her bias against TT (Rosa et al., 1998). The subjects were tested under blind conditions to determine whether they could correctly identify which of their hands was closest to the investigator's hand. The vaguely described recruitment method leaves questions as to whether the practitio-ners were TT professionals, and the gimmicky use of "sensing" an energy field is a nonessential element in the process of performing TT. It is troubling that *JAMA* should have published this methodologically flawed fourth-grade school science project in light of the efforts being made by the NIH to bring to the forefront solid, well-designed research on complementary therapies.

REIKI

The principles that guide Reiki are somewhat similar to those of TT. Reiki was developed by Dr. Mikao Usui, a theologian and the president of the Doshisha University in Kyoto in the mid-1880s, in response to students' queries as to how sick people were healed by Jesus and other spiritual leaders. Like TT, the practitioner begins by focusing or centering him or herself on the intent for the patient's highest good. The practitioner's fingers are placed on or just above the patient's body. During a sequence of hand positions, universal life energy is said to flow from the practitioner's hands to the patient's body. The word *Reiki* comes from two Japanese characters: *rei*, meaning universal, source of life, air, or spirit; and *ki*, meaning life force or vital energy. The patient's energy is said to be attuned or realigned from the session. Studies support the claim that Reiki may support the immune system (e.g., significant IgA salivary elevations), invokes a sense of relaxation and reduces pain symptoms (Olson, 1997; Wardell, 2001). However, these findings are preliminary, and more research is warranted.

POLARITY THERAPY

Polarity Therapy is another energy medicine modality that is akin to Reiki or other touch therapies. Polarity Therapy was developed by Dr. Randolph Stone (1890–1981), who held doctorates in osteopathy, chiropractic, and naturopathy. Stone first published his findings in 1947 in a book entitled *Energy*. He felt that the unseen but empirically known polarity that is manifested in magnetic attraction and repulsion was a reflection of the relationship underlying all physical phenomena, including health. Stone, who derived many of his theories from traditional Eastern religions and medicine, believed that when energy is blocked or unbalanced, disease and other stress-related conditions can occur. He felt that the human energy field could be corrected or brought back to health by several different modalities (e.g., touch, nutrition, exercise, communication), preferably in conjunction with one another. Polarity Therapy is at the core of the treatment. An experienced practitioner places his or her hands on a particular energetic pathway, enhancing the current flowing through the patient. The shift in energy can be experienced by both the therapist and the patient. Stone liked to say "God Geometrizes," meaning that many of the energy pathways in the body form geometric shapes. Polarity Therapy also facilitates the conscious recognition of connections between the mind and the body, while supporting patients to take charge of their own lives and health. Touch, in addition to supportive verbal communication, appears to help clients build inner resources to cope with various emotional issues, even assisting the resolution of posttraumatic syndrome. As far as we have been able to determine, little to no scientific research has been performed on Polarity Therapy. Our literature search yielded one study that showed a decrease in the number of gamma rays measured in a subject's electromagnetic field as a result of receiving polarity therapy, but nothing on treatment efficacy (Benford et al., 1999).

HOMEOPATHY

Dr. Samuel Hahnemann, a German physician, developed homeopathy over many years, beginning in 1790. Hahnemann coined the term *homeopathy* from the Greek words for similar (*omoios*) and feeling (*pathos*) because his medicine produced symptoms in healthy volunteers that were similar to the designated disease symptoms. His philosophy was "let likes be cured by likes," which he called the "principle of similars." He tested 90 substances (plants, minerals, poisons, hormones, bacteria, viruses, and many others) on himself and various volunteers. He then correlated the reaction to the disease or condition that produced the same symptoms. This was an enormous undertaking. Like the founders of TT or Reiki, Hahnemann also believed that homeopathy transferred a vital energy. Homeopathy was brought to the United States by Hans Burch Gram in 1825 and then supported by the immigration of other German homeopaths.

The problem with homeopathy for any type of molecular or chemical scientist is that the remedies are diluted (and then submitted to a process of vigorous shaking or "succussion") to an extent that supersedes Avogadro's number of molecules or theoretical setpoint (10^{-24}). Avogadro's number is the serial dilution point beyond which even an atom of the original substance theoretically could remain in the dilution. Some physicians are so bothered by this that they protest the efficacy of homeopathy in words such as "quackery" or "placebo." The patterns of criticism of homeopathy have actually been statistically documented (Vickers, 2000). Numerous well-designed studies can be found in support of the skeptic's view, illustrating either that homeopathy simply does not work (e.g., Ramelet et al., 2000; Vickers et al., 2001; Walach et al., 2001a) or criticizing the methodological quality of the studies (e.g., Linde et al., 2001). Recent research that leans toward findings of efficacy for homeopathic treatment generally calls for the need for larger studies to support their findings (e.g., Linde and Jobste, 2000 [asthma]; Jacobs et al., 2001 [acute otitis media (earache) in children]). However, some studies clearly have favorable results and are also well designed (e.g., Reilly et al., 1986 [hay fever]; Walach et al., 2001b [chronic headache]; Riley et al., 2001 [respiratory and ear complaints]; Berrebi et al., 2001 [lactation]; Papp et al., 1998 [Oscillococcinum®, which can decrease both symptoms and duration of flu if taken within 24 hours of onset]). The work that is most difficult to dismiss is the oft-cited and landmark study performed by researchers from the lab of Dr. Jacques Benveniste. Benveniste and colleagues took basophils (a type of white blood cell) from human blood, mixed them with the homeopathic dilution of IgE antiserum, and found that the basophils proceeded to release histamine (Davenas et al., 1988; Poitevin et al., 1988). That a solution, which according to Avogadro's theoretical setpoint should be devoid of any molecule, could cause histamine release definitely caused a stir among conventional medical scientists.

So, what is going on here? First, selecting the correct homeopathic remedy for a given individual can be a difficult undertaking, even when one utilizes a combination remedy for a specific disorder (and there is controversy about the use of combination remedies). Furthermore, it is my experience that homeopathy is a very subtle adjustment to the body. So, if the patient, for example, is being blasted with steroids for allergy relief, it is the rare individual who will feel any benefit from a homeopathic remedy at such a time. Unlike some in the field, I do not think that homeopathy is only an art or should be relegated to the status of an art. It is a fact that there are times when homeopathy distinctly works and times when it does not; therefore we need to find out why by expanding our research efforts. Ultimately the issue is that we simply do not know the mechanism of action for homeopathy, so we cannot control for those factors that hinder the efficacy of treatment.

Did you notice that we placed homeopathy in the subtle energy section and not, for instance, next to herbs or other chemical remedies? This is because it is likely that the mechanism of action is not chemical. According to Dr. Bill Gray, author of *Homeopathy: Science or Myth?*, remedies that have been *both* diluted and succussed cause an alignment of molecules in water that is less compact and has regions that are more organized than the simple diffusion that occurs when a molecule is simply dropped in water. It is also known that electrical fields can create polarized groupings that cluster themselves into coherent groups and move about in the water. Therefore, at homeopathic dilutions of 10^{-7} or greater, principles of quantum electrodynamics replace simple chemistry (Gray, 2000). Beverly Rubik, Ph.D., and others have postulated that electromagnetic information from the original substance is stored in the remedy and then released once it is ingested. Rubik believes that it is theoretically feasible that biological information could be encoded into the remedy and then could interact with endogenous electromagnetic fields, resulting in a transfer of discrete information (Rubik, 1995).

The research for this hypothesis has now been performed. Jacques Benveniste and his colleagues in France are once again leading the investigation in this area. Benveniste has shown that homeopathy's efficacy largely results from possessing a discrete electromagnetic field frequency that is transmittable to humans. He illustrated that a type of albumin (plasma albumin being the major blood plasma protein and osmotic transporter) that originates from hen's eggs (ovalbumin), once diluted and succussed, increases the cardiac flow in a guinea pig, even when there is no ovalbumin molecule present. However, he performed this experiment not with the remedy itself but rather by using ordinary water that had been instilled with the electromagnetic digital pattern of the homeopathic ovalbumin. He recorded the "white noise" of the remedy, or what he calls "the specific electromagnetic signature," and transferred it via an oscilloscope (a device that visually displays electrical variations) into a tube with ordinary water. This indicated that the water holds the discrete subtle energy qualities of the remedy. Benveniste then cut the specific electromagnetic signature into a digital electronic file and sent it thousands of miles away via the Internet. When it was "replayed" to water (and other substances such as plasma), the water was able to generate an effect characteristic of the original substance (Benveniste, 2000). Amazing! I find it exciting that there are now some studies available to show the impact that subtle energies have on our health. Of course, this study must be confirmed by other researchers. Yet, what this is saying is that if the remedy matches the frequency or resonance of the illness, healing could occur. We will be discussing such matters in more detail in Chapter 8, but it appears that what Hahnemann created with his principle of similars was a matching of energetic frequencies that permits healing to occur.

HEALING TRADITIONS OF INDIGENOUS PEOPLES

Different healing traditions have arisen from indigenous populations, such as the shamans of the Native American cultures, the kahuna healers of Hawaii, and the curanderos of Latin America. These healing traditions involve practices unique to each distinctive culture. However, underlying every healing tradition are spiritual beliefs that form the basis for both physical healing and a philosophy of life that aids the individual in his or her inner growth or emotional healing. As others have extensively written about the practices of Native Americans, we will not discuss that rich tradition. Rather, we will briefly review the less well-known practices of the Hawaiians and Latin Americans.

Kahuna

The kahuna, known to possess esoteric knowledge about healing and what was once called magic, were originally the spiritual teachers of Polynesia and then later of the indigenous Hawaiian people. The traditions of the ancient Hawaiian Kahuna were nearly extinguished when Europeans invaded the islands in the late 18th century. Assuming that their knowledge was superior to that of the indigenous people, the invaders nearly caused the extinction of a tradition whose sophistication, in some respects, was unparalleled until the latter half of the 20th century. For example, a concept central to the kahuna practice is that an integration of the conscious and unconscious mind, which occurs with a realignment of the ego, can result in healing. This concept was not fully realized or extrapolated upon until Carl Jung's work in the first half of the 20th century and Milton Erickson's publications in the 1960s.

The teachings and treatments of the Hawaiian Kahuna are multifaceted and range from the administration of remedies to esoteric spiritual practices. Knowledge and use of native plants, as well as those brought by Polynesian settlers, is central to the treatment of common ailments (Krauss, 1981). Current research is confirming the presence of pharmacologically active components in some of the commonly used botanicals. One plant that is being actively investigated is noni (*Morinda citrifolia*). Findings of novel glycosides as well as animal studies indicating immune-enhancing white blood cell activity and tumor-destroying properties should encourage further research (Hirazumi and Furusawa, 1999; Liu et al., 2001; Wang et al., 2000). In addition to botanicals, a kahuna typically uses *kahuna lomi lomi*, a deeply relaxing, rhythmical massage; *hooponopono*, a problem-solving technique that focuses on loving communication; and the invocation of *aumakua*, one's personal guardian spirit (Horowitz, 2001).

Underlying all practical treatments and remedies is a philosophy of a way of life that encourages a deep personal growth and spiritual exploration. In a publication that directly explains the practices and teachings of the kahuna, Dr. Laura Yardley reveals a system of Kahuna spiritual understanding that in many ways shares the basic philosophy of traditional Chinese medicine and Indian Ayurveda (Yardley, 1990). Yardley has researched the kahuna beliefs concerning both the physical body and the energetic body (e.g., vital energy or life force) as well as the reciprocal relationship between the two. Yardley reports that in the 1930s, Max Freedom Long, who devoted much of his life to researching the kahuna, uncovered the meanings of secret words used in kahuna chants and rituals. Long determined that the kahuna had an esoteric system of knowledge that emphasized a pursuit of spiritual perfection, a strong code of ethics, and a component that some call magic because it deals with phenomena that are beyond the five senses. Descriptions of the psychological workings of the conscious and unconscious mind and their relationship to the spiritual or "higher self" are prominent. Fundamental to the philosophy is that we harbor within ourselves both healing and harmful energies. It is the job of the kahuna to help keep these in balance.

Curanderos and Curanderas

Some say that the ancient practice of *curanderismo* (from the Spanish verb *curar*, meaning to heal) began with the Mayan, Aztec, and Incan folk healing traditions (Padilla et al., 2001). Other researchers ascribe its origins to the 16th-century Spanish conquistadors, who brought with them women, called *curanderas*, to treat the illnesses that the friars could not. The curanderas then conferred their knowledge upon the indigenous peoples of Latin America, who in turn incorporated these traditions into their own local practices (Harding, 1999). Today, the practice of curanderismo is also interwoven with prayers and rituals of Christian origin. At the center of curanderismo is the belief that the *curandera* (female) or *curandero* (male) is a conduit for divine healing and is spiritually "chosen" to heal others. Curanderos may refer their patients to modern medical clinics and hospitals. However, they also believe that some illnesses are the result of supernatural causes, which are often confused with natural causes and cannot be treated by conventional medicine. Curanderos fault most modern medical physicians for not being capable of recognizing when supernatural causes are in play. One curandera states that "it amazes me that Western medicine still has not realized the importance of the soul and spirit in healing" (Padilla et al., 2001). In turn, there is concern among the medical establishment that Latin Americans with serious medical conditions may not receive the care they need, turning instead to curanderos. Most curanderos would say that their work involves a supportive partnership with the patient's physician, a relationship of which few physicians ever are aware (Trotter, 2001).

Curanderismo is comprised of three different *niveles* or levels of treatment: physical, spiritual, and mental. Treatment at the physical or material *nivele* involves an extensive knowledge and use of herbs (*yerbera*); massage therapy skills (*sobardoras*); midwifery (*parteras*); psychological counseling (*consejeras*); and the use of rituals for supernatural cures. Perhaps the most common of these rituals is spiritual cleansing (*barrida* or *limpia*), which is performed to remove sadness, negative emotions, or physical pain. Negative energies are "swept" from the patient, typically with objects such as a handful of herbs, an egg, or an eagle feather. Curanderos who practice at the spiritual or mental *niveles* have developed the ability to communicate with spirit beings and thus to make known the spirit world to this world. They are said to channel healing vibrations from the spirit world to patients in need of physical or emotional healing (Trotter, 2001).

Curanderismo is practiced more extensively among Latin Americans residing in the United States than generally assumed (Alegria et al., 1977; Padilla et al., 2001). One study estimated that 150 to 200 curanderos and curanderas practice in the Denver metropolitan area. The studied showed that over 63% of the Latino population had visited one of these curanderos in the past 5 years (1996–2001) and that nearly all of the Latinos in the Denver area (91.3%) were aware of the practices of curanderos (Padilla et al., 2001). We were unable to find studies on clinical efficacy. A case report published in the *American Journal of Psychiatry* in the 1970s did claim that two cases of psychosis were successfully treated with an integration of conventional treatment and curanderismo (Kreisman, 1975).

Prayer and Spiritual Healing

Things found to be unaccountable under rigorous scientific scrutiny ought at least to suggest that science's ability to account for everything may be imperfect.

Elmer and Alyce Green, 1977

To omit the spiritual element from our medical worldview is not only narrow and arbitrary, it appears increasingly to be bad science as well.

Larry Dossey, 1995

Jeff Levin, a physician who researches the impact of prayer and spirituality on healing, examined the results of a general social survey that gathered information on 1481 adults over a 15-year period. Levin determined that there was an 86% lifetime prevalence of some type of mystical or paranormal experience among these individuals. That is a large majority, which means that a lot of us are keeping these experiences to ourselves. Larry Dossey, who for years has advocated the power of prayer, tells the story of a woman who came to speak to him after nearly everyone had left the hall where he had just given a lecture. She had had cancer that resolved without medical intervention. She lamented that nobody wanted to hear her story and that people with experiences like hers are never interviewed on *Oprah* (Dossey, 1993). Discussion of mystical or healing experiences frightens most of us, makes us feel uncomfortable, and appears to strike extreme discomfort in the hearts of the vast majority of physicians. Jeff Levin says that his favorite closed-minded comment from a physician came from a peer-reviewed scientific journal in which the physician is quoted as saying, "This is the kind of thing I would not believe even if it existed" (Levin, 2001).

What is it that makes so many people react with such skepticism to the possibility that there is a spiritual or subtle energy that exists outside the realm of the typical experience of the five senses? The truth is that all humans have insecurities, and physicians are constantly faced with the ultimate source of that insecurity, which is the fear of death and what may or may not follow that moment. In the United States, this fear has been escalated by the terrorist attacks of September 11, 2001. As the insightful physician, Andrew Newberg, states: "In its tireless quest to identify and resolve any threat that can potentially harm us, the mind had discovered the one alarming apprehension that can't be resolved by any means—the sobering understanding that everyone dies" (Newberg et al., 2001). It has taken me many years to realize that needless suffering, and not death, is the real enemy of the practicing physician. I have been a witness to numerous stories and experiences—totally unexplainable in everyday terms—that patients have related as they journeyed through an illness. The scientist in me is becoming much more aware of the mystery of life and the fact that there are phenomena that exist and are quite "real" but not yet explainable in scientific terms.

It is now well documented that prayer, spirituality, and religious experiences can have an impact on both our physical and mental well-being. The research has received both unreasonable criticism (as addressed above) and some valid criticism regarding methodological problems. Even the best-designed studies leave some troubling questions about the impact of prayer and spirituality on health. For example, in Levin's review of the general social survey, he curiously found that mystical experiences (i.e., an intrinsically religious experience) were reported more often by those who were not a part of any organized religion, even after controlling for other possible factors (Levin, 2001). And, we cited another work of Levin's in which he explains that the *intrinsically* religious are 20% more likely to have experiences of "absorption" or states of altered consciousness than the *extrinsically* religious (ce., those who are part of an orgainzed religion). Furthermore, Dr. Harold Koenig, a psychiatrist and researcher in the Department of Psychiatry at Duke University's Medical Center and a preeminent scientist in the field of religion and health, has shown a correlation in elderly depressed patients between rate of time to remission and intrinsic religiosity but not in church attendance or private religious activities (Koenig et al., 1998). We have reviewed studies indicating that, for example, loneliness increases the mortality rate in patients with heart disease or that social support increases survival time of women with breast cancer. So, is going to church just a positive source of socializing with associated health effects? Yes, I think this is fully possible. But what is truly exciting and needs to be more fully researched are those intrinsically religious individuals. What are they doing and what lessons do they have for the rest of us?

There is a body of literature that deals with the specific health advantages that are associated with spending time in meditation or prayer. A number of studies, for instance, have looked at the health-related benefits of practicing transcendental meditation (TM). TM is a meditative practice that is done twice a day for 20 minutes and has been shown to calm the mind, as evidenced by increased alpha-wave activity on EEG. There are also reports—verified by lower lipid peroxide levels—that practice of TM decreases blood pressure, improves hemodynamic functioning, and reduces free radical activity (Barnes et al., 1999; Schneider et al., 1998). It is now well known that a number of psychological and psychosocial interventions can affect immune function and the course of a disease (see Simonton and Sherman, 1998, and Spiegel et al., 1998, for reviews.)

Moreover, there are now a handful of studies that cover the issue of religion or spirituality and immune function (Koenig, 2000). The first of these studies, which examined the relationship between frequency of religious service attendance and plasma interleukin-6 (IL-6) levels in 1718 elderly adults, was performed by Harold Koenig. Koenig found that individuals who attended religious services were 42% (when controlled for other health variables) less likely to have high IL-6 levels (high is defined as >5 pg/mL) than those who did not attend (Koenig et al., 1997). High IL-6 has been correlated to cancer, heart disease, arthritis, and other conditions. IL-6 is also a classic marker of emotional and physical stress. This is only speculative, but perhaps the lack of a religious or spiritual belief system increases one's stress level and thus correlates to increased disease, as we discussed in Chapter 3.

Numerous studies have investigated the efficacy of prayer in ameliorating disease in other people. This type of prayer is called *intercessory prayer*, which means praying for others' well-being by asking God's help in the patient's recovery. Dr. Daniel J. Benor has compiled one of the more extensive reviews of the literature on intercessory prayer in his book, *Healing Research*, which covers over 150 studies on healing (some of which were first published in *Complementary Medical Research*). Subjects of healing included everything from live plants and yeast in a test tube to humans with a variety of diseases. Benor found that more than half of the experiments resulted in positive effects (Benor, 1992). John Astin, while at the University of Maryland School of Medicine, performed a meta-analysis of 23 trials involving 2774 patients. He has concluded that while the methodology in many of the studies is poor, the fact that 57% of the trials showed a positive treatment response warrants further research on the topic (Abbot et al., 2001; Astin et al., 2000; Helm et al., 2000; Mackenzie et al., 2000; Meisenhelder and Chandler, 2000; Wiesendanger et al., 2001).

The study that introduced the subject of intercessory prayer to physicians in this country was conducted by a cardiologist, Randolph Byrd, and was published in the *Southern Medical Journal* (Byrd, 1998). Dr. Byrd carried out a well-designed, randomized, double-blind trial that caused many physicians some serious intellectual challenges, to say the least. The results unequivocally showed the benefits of intercessory prayer in the recovery of cardiac patients, and it was not possible to reasonably criticize the study on methodological grounds. Briefly, Byrd randomly assigned 393 patients from the cardiac care unit of a hospital in San Francisco to either a Protestant or Catholic Christian with a history of active devotional life who would regularly pray for the patients or to a control group that was not appointed to pray for the patients. Neither patients nor staff knew to which group the patient was assigned. Patients who had received prayer had statistically fewer complications during the course of their hospital stay. A second, similar study involving 990 cardiac patients was published in *Archives of Internal Medicine* in 1999 (Harris, 1999). Both studies showed that while intercessory prayer did not shorten length of hospital stay, it did significantly decrease the course-of-treatment scores. Patients receiving prayers had fewer complications such as pneumonia, cardiopulmonary arrest, or congestive heart failure. What is remarkable in the 1999 study is that consent forms were avoided, and patients in the study had no knowledge of being participants. In other words, the intercessory prayer was effective, even when the patient was unaware of its occurrence.

Two factors are not controlled for in either of these well-designed studies. The first is that the researchers did not know whether any of the subjects or the controls were already being prayed for by others outside of the study. Perhaps, some of the subjects were getting double doses of prayer or, perhaps, a control subject had a church whose members were keeping constant vigil. Trying to control for how many people are praying for a given patient, however, would never pass an ethics committee. The second factor is who is doing the praying. I believe that Therapeutic Touch, healing, or intercessory prayer are all acquired skills, which, like any skill, can be improved with training and use. It also is possible that some of us are born with a predisposition to these skills (as is true for many vocational or avocational choices in life), but I am convinced that we all harbor the potential. I believe that prayers are good not only for those for whom we pray, but are also good for those who do the praying. Furthermore, I have often wondered what might be the result of a study in which the friends and relatives of a sick person (e.g., a cardiac patient) agreed to spend just 10 minutes a day thinking loving thoughts about that individual—not praying, just thinking loving thoughts. Could this also influence recovery parameters? I think so. While research seems to indicate that some people might be better conduits of healing energy than others, this theory treads on unknown ground. Oral tradition, literature, and perhaps an experience that has somehow touched your own life give testimony to powerful incidences of spontaneous healing and the efficacy of prayer, even from those who do not consider themselves religious.

Russell Targ, physicist and cofounder of Stanford Research Institute (SRI) at Stanford University, reviewed several of the studies mentioned here plus a study that he performed with Fred Sicher. To fully appreciate this study, it is important to understand the distinction between intercessory prayer and distant healing. Distant healing means that someone who is physically remote from the patient is projecting healing energy to that person. The Sicher–Targ study was a double-blind, randomized trial of patients with AIDS who were being treated with triple-drug therapy. Subjects were assigned either to receive 10 weeks of distant healing or to a control group. After 6 months, a blind review of medical charts showed significantly fewer AIDS-related illnesses and fewer hospitalizations in the group that received the distant healing (Sicher et al., 1998). Targ points out that their study took one-tenth the number of patients to achieve statistical significance as compared with the other major studies that had been performed. He attributed the positive results of the study to the fact that the study used only individuals with 5 years or more of healing experience (Targ and Tatra, 2001). Apparently, well-intentioned people without skill and training in distant healing may not be capable of producing the same effect.

The most frequently cited study that is critical of the research on intercessory prayer and distant healing was performed by Sloan and colleagues at Columbia University (Sloan et al., 1999). They cite issues such as not controlling for confounding variables, covariates, and multiple comparisons as typically occurring in research on intercessory prayer and distant healing. Sloan also is critical of the prayer research because it has uncovered conflicting findings, such as the fact that church attendance and lower mortality are predominantly associated with women, not men. I do not see this as a flaw in research findings, but rather an interesting fact. Could this be related to the intrinsic/extrinsic practice of religion of which Levin writes? Or, could it maybe be that women are more effectively hardwired for spiritual experiences?

Sloan, however, makes good points in addressing the need to clearly define what is meant by religious or spiritual activity if we are to subject these topics to conventional research. His concerns about the ethics of discussing issues of spirituality with a patient and not imposing one's own beliefs are valid, but this should not be interpreted as permission to deny patients access to such involvement in their healthcare. Certainly, the rule of thumb should be that the patient's spiritual orientation is respected above all else. It is imperative that the physician or healthcare professional honor the patient's wishes, even in determining whether to enter into or avoid a discussion of spirituality or religion. Sensitivity to the patient's needs and desires is paramount in any discussion of this nature.

If the patient chooses to enter into dialogue, the physician can facilitate the patient's effort to clarify issues and provide a forum in which to verbalize the deep emotions that arise during serious illness. The physician needs to appreciate the sacred ground upon which this discussion is held and to have respect for the patient's viewpoints. The most important words to remember in this type of discussion are *sensitivity*, *respect*, and *appropriateness*. Over the years, I have found this type of discussion to be immensely rewarding for both the patient and myself. However, it requires a completely different set of skills from the patient interviewing process that I was taught in medical school. Harvard Medical School, as well as numerous other medical schools, now offers courses on how to discuss topics of spirituality and religion with patients. The George Washington University Medical School has formed The George Washington Institute for Spirituality and Health with the objective of fostering research on health and spirituality as well as developing programs that address spirituality in both medical education and clinical care.

Sloan, himself, cites a 1996 poll of 1000 adults in the United States showing that 79% of the respondents feel that spiritual faith can help people recover from disease. So, if you are a doctor who is uncomfortable in talking about such matters, could you be harming your patient's recovery by not allowing that person at least to feel permitted to discuss his or her spirituality? It is a difficult question, but one for all physicians to consider. It is my opinion that even as we pursue the science of healing, we must continue to practice the art of healing. While methodological problems will persist as we determine how best to explore this new area for medical application, the answers will be forthcoming by incorporating spirituality into practice, not by keeping it out. There is no doubt in my mind that if physicians are capable of being an emotionally, if not spiritually, caring presence, our patients will fare better no matter what the physical outcome may be. When we present ourselves to our patients as intellectual technicians, there is little room for a truly healing relationship.

So, let us go out on a limb a bit here and ask, "What are the possible mechanisms of action for intercessory prayer, spiritual healing, or distant healing?" It has been proposed that such healing may occur as a result of activating a healing bioenergy, a subtle energy as we have called it. In this paradigm, spiritual healing occurs because the healer is capable of taking energy from the subtle energy realm, using her or his body as a conduit, and then emitting the subtle energy to the ill person, literally giving it to that person. If the ill person is open to receiving it, she or he may benefit physically, emotionally, and spiritually. It is a type of entrainment of subtle energy to a resonance that the patient can access and use to her or his benefit. One can also focus the same kind of healing energy on oneself.

Is there any evidence for such a hypothesis? Yes, actually there is a fair amount. First, there is a principle in physics called *nonlocality* that was proposed by physicist Dr. David Bohm, who felt that there was an error with quantum physics. He believed that particles at the subquantum level, as we know them, ceased to be separated from one another. Therefore, theoretically, a connection between two seemingly separated entities is maintained. In 1964, a physicist, Dr. John Stewart Bell, mathematically proved Bohm's hypothesis, which has come to be known as Bell's theorem. However, the technology was not available to conclusively prove the theorem until 1982, when French physicists at the Institute of Optics at the University of Paris developed the technology and succeeded in proving the theorem (Talbot, 1991). Bell figured out that if two particles that have interacted are sent in different directions (imagine, for instance, a particle of light), they maintain a connection to each other such that what happens to one particle affects the other one, no matter how far apart. So, essentially, our view that objects are separated by space and time is a human experience, perhaps a human illusion, but certainly not an ultimate reality. Why does Western medicine never take this fact into account? Dr. Jeff Levin, who notes medicine's envy of physics, states it well: "While nonlocality is fast becoming old news to a generation of physicists, biomedical science has not yet caught on....The fact is that allopathic medicine is not even being true to its own envy; the physics to which it clings has been out dated for most of the twentieth century" (Levin, 2001).

Dr. Larry Dossey writes about three eras in Western medicine. According to Dossey, the first is the era of "materialistic medicine," and the second is the era of mind–body medicine ushered in by research on psychoneuroimmunology (PNI). The third era, Dossey says, is "nonlocal" and holds "that the mind is not confined to points in space and time." He states that in the third era, "minds are viewed as spread through space and time...and that human consciousness is unbounded—and if unbounded then some aspect of the human psyche must be unified" (Dossey, 1993). So, between current knowledge in physics and Dossey's vision of a third era in medicine, the theoretical groundwork has been laid to acknowledge the existence of prayerful energy that could "travel" from one person to another. In fact, what physics perhaps is telling us is that it does not have to go anywhere; it just has to be effectively directed. Several researchers have scientifically investigated healing phenomena.

Elmer Green (yes, the same father of biofeedback) and his wife, Alyce, have performed some fascinating research on intuitives and distant healers at the Menninger Clinic in Topeka, Kansas, where he directed the psychophysiology laboratory. The Greens used an apparatus developed for biofeedback of the theta state and trained themselves and others to remain in the theta state without falling asleep.

They learned that hypnogogic insights occur in this state, and it appears that it may be the mind state in which information beyond the knowledge of five senses is acquired. In their book, *Beyond Biofeedback*, the Greens recount numerous stories of people who have intuitive abilities and extraordinary capacities to control body regulation (Green and Green, 1977). Elmer Green also worked with well-known healer Mietek Wirkus. In a copper-walled room, designed to avoid electrical or magnetic influences, electrical emissions were measured from Wirkus as he performed distant healing. Electrical surges as high as 80 volts were emitted from Wirkus as he healed. Wirkus says that he is aware of emitting a charge, which corresponds to these recorded peaks.

Dr. William Tiller of the Department of Material Science and Engineering at Stanford University and a preeminent scientist on the structure of matter has done work similar to Green's. The following is his description of what happens when a healer is healing (Tiller, 1994).

> [W]hen a healer emits pulses of subtle energy (not directly observable because they function at levels beyond space-time), a pulse of magnetic vector potential appears at the periphery of this 4-space via interaction between subtle level substance and physical level substance. This magnetic vector potential pulse, in turn, creates an electrical field in the body in the vicinity of the pulse which acts on the electrodes of the tissue fluids to cause electrical charge separation and thus electrical dipole formation. This electrical dipole inside the body of the healer manifests outside the body as a large electrical voltage pulse at an electrode connected to the ear. The body voltage represents a substantial energy effect triggered by the conscious intent of the healer acting through organized subtle/physical body mechanisms.

Tiller writes scientifically, but what he has to say speaks to the theoretical workings of prayer and a transfer of energy. In the quotation above, he reports on a scientific experiment that he has performed, showing the very specific exchange of electrical current that occurs as the healer performs his or her work. In this same article, Tiller also says that he thinks that as spirit increases in dense matter (i.e., as we allow ourselves the experience of the spiritual or subtle energy), so does consciousness. So, as we permit spiritual experiences to be more a part of our lives, our bodies (dense matter) are infused with more consciousness. Tiller believes that with implied intentionality, or what others call "will," "focused attention," or "awareness," we can open our hearts to allow "spirit substance to enter the body." Consciousness comes in through opening the heart and is important because it activates the imprinting of patterns on both our emotions and on the etheric or spiritual energy surrounding our bodies. The pattern of emotion can allow the etheric or spiritual to enter and affect the physical body, activating hormones, neurons, and more. As Tiller explains, "*Consciousness* initiated the process but various levels of *energy/matter* stuff cooperated to materialize the effect" (Tiller, 1994). So, as our bodies undergo what Tiller calls "structural refinement," we are capable of effectively sending healing energy as well as receiving it to our benefit.

Another piece of research that supports the idea that prayer is a transference of energy is Russell Targ's work at SRI. For years, the CIA funded Targ and his colleagues to perform secret research to learn how information is acquired psychically (also called *remote viewing*) and then to use psychics to obtain information about the Soviet Union. I know this must sound like a Tom Clancy novel, but it was in 1972, at the height of the Cold War, and it truly is factual. Targ has conducted numerous experiments that confirm, far beyond chance, the existence of psychically procured information. Targ's work showed that people are capable of learning rather quickly how to do remote viewing and then, with practice, learn to distinguish between what he calls the psychic signal and other mental information, such as memory or imagination (Targ and Katra, 2001).

Targ admits that the physics behind what permits intuitive acquisition of knowledge is not yet understood, but what is clear from all the research is that time, in this realm of acquiring information, does not correspond to our sense of time. An intuitive can just as easily describe something in the near future as in the present. Targ notes that the Eastern philosophers have, for thousands of years, said that human perception of separation, or what could be called *singularity*, is an illusion. In an interesting paper, Dr. Edward Garbacz has laid out a theoretica, but sound, comparison between the main facets of Taoist philosophy and modern physics. While his descriptions of Taoism are stronger than those of physics, he makes some interesting comparisons. Garbacz describes of the Yin–Yang aspect of Taoism as "the qualitative representation of polarity, or the relationship of opposite but related constituents...the immutable duality, mutuality, and balance between events, actions, and individuals; indeed, within or between any and all phenomena" (Garbacz and Marshall, 2001). All of this certainly sounds consistent with Bell's theorem to me. We will discuss this topic in more detail in the final chapter.

I sometimes work with Lesley Carmack, who is an intuitive practitioner. One patient of mine, Sam, who is a 30-year-old successful architect, came to my office with a fever and elevated white blood cell count. A standard digital rectal examination indicated severe prostatitis. Lesley, with no more than the patient's name, told me that there were hot spots not only in his pelvis but in his neck as well. I had seen no evidence of a throat or thyroid problem. Trusting her, I ordered a blood thyroid hormone level, which came back quite elevated—a finding consistent with hyperthyroidism. Further examination revealed that Sam had a rare form of thyroiditis called *Savoie's syndrome*, also called *silent thyroiditis* because of its lack of presentation of thyroid tenderness. If it were not for Lesley's intuitive reading, I never would have investigated for a thyroid disorder or have been able to assist Sam in such a comprehensive manner. Since that time, I have had the opportunity to share numerous, complex cases with Lesley. The information that Lesley has given to me has greatly enhanced my ability to treat these patients. I do not pretend to understand the physiological mechanisms underlying Lesley's intuitive observations, but I have come to fully believe in her ability to make accurate observations—repeatedly.

Stories like these may make us uncomfortable, and we try to dismiss them as simply not scientifically possible or as anecdotal. Remember that, according to Levin, 86% of us experience these "anecdotal" events. Such experiences, however, can require living with a profound duality, a foot in two worlds. Oddly, it requires a solid groundedness in this realm of linear time and separation of objects to effectively operate in the world outside of singularity and time and then to "come back" again. In indigenous cultures, I believe that it was the shaman who held this duality for the whole community. He or she was the one who could move gracefully between the two worlds and bring understanding of the spiritual world back to the community. Experiences of subtle energy can be frightening to some people, as if they are experiencing a little piece of death from which they might not come back. Perhaps, it is also frightening because our culture views people who have these experiences as being a little addled. Yet, the majority of intrinsically religious persons appear to have a higher level of emotional and mental stability (Levin, 2001). The issues are made more complex by the fact that so little research has been done to understand what happens as people enter healing or intuitive states. In this country, such phenomena are spoken of dubiously or woven into ghost stories by children at slumber parties. It is my contention that it is far more valuable to support research in this area than to reject the phenomenon outright—the need to reject perhaps originating from the discomfort within us. The art of medicine is still a mystery. Those in the medical field need to embrace empiric observations even if, as yet, there is no scientific context in which to hold them. Today's mystery may be tomorrow's science. So for today, we must simply embrace the mystery.

In the last chapter of his book, *God, Faith, and Health*, Jeff Levin concludes: "According to the scientific evidence presented in this book, th[e] new era of medicine is no longer hypothetical. Research findings suggest that we are on the verge of a medical revolution....The emerging medical model postulates that body, mind, and something beyond mind—call it 'spirit'—work together to promote health, prevent illness, and produce healing" (Levin, 2001). These words are an excellent segue to a more detailed discussion of subtle energy in Chapter 8. Ultimately, I think you will see that we are spiritual beings having a human experience, and not predominantly human beings occasionally having spiritual experiences.

The most beautiful thing we can experience is the mysterious. It is the source of all true art and science. He to whom this emotion is a stranger, who can no longer pause to wonder and stand rapt in awe, is as good as dead: his eyes are closed. This insight into the mystery of life, coupled though it be with fear, has also given rise to religion. To know that what is impenetrable to us really exists, manifesting itself as the highest wisdom and the most radiant beauty which our dull faculties can comprehend only in their most primitive forms—this knowledge, this feeling, is at the center of true religiousness. In this sense and in this sense only, I belong to the ranks of devoutly religious men.

Albert Einstein, 1950

REFERENCES

Abbot, N.C., Harkness, E.F., Stevinson, C., Marshall, F.P., Conn, D.A., and Ernst, E., Spiritual healing as a therapy for chronic pain: a randomized, clinical trial, *Pain*, 91 (1–2), 79–89, 2001.

Ai, A.L. et al., Designing clinical trials on energy healing: ancient art encounters medical science, *Alternative Ther. Health Med.*, 7 (4), 83–90, 2001.

Alegria, D., Guerra, E., Martinez, Jr., C., and Meyer, G.G., El hospital invisible: a study of Curanderismo, *Arch. Gen. Psychiatry*, 34 (11), 1354–1357, 1977.

Astin, J.A., Harkness, E., and Ernst, E., The efficacy of "distant healing": a systematic review of randomized trials, *Ann. Intern. Med.*, 132 (11), 903–910, 2000.

Barnes, V.A., Treiber, F.A., Turner, J.R., Davis, H., and Strong, W.B., Acute effects of transcendental meditation on hemodynamic functioning in middle-aged adults, *Psychosomatic Res.*, 61 (4), 525–531, 1999.

Benford, M.S., Talnagi, J., Doss, D.B., Boosey, S., and Arnold, L.E., Gamma radiation fluctuations during alternative healing therapy, *Alternative Ther. Health Med.*, 5 (4), 51–56, 1999.

Benor, D.J., *Healing Research: Holistic Energy Medicine and Spirituality*, Vol. 1, *Research in Healing*, Helix, Munich, 1992.

Benveniste, J., Lecture delivered at 11th International Congress on Stress, HI, 2000.

Berrebi, A. et al., Treatment of pain due to unwanted lactation with a homeopathic preparation given in the immediate post-partum period, *J. Gynecologie, Obstetrique Biologie reproduction*, 30 (4), 353–357, 2001.

Byrd, R.C., Positive therapeutic effects of intercessory prayer in a coronary care unit population, *South. Medical J.*, 81 (7), 826–829, 1998.

Callahan, R.J., *Five Minute Phobia Cure*, Enterprise, Wilmington, DE, 1985.

Callahan, R.J., A Thought Field Therapy (TFT) Algorithm for Trauma: a Reproducible Experiment in Psychology, paper presented at Annual Meeting of the American Psychological Association, New York, 1995.

Davenas, E. et al., Human basophil degranulation triggered by very dilute antiserum against IgE, *Nature*, 333 (6176), 816–818, 1988.

Dossey, L., *Healing Words*, HarperCollins, San Francisco, 1993.

Eckes Peck, S.D., The effectiveness of therapeutic touch for decreasing pain in elders with degenerative arthritis, *J. Holistic Nursing: Off. J. Am. Holistic Nurses Assoc.*, 15 (2), 176–198, 1997.

Francomano, C.A. and Jonas, W.B., *Proceedings: Measuring the Human Energy Field: State of the Science*, Chez, R.A., Ed., Samueli Institute, Corona Del Mar, CA, 2003.

Gallo, F.P., *Energy Psychology*, CRC Press, Boca Raton, FL, 1999.

Garbacz, E.S. and Marshall, S.C., Classical Chinese medicine: the science of biological forces, *Medical Acupuncture*, 12 (2), 21–28, 2000/2001.

Giasson, M. and Bouchard, L., Effect of therapeutic touch on the well-being of persons with terminal cancer, *J. Holistic Nursing: Off. J. Am. Holistic Nurses Assoc.*, 16 (3), 383–398, 1998.

Gray, B., *Homeopathy: Science or Myth?* North Atlantic Books, Berkeley, CA, 2000.

Green, E. and Green, A., *Beyond Biofeedback*, Delta, New York, 1977.

Harding, S., Curanderas in the Americas, *Alternative Complementary Theories*, Oct., 309–316, 1999.

Harris, W.S. et al., A randomized controlled trial of the effects of remote, intercessory prayer on outcomes in patients admitted to the coronary care unit, *Arch. Intern. Med.*, 159 (19), 2273–2278, 1999; published erratum, *Arch. Intern. Med.*, 160 (12), 1878, 2000.

Heidt, P.R., Openness: a qualitative analysis of nurses' and patients' experiences of therapeutic touch, *Image: J. Nursing Scholarship*, 22 (3), 180–186, 1990.

Helm, H.M., Hays, J.C., Flint, E.P., Koenig, H.G., and Blazer, D.G., Does private religious activity prolong survival? A six-year follow-up study of 3,851 older adults, *J. Gerontol. Ser. A, Biological Sci. Medical Sci.*, 55 (7), M400–M405, 2000.

Herdtner, S., Using therapeutic touch in nursing practice, *Orthopedic Nursing/Natl. Assoc. Orthopedic Nurses*, 19 (5), 77–82, 2000.

Hirazumi, A. and Furusawa, E., An immunomodulatory polysaccharide-rich substance from the fruit juice of *Morinda citrifolia* (noni) with antitumour activity, *Phytother. Res.: PTR*, 13 (5), 380–387, 1999.

Horowitz, S., Traditional Hawaiian healing arts enrich conventional medical practices, *Alternative Complementary Therapies*, 7 (2), 68–73, 2001.

Jacobs, J., Springer, D.A., and Crothers, D., Homeopathic treatment of acute otitis media in children: a preliminary randomized placebo-controlled trial, *Pediatric Infect. Dis. J.*, 20 (2), 177–183, 2001.

Jahnke, R., *The Healer within: the Four Essential Self-Care Methods for Creating Optimal Health*, HarperCollins, San Francisco, 1997.

Koenig, H.G., Psychoneuroimmunology and the faith factor, *J. Gender-Specific Med.*, 3 (5), 37–44, 2000.

Koenig, H.G., Cohen, H.J., George, L.K., Hays, J.C., Larson, D.B., and Blazer, D.G., Attendance at religious services, interleukin-6, and other biological parameters of immune function in older adults, *Int. J. Psychiatry Med.*, 27 (3), 233–250, 1997.

Koenig, H.G., George, L.K., and Peterson, B.L., Religiosity and remission of depression in medically ill older patients, *Am. J. Psychiatry*, 155 (4), 536–542, 1998.

Korotkov, K.G., *Human Energy Field: Study with GDV Bioelectrography*, St. Petersburg Technical University, St. Petersburg, Russia, 2001.

Korotkov, K.G., *Human Energy Field: Study with GDV Bioelectrography*, Backbone Publishing, Fairlawn, NJ, 2002.

Kramer, N.A., Comparison of therapeutic touch and casual touch in stress reduction of hospitalized children, *Pediatric Nursing*, 16 (5), 483–485, 1990.

Krauss, B.H., *Native Plants Used as Medicine in Hawaii*, 2nd ed., University of Hawaii at Manoa, Honolulu, 1981.

Kreisman, J.J., The curandero's apprentice: a therapeutic integration of folk and medical healing, *Am. J. Psychiatry*, 132 (1), 81–83, 1975.

Krieger, D., Therapeutic touch: the imprimatur of nursing, *Am. J. Nursing*, 75 (5), 784–787, 1975.

Krieger, D., Alternative medicine: therapeutic touch, *Nursing Times*, 72 (15), 572–574, 1976.

Krieger, D., *The Therapeutic Touch: How to Use Your Hands to Help or to Heal*, Simon and Schuster, New York, 1979.

Lafreniere, K.D. et al., Effects of therapeutic touch on biochemical and mood indicators in women, *J. Alternative Complementary Med.*, 5 (4), 367–370, 1999.

Larson, D., The role of connective tissue as the physical medium for the conduction of healing energy in acupuncture and Rolfing, *Am. J. Acupuncture*, 18 (3), 251–266, 1990.

Lee, R.H., *Scientific Investigations into Chinese Qigong*, China Healthways Institute, San Clemente, CA, 1999.

Lei, X.F., Bi, A.H., Zhang, Z.X., and Cheng, Z.Y., The antitumor effects of qigong-emitted external Qi and its influence on the immunologic functions of tumor-bearing mice, *J. Tongji Medical Univ.*, 11 (4), 253–256, 1991.

Levin, J., *God, Faith, and Health: Exploring the Spirituality–Health Connection*, John Wiley & Sons, New York, 2001.

Linde, K. and Jobst, K.A., Homeopathy for chronic asthma, *Cochrane Database Systematic Rev. (Online Update Software)*, (2), CD000353, 2000.

Linde, K., Jonas, W.B., Melchart, D., and Willich, S., The methodological quality of randomized controlled trials of homeopathy, herbal medicines and acupuncture, *Int. J. Epidemiol.*, 30 (3), 526–531, 2001.

Litscher, G., Wenzel, G., Niederwieser, G., and Schwarz, G., Effects of QiGong on brain function, *Neurological Res.*, 23 (5), 501–505, 2001.

Liu, G., Bode, A., Ma, W.Y., Sang, S., Ho, C.T., and Dong, Z., Two novel glycosides from the fruits of *Morinda citrifolia* (noni) inhibit AP-1 transactivation and cell transformation in the mouse epidermal JB6 cell line, *Cancer Res.*, 61 (15), 5749–5756, 2001.

Mackenzie, E.R., Rajagopal, D.E., Meibohm, M., and Lavizzo-Mourey, R., Spiritual support and psychological well-being: older adults' perceptions of the religion and health connection, *Alternative Therapies*, 6 (6), 37–45, 2000.

Meisenhelder, J.B. and Chandler, E.N., Prayer and health outcomes in church members, *Alternative Therapies*, 6 (4), 56–60, 2000.

Newberg, A., D'Aquili, E., and Rause, V., *Why God Won't Go Away: Brain Science and the Biology of Belief*, Ballantine Publishing Group, New York, 2001.

NIH consensus statement, *Acupuncture*, 15 (5), 1–34, 1997.

Olson, K. and Hanson, J., Using Reiki to manage pain: a preliminary report, *Cancer Prev. Control*, 1 (2), 108–113, 1997.

Padilla, R., Gomez, V., Biggerstaff, S.L., and Mehler, P.S., Use of curanderismo in a public healthcare system, *Arch. Intern. Med.*, 161 (10), 1336–1340, 2001.

Papp, R. et al., Oscillococcinum® in patients with influenza-like syndromes: a placebo-controlled double-blind evaluation, *Br. Homeopathic J.*, 87 (2), 69–76, 1998.

Poitevin, B., Davenas, E., and Benveniste, J., *In vitro* immunological degranulation of human basophils is modulated by lung histamine and *Apis mellifica*, *Br. J. Clinical Pharmacol.*, 25 (4), 439–444, 1988.

Quinn, J.F., Therapeutic touch as energy exchange: replication and extension, *Nursing Sci. Q.*, 2 (2), 79–87, 1989.

Quinn, J.F. and Strelkauskas, A.J., Psychoimmunologic effects of therapeutic touch on practitioners and recently bereaved recipients: a pilot study, *ANS, Adv. Nursing Sci.*, 15 (4), 13–26, 1993.

Ramelet, A.A., Buchheim, G., Lorenz, P., and Imfeld, M., Homeopathic *Arnica* in postoperative haematomas: a double-blind study, *Dermatology*, 201 (4), 347–348, 2000.

Reilly, D.T., Taylor, M.A., McSharry, C., and Aitchison, T., Is homoeopathy a placebo response? Controlled trial of homoeopathic potency, with pollen in hayfever as model, *Lancet*, 2 (8512), 881–886, 1986.

Riley, D., Fischer, M., Singh, B., Haidvogl, M., and Heger, M., Homeopathy and conventional medicine: an outcomes study comparing effectiveness in a primary care setting, *J. Alternative Complementary Med.*, 7 (2), 149–159, 2001.

Rosa, L., Rosa, E., Sarner, L., and Barrett, S., A close look at therapeutic touch, *J. Am. Medical Assoc.*, 279 (13), 1005–1010, 1998.

Rosch, P.J., Stress and subtle energy medicine, *Stress Med.*, 10 (1–3), 1–3, 1994.

Rubik, B., Energy medicine and the unifying concept of information, *Alternative Therapies*, 1 (1), 34–39, 1995.

Sancier, K.M., Therapeutic benefits of qigong exercises in combination with drugs, *J. Alternative Complementary Med.*, 5 (4), 383–389, 1999.

Schneider, R.H. et al., Lower lipid peroxide levels in practitioners of the Transcendental Meditation program, *Psychosomatic Med.*, 60 (1), 38–41, 1998.

Sicher, F., Targ, E., Moore, D., and Smith, H.S., A randomized double-blind study of the effect of distant healing in a population with advanced AIDS; report of a small scale study, *West. J. Med.*, 169 (6), 356–363, 1998.

Simonton, S.S. and Sherman, A.C., Psychological aspects of mind-body medicine: promises and pitfalls from research with cancer patients, *Altern. Therapies*, 4 (4), 50–67, 1998.

Sloan, R.P., Bagiella, E., and Powell, T., Religion, spirituality and medicine, *Lancet*, 353 (9153), 664–667, 1999.

Spiegel, D., Sephton, S.E., Terr, A.I., and Stites, D.P., Effects of psychosocial treatment in prolonging cancer survival may be mediated by neuroimmune pathways, in *Annals of the New York Academy of Sciences*, Vol. 840, McCann, S.M., Sternberg, E.M., Lipton, J.M., Chrousos, G.P., Gold, P.W., and Smith, C.C., Eds., New York Academy of Sciences, New York, 1998, pp. 674–683.

Talbot, M., *The Holographic Universe*, HarperCollins, New York, 1991.

Targ, R. and Katra, J., The scientific and spiritual implications of psychic abilities, *Alternative Therapies*, 7 (3), 143–149, 2001.

Tiller, W., But is it energy? Reflections on consciousness, healing and the new paradigm. Commentary on: healing, energy and consciousness: into the future or a retreat to the past? *Subtle Energies*, 5 (3), 253–258, 1994.

Trotter, R.T., Curanderisimo, in *Fundamentals of Complementary and Alternative Medicine*, 2nd ed., Micozzi, M.S., Ed., Churchill Livingston, New York, 2001.

Vickers, A.J., Clinical trials of homeopathy and placebo: analysis of a scientific debate, *J. Alternative Complementary Med.*, 6 (1), 49–56, 2000.

Vickers, A.J., van Haselen, R., and Heger, M., Can homeopathically prepared mercury cause symptoms in healthy volunteers? A randomized, double-blind placebo-controlled trial, *J. Altern. Complement. Med.*, 7 (2), 141–148, 2001.

Walach, H., Koster, H., Hennig, T., and Haag, G., The effects of homeopathic belladonna 30CH in healthy volunteers: a randomized, double-blind experiment, *J. Psychosomatic Res.*, 50 (3), 155–156, 2001a.

Walach, H. et al., The long-term effects of homeopathic treatment of chronic headaches: one year follow-up and single case time series analysis, *Br. Homeopathic J.*, 90 (2), 63–72, 2001b.

Wang, M. et al., Novel glycosides from noni (*Morinda citrifolia*), *J. Nat. Prod.*, 63 (8), 1182–1183, 2000.

Wardell, D.W. and Engebretson, J., Biological correlates of Reiki Touch[SM] healing, *J. Advanced Nursing*, 33 (4), 439–445, 2001.

Wiesendanger, H., Werthmuller, L., Reuter, K., and Walach, H., Chronically ill patients treated by spiritual healing improve in quality of life: results of a randomized waiting-list controlled study, *J. Altern.e Complement. Med.*, 7 (1), 45–54, 2001.

Wirth, D.P., The effect of non-contact therapeutic touch on the healing rate of full thickness dermal wounds, *Subtle Energies*, 1 (1), 1–20, 1992.

Wu, W.H. et al., Effects of qigong on late-stage complex regional pain syndrome, *Altern. Therapies Health Med.*, 5 (1), 45–54, 1999.

Yardley, L.K., *The Heart of Huna*, Advanced Neuro Dynamics, Honolulu, 1990.

ADDITIONAL RESOURCES

Benson, H. and Stark, M., *Timeless Healing: the Power and Biology of Belief*, Scribner, New York, 1996.

Dossey, L., Whatever happened to healers? *Alternative Therapies Health Med.*, 1 (5), 6–13, 1995.

Gerber, R., *Vibrational Medicine: New Choices for Healing Ourselves*, Bear and Co., Santa Fe, NM, 1988.

Eden, J., *Energetic Healing: the Merging of Ancient and Modern Medical Practices*, Plenum Press, New York, 1993.

Koenig, H.G., *The Healing Power of Faith: Science Explores Medicine's Last Great Frontier*, Simon & Schuster, New York, 1999.

Matthews, D.A. and Clark, C., *The Faith Factor: Proof of the Healing Power of Prayer*, Viking Penguin, New York, 1998.

Schlitz, M. and Braud, W., Distant intentionality and healing: assessing the evidence, *Alternative Therapies Health Med.*, 3 (6), 62–73, 1997.

Targ, E., Evaluating distant healing: a research review, *Alternative Therapies Health Med.*, 3 (6), 74–78, 1997.

Wallace, R.K., Physiological effects of transcendental meditation, *Science*, 167 (926), 1751–1754, 1970.

8 Soul Medicine: Crossing the Border

CONTENTS

WE ARE ENERGY

In the course of writing this book, the authors discussed the fact that, from a very young age, we both remember asking the question: "Who is God?" We really wanted to know; however, we found the answers to be wholly unsatisfying. We came from different types of Western religious traditions, but in both cases, the information did not satisfy our analytical minds. We wanted to know *what* God is. What is that energy that ends at death; what is that energy that allows for spontaneous healing; and what is that energy that is referred to as our "higher self"? When the Eastern and Western mystics claim to be "one with all beings," or "one with God," or "one with the universe," what is happening in their bodies and minds? Is there a physiology of spirituality?

Chapter 2 provided an overview of psychoneuroimmunology (PNI) and the interactions of body systems previously thought to be pristinely separate, demonstrating that the field of medicine can no longer refute the inextricable integration of the mind and the body. In Chapter 4, compelling indications of a relaxation system and distinct features of its hormonal cascade were proposed. Now we must ask whether there is enough medical evidence to begin to speculate about the physiological events that occur during experiences that transcend, yet inform, the five senses. These experiences, which traditionally have been relegated to mystics and spirituality, are currently finding their way into medical research and are typically referred to as *subtle energy medicine*.

Subtle energy is the final component to the paradigm of *integral physiology*—a system of medicine that incorporates not only the body and the mind/emotions, but that also addresses the impact of subtle energy on an individual's overall health. In this chapter, we begin by introducing a theoretical construct of subtle energy, and then we present some compelling research that evaluates physiological responses to experiences that traditionally have been called *spiritual* or *transcendent* but are increasingly referred to as *subtle energy*. We have chosen a set of thinkers to explain the subtle-energy component of integral physiology, but we firmly believe that four or five other well-chosen individuals would have allowed us to arrive at the same understanding. We encourage the reader to engage intuitively, not just intellectually, while reading this chapter.

THE SCIENCE OF SUBTLE ENERGY: A THEORY

In his General Theory of Relativity, Einstein gave us the now famous theorem: $E = mc^2$, or energy (E) equals mass (m) times a constant (c), which Einstein designated as the speed of light, squared (c^2). Einstein asserted that the speed of light is an absolute constant that unites time and space in a continuum and, therefore, that time, space, and matter can be compressed or expanded. Einstein demonstrated that time cannot be separated from matter and that all matter is energy.

Energy and mass (i.e., matter) are thought to be different forms of the same basic substance from which all existence is constructed. They are different parts of a spectrum of vibrating molecules. Just as we know that light and electromagnetic energy have a frequency spectrum, similarly all matter has a frequency of oscillation that varies depending upon the density of the matter. The more dense the matter, the slower is the vibration, and theoretically, the more subtle the matter, the higher or faster is the frequency of oscillation (Table 8.1). As energy becomes subtler and the frequency of oscillation increases significantly, the five common senses are no longer able to cognitively experience the "matter." However, this does not mean that such energy does not affect the physical body. In fact, it is our contention that this form of energy informs, but transcends, the five common senses.

TABLE 8.1
Energy Continuum

Slower vibration (matter is more dense) $\longrightarrow$ **Faster vibration** (matter is less dense)

Out of necessity, Einstein also developed a theory of antigravity. In order for the predictions of his relativity theory to be accurate and to match what astronomers thought the universe looked like, there had to be antigravity. Einstein called this the "cosmological term." In the 1920s, when it was discovered that the universe was expanding, Einstein called his antigravity theory "my greatest blunder." Yet, scientists have recently shown that there is antigravity. By measuring the changing brightness of supernovas and their distances from earth, scientists have determined that the forces of antigravity now have exceeded the gravitational forces, causing the expansion of the universe to occur ever more quickly (Lemonick, 2001).

Physicists have generally concurred that matter cannot be moved at a velocity beyond the speed of light. The newly illustrated existence of antigravity reverses this doctrine in principles of physics too complex to include here (see Tiller et al., 2001). Scientist call antigravity, "dark matter" because it is so poorly understood and largely remains a mystery. However, it is known that Einstein's relativity theory accommodates the existence of antigravity and that antigravity is equivalent to nonphysical matter.

The discovery of antigravity dovetails with, and perhaps someday will confirm, the work done by Dr. William Tiller of the Department of Material Science and Engineering at Stanford University, who has postulated a theory of nonphysical matter or subtle energy. His theories are shared here only insofar as they help to convey the subtle-energy component of integral physiology. Tiller's writing incorporates evidence of subtle energy, via various principles of physics, to an extent that is beyond the scope of this book. However, if you are inclined to read further in this area, you might want to acquire his text, *Science and Human Transformation* (Tiller, 1997).

Long ago, Tiller postulated that there are various subtle energies arising from magnetic, monopole substance, having an indiscernible form and traveling at a velocity greater than the speed of light. Furthermore, he determined that subtle energies are part of a continuum of energy. In an analogy of numbers or temperatures that lie above or below zero, subtle energies would be the nonphysical matter that lies below zero. Tiller describes subtle energies as different from those arising from the four accepted fundamental forces (forces commonly known to any physicist) and lacking the features that are accessible to the five common senses. Because subtle energy exists beyond the speed of light, it therefore exists outside of time as we experience it. (Einstein's $E = mc^2$ is used to deduce this.) Our physical world is in the arena of electrical energy, which travels at a velocity slower than or equal to the speed of light (see Table 8.2). Therefore, according to some scientists, matter can be thought of as condensed light.

TABLE 8.2
Properties of Subtle Energy, Physical Energy, and Deltrons

Subtle energy:
magnetic energy traveling at a velocity greater than the speed of light ($v > c$)
Physical energy:
electrical energy traveling at a velocity slower than the speed of light ($v < c$)
Deltrons:
particles capable of interacting between physical and subtle energies ($v = c$)

Tiller asserts that the dividing line between physical and subtle energy is v (velocity) $= c$ (constant), or the point at which velocity reaches the speed of light (Einstein's constant). It would be a hypothetical "zero" point in our analogy of

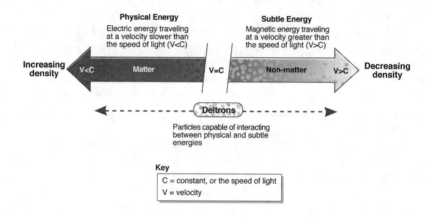

FIGURE 8.1 Deltrons.

numbers on a thermometer. Tiller explains that "because of the light barrier at v = c, the two systems are designed to stay isolated from each other" (Tiller, 1997). He postulates that any communication between the physical and subtle energies occur via special particles "from a higher dimensional domain than space time," which he has named *deltrons* (see Figure 8.1). Deltrons can interact with particles whose velocity is greater or less than the speed of light (v > c or v < c), permitting communication between the physical and the subtle types of substance. It is possible for the "light barrier" to be broken, causing what many people would call a spiritual experience. In other words, it is what occurs when humans experience the realm of subtle energy.

Humans are made up of both relatively dense matter as well as subtle matter. We have an innate ability to tap into subtle energy, which historically has been referred to as a "transcendent experience," "intuition," "our higher self," "God," or just "spirituality." Understanding the concept of subtle energy allows us to step well beyond a mechanistic view of physically repairing the body and allows responsible exploration of new modalities for curing disease. Energy fields literally influence cellular growth. Subtle energy is known to assist healing (e.g., see the studies on prayer or therapeutic touch that we reviewed). When the physical body cannot be healed, spiritual or subtle energy also can assist the individual to reach a state of peace, both emotionally and intellectually. There is a synergistic interplay between our subtle and mundane (i.e., physical) energies, which can work to promote optimum health and expand the types of awareness that can be available to us.

Tiller believes that by focusing our "intentionality" (which, for example, occurs during meditation, deep relaxation, or other transcendent states of awareness), we can encounter the field of subtle energy. It is my feeling that we can create a receptive or hostile atmosphere for subtle energy, depending upon the health of our bodies and the soundness of our minds. Self-judgment, for example, can completely close off the vibrational resonance at which we can experience subtle energy. Emotional soundness supports "returning to" and living in the everyday world after an experience of subtle energy. If we can hold the duality of our physical life and our subtle energy experiences, without needing to dismiss or fear them, we potentially can develop both a keener understanding of life as well as obtain our personal optimum health.

THE INTERFACE OF HUMAN PHYSIOLOGY AND SUBTLE ENERGY

According to Eastern Indian tradition, the body has seven major chakras or energy centers that are conduits for subtle energy. The word *chakra* actually comes from a Sanskrit word meaning *wheel*. Chakras are the openings or pathways by which spiritual or subtle energy is taken into the body and translated into a form of energy that the body can use, literally use, at the cellular level. Just as the pineal gland is the energy transducer for our bodily experience, the chakras are the energy transducers for subtle energy. They convert the subtle energy to a resonance that the body can use, which means that the subtle energy is transduced into hormones and neurotransmitters. Each chakra is correlated to actual physiological structures, such as endocrine glands and major nerve areas, resulting in a complex network of energy that courses through the body. This is the energy that is referred to in Chinese medicine as *Qi* and is loosely translated as "vital energy" or "life force." Chakras, speculatively, open and connect into the autonomic nervous system (ANS), interacting richly with the endocrine system.

Although different belief systems have slight variations, the seven chakras generally are conceptualized as follows (see Figure 8.2):

1. The first chakra, also called the *root chakra*, is located near the coccyx or sacral plexus. It is associated with the kidneys and the adrenal glands.
2. The second chakra is located just below the umbilicus at the pelvic plexus. It is associated with the reproductive system.
3. The third chakra is located in the upper part of the abdomen at the solar plexus. It is associated with the pancreas and the digestive system.
4. The fourth chakra is located in the middle of the sternum, near the heart. It is also called the *heart chakra*. It is associated with the thymus and the circulatory system.
5. The fifth chakra is located in the throat just below the Adam's apple. It is associated with the thyroid and the respiratory system.
6. The sixth chakra is located above the bridge of the nose. As discussed in the chapter on the pineal gland, it is also called the *third eye*. It is associated with the pituitary and the ANS.
7. The seventh chakra is located at the crown of the head. It is associated with the pineal and the central nervous system (CNS).

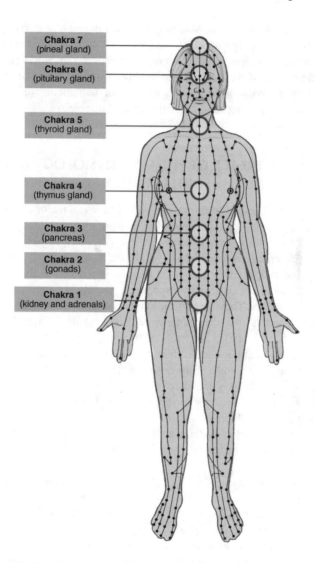

Chakra 7
(pineal gland)

Chakra 6
(pituitary gland)

Chakra 5
(thyroid gland)

Chakra 4
(thymus gland)

Chakra 3
(pancreas)

Chakra 2
(gonads)

Chakra 1
(kidney and adrenals)

FIGURE 8.2 Chakras and acupuncture meridians.

The "principal meridians" are pathways within the body along which Qi flows. They intersect both with the chakras and with acupuncture points. Qi is subtle energy, the invisible but wholesome energy that flows through the meridians, nourishing both the body and the mind.

Speculatively, in Tiller's terms, Qi is the deltron interface, an energy interchange between $v > c$ and $v < c$. It is non-matter; indeed, it is subtle energy interacting with matter. According to the Chinese system of medicine, any blockage in the flow of Qi will result in dysfunction, physical or emotional, to the area of the body that is associated with the part of the body that is blocked.

According to Chinese medicine, there are actually various types of Qi. For example, *wei Qi* is a coarse energy that circulates on the outside of the body and is protective during the awakened state. It is the energetic equivalent of the immune system. It is part of the body's inner clock and circulation of energy. If an emotional or physical trauma occurs, the *wei Qi* surrounds the corresponding organ and reverberates in that area while we sleep. It is my feeling that any trauma is stored in the fascia (connective tissues) and in the limbic system during those sleeping hours. The limbic system encodes the various memories, including repressed memories. Through modalities, such as those described in Chapters 5 and 7, the repressed memories can be released from the fascia as well as from the limbic system. They can be released through bodywork, but the optimal method is through work both on the body and the mind.

Another type of Qi is called *yuan Qi*, which is said to represent the energy we brought with us into this life, including ancestral energy and the energy of the soul. In systems that possess a belief in reincarnation, it represents the essence of who we were, are, and that which we will bring into our next life. *Long Qi* is derived from the food we eat and the air we breathe, that is, from our environmental surroundings. We also take in this type of Qi while we sleep and during sexual orgasm. For certain people, their only interaction with subtle energy will occur from elements taken from the environment, such as dreams. In other words, even without a conscious effort, humans are nurtured by subtle energy. *Yuan Qi* is housed in deeper meridians, called the *extraordinary* or *curious* meridians. When *yuan Qi* flows through the principal meridians, it is an indication that the chakras have opened to allow subtle energy to permeate the body.

As one takes the requisite step of clearing repressed or known emotional issues through work on the body and the mind, a shift occurs by which the principal meridians become infused with *yuan Qi*, a type of subtle energy. This event causes the chakras to open, allowing yet more *yuan Qi* to enter the body and to increase our conscious awareness of experiencing subtle energy, which is manifested as increased mental clarity, heightened creativity, or, perhaps, emotional calmness. It is my contention that the greater the development of personal serenity or equanimity, the greater is the infusion of subtle energy from the curious meridians into the principal meridians. Curiously, there is also a striking correlation between the increased amount of energy attributed to a chakra (as represented in drawings by the number of lotus petals assigned to it, moving from the root or lowest chakra to the crown or highest chakra) and the energetic output of the hormone for the gland designated to that chakra.

IS THERE A PHYSIOLOGY OF SPIRITUALITY?

There is no question in my mind that we can teach ourselves to perceive subtle energy. It is my experience (and apparently that of Tiller as well) that the heart chakra is the site at which humans most easily open to subtle energy, and human feelings of love and compassion are most similar to the vibration of subtle energy. But the spectrum of emotions that we call "love" can include a wide variety of emotions, including less wholesome aspects that are predominantly involved with cravings. These are not vibrations that are conducive to connecting with subtle energy.

For those who are curious or so inclined, a simple exercise may offer you the opportunity to experience subtle energy. Start by bringing your attention to the heart chakra and letting yourself experience sensations of openness, as if your heart is breathing (as in the HeartMath technique; see the modalities section of Chapter 5). Next, let yourself experience deep feelings of appreciation, almost like love but deep appreciation, such as appreciation for the beauty of the magnolia or the trout lily in springtime. Let your heart "breathe" this sense of appreciation. It is possible that you will have an experience of subtle energy of which you are consciously aware.

The Buddha, Jesus, Mohammad, Abraham, Confucius, and other spiritual leaders through the ages have left us with stories about the knowledge they gained during prayer or meditation. These stories, theoretically, are insights gained during their personal encounters with subtle energy and have become the cornerstones of their respective religions. The stories often incorporate a benevolent or loving "God," reflecting the nature of the subtle energy that they had experienced. Stories are used to attempt to express experiences that are not particularly conducive to being verbalized. Analogously, think how difficult it can be to convey the contents of a dream. Their stories are the anthropomorphic expression of the experience of subtle energy via the heart chakra.

RESEARCH SUPPORTING A PHYSIOLOGY OF SPIRITUALITY

In the chapter on relaxation (Chapter 4), biochemical windows that may facilitate experiences of deep relaxation were identified based on current research. Similarly, there are medical studies that begin to identify discrete biochemical and physiological changes that occur when an individual experiences subtle energy, that is when an individual has an experience that transcends, yet informs, the five senses.

BRAIN SCANS OF SPIRITUAL EXPERIENCES

Two physicians, friends, and research partners, Dr. Andrew Newberg and Dr. Eugene D'Aquili, performed intriguing research in which they captured brain images of individuals in the midst of transcendent spiritual experiences. Their subjects were long-time Tibetan meditators and Franciscan nuns. Before the experiment, the subjects reported having broadly similar experiences during meditation or prayer. These included the impression of being on a deep, inner journey; a feeling of unity with God or with all beings; a sense of the self as limitless or of no self; and experiences of space and time as limitless. Such mystical experiences of the dissolution of the self are common to religions worldwide.

Newberg's and D'Aquili's subjects were asked to meditate or pray until they felt that they were at a moment of peak experience. At that point, their instructions were to tug on a string to alert the researchers to begin injecting a small amount of radioactive material via an intravenous line. The line traveled into the subject's room, where it was hooked up to a vein in the subject's arm. Moments later, the meditator was given a brain scan with a camera that detects radioactive emissions. The radioactive isotope, or tracer, emits a single photon of light, which can be photographed by a SPECT (single-photon-emission computed tomography) camera and converted into a three-dimensional image of the brain. This type of isotope follows the path of the blood to various areas of the brain. The technique provides an image of blood flow patterns and thus a picture of how the brain is functioning; it does not provide a picture of brain structures. This research created the first pictures of what the brain looks like during a spiritual experience (D'Aquili and Newberg, 1999; Newberg et al., 2001).

Simplifying the researchers' findings, it is apparent that two key events occur during a spiritual experience. First, the imaging showed that the prefrontal cortex, which they dub the attention association area (AAA), has increased activity. Among various other activities, the AAA is the part of the brain that processes emotions and allows us to be goal-oriented, to form intentions, and to concentrate. Zen meditators show pronounced electrical activity in this region during meditation, as measured by electroencephalogram (EEG). So what this tells us, which Eastern meditators have known for centuries, is that the mind must be concentrated, focused, and quiet to allow a spiritual experience to occur.

Second, the imaging showed quiescence in an area of the brain (corresponding to posterior superior partietal lobe) that orients a person as a three-dimensional being in physical space and, thus, is typically extremely active. The researchers call this area the orientation association area (OAA). It integrates visual, auditory, and somaesthetic (i.e., body position and touch) information. It is actually the left side of this area that has the least activity during meditation. The left portion of the OAA gives us the sense of ourselves as a limited, physically separate entity: I am here; you are there. It is the job of the OAA "to sort out the you from the infinite not-you that makes up the rest of the universe" (Newberg et al., 2001). Neural input to this area is limited or blocked during a deep spiritual experience. The OAA no longer receives the neural information that distinguishes self from other and, according to Newburg, "would have no choice but to perceive that the self as endless and intimately interwoven with everyone and everything" (Newberg et al., 2001). This reflects the descriptions of Christian mystics, Buddhist meditators, and others who describe experiences of feeling one with an absolute reality and a connectedness to all.

The researchers found a strong inverse association between increased activity in the AAA and decreased activity in the OAA. In other words, the more the meditator is able to concentrate, the greater is the neural blockage to the OAA, and, consequently, the stronger is the experience of unity or no self. Newberg and D'Aquili refer to this as a "unitary continuum" that "links the most profound experiences of the mystics with the smaller transcendent moments most of us experience" (Newberg et al., 2001). Their language is reminiscent of Tiller's description of subtle energy being part of a continuum.

In addition, the researchers identified areas of the brain concerned with language and visual associations that are important to spiritual experiences. An area of the brain that they call the verbal conceptual association area is positioned at the bottom of the parietal lobe at a junction with the temporal and occipital lobes—an area of highly integrated verbal function that permits the conceptualization and expression of religious experience. The visual association area, which is located toward the bottom of the temporal lobe but receives information from the occipital lobes, facilitates spontaneous visions. It is the area of most highly integrated visual function. Because the visual association area has exhaustive interconnections with the limbic system, meditation can correlate to experiences of emotion and memory (D'Aquili and Newburg, 1999).

Newberg and D'Aquili deduce that our biology compels us to seek an answer to the unanswerable question of what happens when we die. They write that the spiritual urge is a "biologically driven need to make sense of things through the cognitive analysis of reality," which they call the "cognitive imperative." Although mystics and others who have profound spiritual experiences have historically been ridiculed as being a little addled, if not suffering from a mental illness, Newberg and D'Aquili point to research showing that these individuals actually are psychologically more stable than others. Other researchers have found a correlation to well-being, greater purpose, and optimism among individuals having paranormal experiences (Kennedy et al., 1994; Kennedy and Kanthamani, 1995). The SPECT scans of transcendent spiritual experiences confirm that these individuals are coherently describing what they have experienced. Furthermore, the researchers claimed to have established that mystical experiences are "biologically observable" and thus "scientifically real." Newberg (D'Aquili died before the book was written) courageously pushes the issue and asks the question: "Are these unitary experiences a result of neurological function—which would reduce mystical experience to a flurry of neural blips and flashes—or are they genuine experiences that the brain is able to perceive?"

BRAIN SCANS OF EMOTIONAL EXPERIENCES

Another neuroscientist, Dr. Antonio Damasio, has performed some research that is much like Newberg's, except that he uses positron emission tomography (PET) instead of SPECT and emotions instead of spiritual experiences. Damasio found that the induction or recall of experiences of sadness, happiness, anger, or fear engaged the somatosensory cortices and the upper brainstem nuclei that are involved in the regulation of these internal states. Furthermore, each emotion had a discrete neural mapping pattern. For instance, sadness consistently constructs a pattern or map that reveals activation of the ventromedial prefrontal cortex, hypothalamus, and brainstem. This research strongly supports the idea that the subjective process of feeling emotions is partly grounded (neurotransmitters and hormones would also influence such events) in dynamic neural maps (Damasio, 1999, 2000). If Damasio's research is widely accepted as an objective mapping of a specific emotion, then is there not persuasive and logical reason to accept Newberg's work as a reliable mapping of a spiritual experience?

N,N-DIMETHYLTRYPTAMINE (DMT) REVISITED

DMT, as mentioned in Chapter 4 on the relaxation system, is an endogenous molecule with hallucinogenic properties (Strassman, 2001). Recall Rick Strassman's research describing how the monoamine oxidases (MAOs) enzymes quickly break down DMT and prevent its hallucinogenic effects. Strassman injected DMT into volunteers (to bypass the MAOs), which resulted in their having classic stress responses and almost no meaningful spiritual insights. Although Strassman remained convinced that DMT was "the spiritual molecule," he saw that it had no therapeutic value.

Strassman reasoned that the pineal gland is the endogenous source of DMT. It does seem plausible that there could be a synergistic relationship in which melatonin reaches a threshold that triggers the synthesis of DMT. It has already been established that melatonin is secreted during meditation. Could it be that DMT is released during deeper states of meditation, such as those described by Newberg's Tibetan meditators and Christian nuns? Could it also be that DMT is the molecule that is released when an individual's concentration (and increased blood flow to AAA) intensifies enough to switch off the area of the brain that orients us to space and time (i.e., the OAA)? Yes, I think so. Endogenous DMT, seemingly, is the first hormone identified as belonging to the subtle energy system.

In Chapter 4 on the relaxation system, we talked about β-carbolines, which are synthesized in the pineal. They increase melatonin production and inhibit MAOs from breaking down DMT (recall that β-carbolines keep ayahuasca, the South American drink, psychoactive after ingestion). The β-carbolines probably also contribute to keeping our bodies from hallucinogenic-type experiences. Speculatively, β-carbolines also may be the chemical, and ultimately the energetic, gatekeepers to the barrier between the matter and non-matter realms of which Tiller writes.

INTEGRAL PHYSIOLOGY: INTEGRATION OF THE BODY, MIND/EMOTIONS, AND SPIRIT

In developing the theory of *integral physiology*, we have often utilized the image of the Rosetta stone. Deciphering the Rosetta stone of ancient Egypt unlocked enormous knowledge. Each part of the stone revealed a portion of the information crucial to deciphering the whole. Analogously, integral physiology incorporates the "language" of physiology, of the mind and emotions, and of subtle energy—the various sides to our stone. Interactions between the body and the mind/emotions are now a well-established fact of medical research. Integral physiology takes the bold step beyond the so-called body–mind connection to recognize the importance of experiences traditionally called *intuitive* or *spiritual* and to begin to verify their impact on both the body and the mind/emotions. In fact, there is now evidence that our bodies not only are hard wired, but are also are chemically designed, to permit interactions with subtle energy.

The manner in which the human body functions is more complicated and extensive than scientists have previously identified. Deciphering the Rosetta stone of integral physiology may require shattering beliefs as we have held them, only to bring us back to the essence of those beliefs that we held most dear. Perhaps, in this book, you have come to understand that, reduced to a common denominator, everything and everyone arises from energy of one sort or another. Subtle energy can explain and be incorporated into any belief system—from scientific to religious. Ultimately, it is a language of the heart embedded in the stories that spiritual leaders, mystics, philosophers, scholars, physicians, and others have left us.

My silence, like an expanding sphere, spreads everywhere.... My silence spreads like a wildfire of bliss. The dark thickets of sorrow and the tall oaks of pride are all burning up. My silence, like the ether, passes through everything, carrying the songs of earth....

Swami Yogananda

Small is the number of them that see with their own eyes and feel with their own hearts.

Albert Einstein

REFERENCES

Damasio, A.R., *The Feeling of What Happens: Body and Emotion in the Making of Consciousness*, Harcourt Brace, New York, 1999.

Damasio, A.R., Subcortical and cortical brain activity during the feeling of self-generated emotions, *Nat. Neurosci.*, 3 (10), 1049–1056, 2000.

D'Aquili, E.G. and Newberg, A.B., *The Mystical Mind: Probing the Biology of Religious Experience*, Augsburg Fortress Press, Minneapolis, MN, 1999.

Kennedy, J.E. and Kanthamani, H., An exploratory study of the effects of paranormal and spiritual experience on people's lives and well-being, *J. Am. Soc. Psychical Res.*, 89, 249–264, 1995.

Kennedy, J.E., Kanthamani, H., and Palmer, J., Psychic and spiritual experiences, health, well-being, and meaning in life, *J. Parapsychol.*, 58, 353–383, 1994.

Lemonick, M. D., "Einstein's Repulsive Idea," *Time Magazine*, 16 April, 2001.

Newberg, A., D'Aquili, E., and Rause, V., *Why God Won't Go Away: Brain Science and the Biology of Belief*, Ballantine Publishing Group, New York, 2001.

Strassman, R., *DMT: The Spirit Molecule*, Park Street Press, Rochester, VT, 2001.

Tiller, W.A., *Science and Human Transformation: Subtle Energies, Intentionality and Consciousness*, Pavior Publishing, Walnut Creek, CA, 1997.

Tiller, W.A., Dibble, W.E., and Kohane, M.J., *Conscious Acts of Creation: The Emergence of a New Physics*, Pavior Publishing, Walnut Creek, CA, 2001.

ADDITIONAL RESOURCES

Damasio, A.R., *Descartes Error: Emotion, Reason, and the Human Brain*, Avon Books, New York, 1994.

Eden, J., *Energetic Healing: the Merging of Ancient and Modern Medical Practices*, Plenum Press, New York, 1993.

Gallo, F.P., *Energy Psychology*, CRC Press, Boca Raton, FL, 1999.

Szara, S., Are hallucinogens psychoheuristic? *NIDA Res. Monogr.*, 146, 331–351, 1994.

Index